The Sick Newborn Baby

13.

9ª

We dedicate this book to our fathers – to Duncan Simpson, and in memory of John Kelnar and Cyril Harvey.

— THIRD EDITION —————————————————————

The Sick Newborn Baby

Christopher J. H. Kelnar

MD, FRCP, DCH
Consultant Paediatrician
The Royal Hospital for Sick Children, Edinburgh
Senior Lecturer, Department of Child Life and Health
University of Edinburgh

David Harvey

MB, FRCP, DCH, DObstRCOG
Senior Lecturer in Paediatrics
Royal Postgraduate Medical School
Queen Charlotte's and Chelsea Hospital, London

Carol Simpson

RGN, RM, ENB Course 405
Family Care Midwife
St Michael's Hospital, Bristol

Foreword by Barbara Weller

Baillière Tindall
London Philadelphia Toronto Sydney Tokyo

<u>Baillière Tindall</u>   24–28 Oval Road
London NW1 7DX

The Curtis Center
Independence Square West
Philadelphia PA 19106–3399, USA

Harcourt Brace & Company
55 Horner Avenue
Toronto, Ontario, M8Z 4X6, Canada

Harcourt Brace & Company, Australia
30–52 Smidmore Street
Marrickville
NSW 2204, Australia

Harcourt Brace & Company, Japan
Ichibancho Central Building
22–1 Ichibancho
Chiyoda-ku, Tokyo 102, Japan

© 1995 Baillière Tindall

First published 1981
Second Edition 1987
Reprinted 1988
Third Edition 1995

This book is printed on acid-free paper

A catalogue record for this book is available from the British Library

ISBN 0–7020–1647–0

Typeset by J&L Composition Ltd, Filey, North Yorkshire
Printed and bound in Great Britain by The University Printing House, Cambridge.

Contents

Foreword

It has perhaps become a cliché to describe neonatology as being on the frontier of medical developments or that it combines scientific knowledge and understanding with 'state-of-the-art' technology. Both these statements are true. But the delivery of high quality neonatal care is also about so much more, bringing, as it does, new techniques, skills and knowledge with an awareness of current social issues against a background of changing health care services. It is also about providing for the future as most babies grow up into adults. Appropriate and sensitive health promotion can often be an important influence for the parents at this time, thus having a long term effect for the family and the nation's future health and well being.

Primarily, neonatology is about bringing together all these aspects of care, but newborn babies do not exist in isolation. They are dependent on parents for existence. Sick newborn babies have also other special needs for the nurture of life which includes the need for love, contact and recognition. There is no automatic affection between parents and their baby, both need the opportunity to build up a relationship even in the neonatal intensive care unit. The contribution that parents and the family can make to care is part of the uniqueness of a high quality neonatal service. Can neonatology perhaps be described as the first holistic medical science embracing, as it does, all aspects of life?

Just as the baby does not exist in isolation neither does any one health care professional. Interdisciplinary care is one of the hallmarks of such a service bringing together the skills of many professionals. Those working in the community setting have an increasing role in providing neonatal care and family support because babies are staying in neonatal intensive care and special baby care units for shorter periods of time. This book, skillfully and in a user friendly way, provides the neonatal caring team with new information and data that will be appropriate for all working in this field of care. Any one of the team will find within the text much to refresh old ideas and concepts whilst providing new thoughts and ideas to reflect and ponder on.

As we move neonatal care forward into the next millenium, against a backdrop of clinical and organisational audit, value for money and efficiency savings, the care of our smallest and most vulnerable patients must continue to be based on research, skills, compassion and commitment. This text now in its third edition continues to help health care professionals in the neonatal field provide this service.

Barbara F. Weller MSc., RSCN. RGN., RNT
Professional Officer, Neonatal Nurses' Association

Preface to First Edition

Infant mortality has improved greatly over the last eighty years, so that deaths in the neonatal period now form a larger proportion of the total. It is therefore not surprising that the last ten to twenty years have seen an explosion of interest in the newborn baby, particularly the ones who are born early and liable to die from respiratory disorders. The perinatal mortality in the United Kingdom is now dropping faster than at any time since it was first recorded; however, the rate could be much lower—fewer babies die in many European countries than in the UK.

The House of Commons Select Committee on Social Services recently issued a report on perinatal mortality. They estimate that the deaths of about 5000 newborn babies could be avoided every year, if existing knowledge about illness in the newborn baby was applied in practice. The enormous discrepancy between centres with intensive care units for the newborn and other hospitals, without modern facilities, shows that many lives could be saved.

We have all been concerned about the long-term outlook for babies who survive today but would have died in the past. Recent follow-up studies suggest that babies weighing over 1000 g have an extremely good outlook if death from respiratory disease or intraventricular haemorrhage can be prevented. This is probably true also for babies under 1000 g although there is still a question mark over those as small as 600 g. The first day of life is the most dangerous and good care at birth and subsequently can prevent many deaths.

There are a number of books on the very simple care of newborn babies and also on highly intensive care. This book aims to be between those two extremes and to provide a guide to the care of both normal babies and those requiring special care. Some aspects of more intensive care (for example mechanical ventiliation) have also been included where this has seemed appropriate. We have tried to be as practical as possible but it is not always sufficient to know how to do something unless you also know why it is being done. We have been very lucky in Britain in having the advice of physiologists, who have shown us the basic principles of care from careful physiological research on newborn babies. It would be a shame not to have included some of this information as a guide to our work.

Modern care of the newborn depends on building up a multidisciplinary team of doctors, nurses, social workers and laboratory staff to provide expert technical care for the many physical disorders of newborn babies, as well as to give them and their families as much loving care as possible, and we have tried to emphasize this team approach to the care of the newborn.

We hope therefore that the book will interest many different members of this team. It is very important that special and intensive care units and postnatal wards throughout the country should be staffed by those with experience and understanding of newborn babies and their problems. The Joint Board of Clinical Nursing Studies has drawn up syllabuses for nurses training in special and intensive care of the newborn. Course 402 is for those planning to work in special or intensive care; Course 400 is for those who expect to take charge of such units. We hope that this book will be of particular use to nurses on these courses.

We constantly recognize the difficulties of a new houseman or nurse faced with the intensive care of the newborn. It is a very frightening experience, because the babies seem so fragile and precious. They are not able to explain what symptoms they have and the principles of their care can often mystify. Many young doctors have told us how traumatic it is to work for the first few weeks in a neonatal special or intensive care unit. Our aim in this book is to give a basis for such doctors by including information on important techniques that are now used, perhaps for only short periods, in district general hospitals. For instance, it is now common for a baby to need mechanical ventilation for several hours before a team can come from the regional intensive care unit to collect the baby for more prolonged care. Every young paediatrician must know the basic principles of neonatal care, both for normal babies and for those who are ill, and we hope that this book provides both a practical and readable guide.

Laboratory technicians and social workers do not always have the background medical knowledge to disentangle the complicated jargon that many doctors use. It is our hope that this book will also help them to understand what is being said on the ward rounds so that they can ask questions more frequently without feeling embarrassed. It is only by a constant stream of discussion that our care of the newborn will improve.

We do not think that undergraduates need spend very much time in a neonatal intensive care unit but should spend more time on the ordinary postnatal wards understanding problems such as jaundice or the establishment of breast feeding. Our aim has been to make this section of the book sufficiently straightforward to interest them. Most of the people reading this book will plan to work in an industrial society. However, most babies are born in rural societies or in the sprawling cities of the third world, and tetanus is probably more important as a cause of neonatal death worldwide than all the conditions we see in our unit. We believe that the principles of neonatal care can be adapted to any society or situation if the right priorities are recognized; we have included one chapter on care in the developing world where it is vital not to become too dependent on modern technology but to do the most possible with few resources.

We are grateful to Miss M. Adams for writing the foreword and to her and her staff for their constructive criticisms, and to Dr Eric Hurden for his survey of the literature on drugs in breast milk. We thank all those who have provided illustrations (acknowledged in the text), Miss Barbara Hulme for typing the manuscript; and the staff of Baillière Tindall for their encouragement.

July 1981   *C. J. H. Kelnar*
                                                      David Harvey

Preface to Second Edition

Since the first edition of this book there has been further progress in the care of sick newborn babies. The perinatal mortality rate is even lower than five years ago and it is now not unusual to see the survival of a baby weighing less than 700 g at birth. The management of sick newborn babies continues to increase in complexity. We must always look critically at the possible effects of new treatments and strive to support parents during this very stressful period.

This book was intended to be an introduction for nurses and house officers to the care of newborn babies and we have been very pleased that many have found it useful. We hope that the changes we have made reflect the trends of the last few years and will allow it to be used for the English National Board Course 405 which has replaced the two previous neonatal nursing courses.

We are grateful to Karissa Jowaheer and Anna Preston-Jones for thier help with this edition and to our colleagues in Edinburgh and in London for their suggestions and corrections.

August 1986   *Christopher Kelnar*
David Harvey

Preface to Third Edition

There have been considerable advances in neonatal care since the second edition of this book. The large controlled trials of surfactant are one example of advances which now allow more babies to survive. More and more time is taken up on neonatal units providing prolonged intensive care for very preterm and extremely low birth weight infants. This provides good outcomes in many cases, but we are faced with more babies requiring prolonged oxygen therapy, particularly at home.

The changes in this book reflect the modern care of the newborn, and the text is now fully referenced, reflecting the welcome trend to researched-based practices. A neonatal nurse/midwife is now one of the three authors. We hope this book will continue to be useful to nursing, medical and other professional staff in neonatal units, particularly those in training, such as ENB courses 405 and 904 students.

This book reflects the results of many discussions on ward rounds and in seminars, and we thank our colleagues from Edinburgh, London and Bristol for their support, helpful suggestions and contributions.

We also thank Sarah James and the staff at Baillière Tindall for their relentless support and encouragement with this edition.

January 1995   *Christopher Kelnar*
David Harvey
Carol Simpson

1

The Challenge for Perinatal Care

Causes of Death

The end of pregnancy and the first few days of independent life are a dangerous time for a baby. Many deaths occur then and an illness can easily lead to serious consequences, such as brain damage, which may affect the whole of the baby's life. Many couples now expect to have only two children and it is important for them and their families that the children should be born alive and should be left without disability; this is the reason for the great concentration of medical and nursing care in the perinatal period. It is essential that any newborn baby should have a careful examination shortly after birth and should receive good basic care during the first few days. A baby who is ill, or is born very early, will need special or even intensive care. We find it useful to review the newborn baby's needs and problems with a problem list (Table 1.1).

Definitions

Many terms which need defining will be used throughout this book. They conform to the *World Health Organisation (WHO) International Classification of Disease (1977)*.

Table 1.1 Problem list for reviewing the needs of a newborn baby.

General	Special
1 Food	1 Respiratory
2 Warmth	2 Cardiovascular
3 Comfort	3 Fluid balance and renal function
4 Love	4 Weight, nutrition and intestinal function
	5 Haematology – blood counts and clotting
	6 Infection
	7 Bilirubin
	8 Glucose
	9 Neurological function and imaging
	10 Drugs
	11 Parents

Live birth. The complete expulsion or extraction from its mother of a product of conception, irrespective of the duration of the pregnancy, which, after such separation, breathes or shows any other evidence of life, such as beating of the heart, pulsation of the umbilical cord, or definite movement of voluntary muscles, whether or not the umbilical cord has been cut or the placenta is attached. Each product of such a birth is considered live-born.

Fetal death. The death prior to the complete expulsion or extraction from its mother of a product of conception, irrespective of the duration of the pregnancy. Death is indicated by the fact that after such separation the fetus does not breathe or show any other evidence of life, such as beating of the heart, pulsation of the umbilical cord, or definite movement of voluntary muscles.

Birthweight. The first weight of the fetus or newborn obtained after birth. This weight should be measured preferably within the first hour of life before significant postnatal weight loss has occurred.

Low birthweight. Less than 2500 g (up to and including 2499 g). (NB This is not yet the formal definition in the UK as, at present, the definition includes babies weighing exactly 2500 g.)

Gestational age. The duration of gestation is measured from the first day of the last normal menstrual period. Gestational age is expressed in completed days or in completed weeks (e.g. events occurring 280–286 days after the onset of the last normal menstrual period are considered to have occurred at 40 weeks gestation). Measurements of fetal growth, as they represent continuous variables, are expressed in relation to a specific week of gestational age (e.g. the mean birth weight for 40 weeks is that obtained at 280–286 days of gestation on a weight for gestational age curve).

Preterm. Less than 37 completed weeks (less than 259 days).

Term. From 37 to less than 42 completed weeks (259–293 days).

Post-term. 42 completed weeks or more (294 days or more).

The definitions of mortality rates are shown in Table 1.2 and Fig. 1.1.

Table 1.2 Definitions of stillbirth and infant mortality rates.

$$\text{Stillbirth rate} = \frac{\text{Stillbirths} \times 1000}{\text{Live births} + \text{stillbirths}}$$ (Stillbirths are fetal deaths after 24 weeks gestation)

$$\text{Perinatal mortality rate (PMR)} = \frac{(\text{Stillbirths} + \text{deaths at 0–6 days after live birth}) \times 1000}{\text{Live births} + \text{stillbirths}}$$

$$\text{Early neonatal mortality rate} = \frac{\text{Death at 0–6 days after live birth} \times 1000}{\text{Live births}}$$

$$\text{Late neonatal mortality rate} = \frac{\text{Deaths at 7–27 days after live birth} \times 1000}{\text{Live births}}$$

$$\text{Neonatal mortality rate} = \frac{\text{Deaths at 0–27 days after live birth} \times 1000}{\text{Live births}}$$

$$\text{Post-neonatal mortality rate} = \frac{\text{Deaths at 1–11 months after live birth} \times 1000}{\text{Live births}}$$

$$\text{Infant mortality rate} = \frac{\text{Deaths under the age of 1 year after live birth} \times 1000}{\text{Live births}}$$

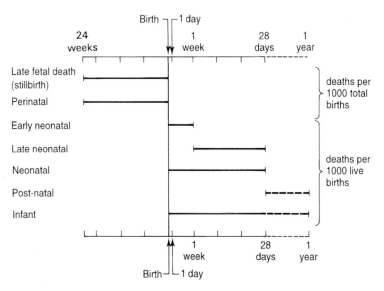

Fig. 1.1 Definitions of mortality rates

The WHO made some recommendations about perinatal mortality rate. The problem is that a baby born at less than 28 weeks gestation is at present included in perinatal mortality figures if born alive but later dies, but is not included if born dead. Practice varies from country to country and some of the differences in perinatal mortality rate from one developed country to another may be the result of a local rule to exclude some babies from statistics. The WHO now recommends that two different sets of statistics should be kept. One set of national figures would include all babies weighing at least 500 g (or at least 22 weeks gestation or 25 cm crown–heel length when a weight is not available), whether the baby was alive or dead at birth. The second set of statistics would be produced for international comparisons. These would include only those babies weighing 1000 g at birth (with a gestational age of 28 weeks or 35 cm crown–heel length when weight had not been recorded). (If one subtracted babies weighing under 1000 g from British perinatal mortality figures in 1970, the PMR would have been reduced from 23.7 per 1000 to around 20 per 1000.) The deaths of babies under 1000 g become proportionately even more important with a lower perinatal mortality; the British PMR is now around 7.6 per 1000; it is possible that it could be as low as 7.5, if one excluded the tiny babies.

There are some other useful definitions not included in the WHO book:

Very low birthweight.   Less than 1500 g (up to and including 1499 g).

Extremely low birthweight.   Less than 1000 g (up to and including 999 g).

Babies under 750 g now often survive. A definition for this group may be needed in the future.

Changes in Mortality Statistics

There have been major changes recently both in the numbers of children born in Great Britain and other developed countries and in the frequency of their deaths. The number of deaths is measured as the PMR. This rate has dropped remarkably since it was first recorded in the 1920s; in fact, it has fallen by a third since the first edition of this book. Even so, of all the deaths of those under 15 years in the UK, about 1 in 5 still occurs within the first 24 hours after birth. The

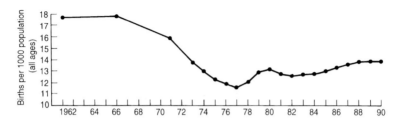

Fig. 1.2 Birth rate (England and Wales) for selected years since 1961. (OCPS)

present perinatal mortality is about 7500 deaths each year. Not all the survivors are normal: any disability, whether physical, intellectual or emotional, may cause significant handicap in adult life.

In Britain there has been a trend to smaller families, although the reduction in birth rate has not been as great as in some European countries. Figure 1.2 shows the birth rate in selected years from 1961 to 1990. We are very nearly at the point where births only just replace deaths and there may be a decline in population by the end of the century. However, there was an increase in the birth rate in the late 1970s.

Figure 1.3 shows the PMR in Great Britain over the last 60 years. The scale is logarithmic, and therefore shows the increasing rate of fall of perinatal mortality in the last few years. The PMR in England and Wales in 1992 was 7.6. One can be very proud of figures such as these, but there has been concern that the mortality is not as low as that in some other countries. PMR has dropped as fast, or even faster, than in most developed countries; it is infant mortality, particularly the deaths after the neonatal period, that shows a lagging Britain. Figure 1.4 shows how infant mortality (deaths of live-born children within the first year of life) has fallen more slowly than in other countries. However, there is still room for improvement in perinatal care.

The British Perinatal Mortality Surveys of 1958 and 1970 helped considerably in the identification of causes of perinatal mortality and the effect of social conditions and other factors. Table 1.3 sets out the major findings in perinatal deaths in the two surveys. There were remarkable changes in the 12 years between the two surveys, which are now over 20 years old. Deaths caused by birth trauma dropped by

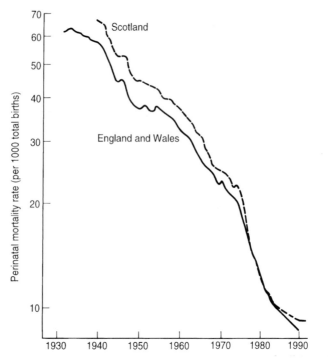

Fig. 1.3 Perinatal mortality in Great Britain 1931–1990. (OPCS)

87% and this was probably due to better obstetrics: difficult forceps deliveries became extremely rare and were replaced by caesarean sections. Pneumonia also became less common; it is difficult to be certain of the reason for this, but the use of antibiotics probably played a part. There are some causes of death which did not change at all. It is not surprising that congenital malformations produced the same number of deaths in 1970. In the UK, neural tube defects had been the commonest fatal congenital malformations. They now account for a smaller proportion of perinatal mortality, partly because more terminations of pregnancies are performed as a result of detection of these abnormalities by screening tests in mid-pregnancy (Fig. 1.5).In the 1990s, respiratory distress syndrome (RDS) less commonly results in death because of prevention by good care in

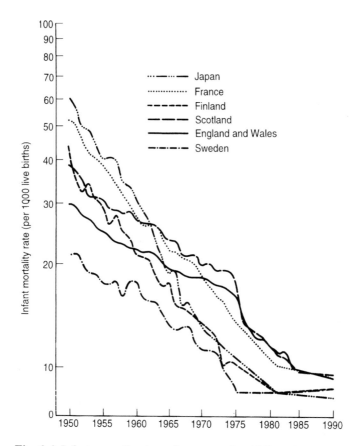

Fig. 1.4 Infant mortality in various countries 1950–1984. (OPCS)

premature labour, and treatment after birth with ventilation and surfactant.

A major problem today is the death rate of very immature babies under 28 weeks or 1000 g. These infants used to be regarded as 'near abortions' and many lived only a very short time after birth. There is evidence that in some areas the number of registered live births under 1000 g has increased recently, probably because babies of 24 weeks gestation or more are now seen as having a chance of life. Intensive care may actually increase the PMR if small babies are kept alive for a short while and then die. A baby born dead before 24 weeks

Table 1.3 Major findings about perinatal deaths (British Births Survey 1970; Perinatal Mortality Survey 1958).

Major findings	Singletons and twins 1970			Singletons and twins 1958		
	% All deaths	Incidence per 1000 deliveries	Order	% All deaths	Incidence per 1000 deliveries	Order
Stillbirths with intrauterine asphyxia	26.3	6.1	1	29.9	10.0	1
Congenital malformation	21.5	5.0	2	15.1	5.0	3
Stillbirths without anatomical lesions	14.9	3.4	3	15.4	5.1	2
Respiratory distress syndrome	13.7	3.1	4	9.1	3.1	4
First-week deaths with intrauterine asphyxia	7.6	1.7	5	4.3	1.4	6
Immaturity	6.8	1.6	6	–	–	–
Blood group incompatibility	2.8	0.6	7	4.0	1.3	7
Intracraneal birth trauma	1.8	0.4	8	8.9	3.0	5
Intraventricular haemorrhage	1.8	0.4	9	2.4	0.7	11
Massive pulmonary haemorrhage	0.8	0.2	10	2.7	0.9	10
Pneumonia	0.5	0.1	11	4.0	1.3	8
Extrapulmonary haemorrhage (first-week deaths)	0.5	0.1	12	0.3	0.1	12
No anatomical lesions	–	–	–	2.7	0.9	9
Miscellaneous	1.0	0.2	13	1.2	0.3	13
Total	100.0	23.0		100.0	33.1	

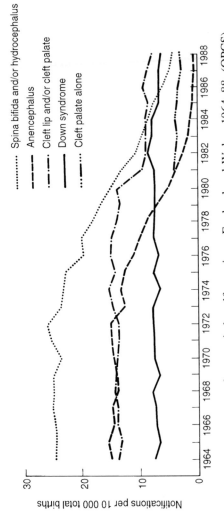

Fig. 1.5 Notifications of congenital malformations, England and Wales, 1964–88. (OPCS)

gestation is at present counted as an abortion and does not enter mortality figures, but if the baby is born alive, and then dies, it does. It is clear that short gestation and low birthweight are major factors in death during the first week. These will be discussed further in Chapter 2.

The causes of perinatal death in developing countries are very different from those seen in Europe and North America. The PMR is much higher and is dominated by death from trauma and infection; RDS appears to be less common. Neonatal tetanus, which is hardly ever seen now in Britain, is the major cause of perinatal mortality in some parts of the world. The use of tetanus toxoid, and the instruction of village midwives in the use of clean instruments to cut the cord and the avoidance of dirty dressings on the umbilicus, would save more babies than most of the sophisticated techniques mentioned in this book (see Chapter 20).

PMR varies not only from one country to another, but also within a country. This is shown by an analysis of the figures for perinatal mortality from the different Regional Health Authorities (RHA) (OPCS). In 1992 there were wide variations between the different regions in England, from as high as 9.2 in the West Midlands RHA to as low as 6.2 in East Anglia. Some of the differences might result from differing standards of medical care, but it is more likely that they arise from social differences; it is well recognised that PMR is higher in less advantaged socio-economic groups. The social class classification based on the occupation of the father is shown in Table 1.4; the classification is not as useful at it used to be because of the increase of single-parent families and unemployment. In 1990 28% of births were outside of marriage, but over 70% of these were registered jointly. The extent of the drop in birth rate varies in different

Table 1.4 Classification of social classes (OPCS).

Class	Definition
Non-manual	
Class I	Professional occupations (e.g. lawyers, doctors)
Class II	Managerial and technical occupations (e.g. sales managers, teachers, nurses)
Class IIIN	Non-manual skilled occupations (e.g. clerks, shop assistants)
Manual	
Class IIIM	Skilled manual occupations (e.g. bricklayers, underground miners)
Class IV	Partly skilled occupations (e.g. bus conductors, postmen)
Class V	Unskilled occupations (e.g. porters, labourers)

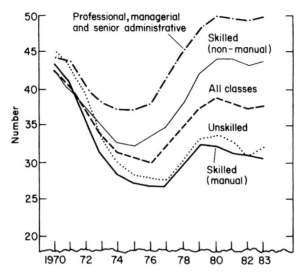

Fig. 1.6 Legitimate live births per 1000 married women aged 30–44 by social class of husband (England and Wales). (OPCS)

parts of our community. Figure 1.6 shows the changes in birth rates in different social classes. In 1975, the number of births in social classes I and II was 96% of the number in 1970; in contrast, there was a major drop in births in social classes IV and V as they were only 67% in 1975 of the number in 1970, and the rise since then has widened the gap. Social changes such as these underlie the recent improvement in PMR since the babies who might have been born in social classes IV and V would have been at greater risk than those in social classes I and II. Many other factors may affect perinatal mortality (see Chapter 2).

The persistent high levels of unemployment might be expected to increase the gap between the deprived and wealthier sections of the community. Nearly 50% of perinatal mortality is associated with the 1% of infants who are of very low birthweight, (less than 1500 g).

Organization of Perinatal Care

The last 20 years have shown a continuation of the major trend away from home births. There has been a recent swing back to home

Table 1.5 Place of confinement: 1964, 1974. 1984 and 1989 (OPCS).

Year	Maternities (thousands)	Percentage distribution of maternities by place of confinement		
		NHS Hospitals	Home	Other
1964	890.5	67.1	28.4	4.5
1974	640.8	94.0	4.1	1.9
1984	634.0	97.8	1.0	1.2
1989	652.4	97.8	1.1	1.1

deliveries, but, nevertheless, almost 99% of babies are now born in hospital (see Table 1.5). It is difficult to produce figures which show convincingly that hospital births are safer than births at home for uncomplicated term deliveries. The Netherlands have one of the lowest PMRs in the world despite a high proportion of home deliveries, but even in that country there has been a trend towards hospital delivery.

The mortality of small babies is heavily influenced by their place of birth and there should be no excuse for knowingly delivering a preterm baby at home. The best place for the birth of a preterm baby is in a hospital with a fully equipped intensive care unit. There is an argument in favour of the home delivery of full-term babies following uncomplicated pregnancies, since they are at very low risk. The last UK study of home births was in 1979 (Campbell). Following the report of the Department of Health's Expert Maternity Group (1993), the National Birthday Trust have just undertaken a study into home births in the UK in 1994. There are clearly some emergencies such as a prolapsed cord in the first stage of labour which are very difficult to manage at home since it would be impossible to do a caesarean section there. A reasonable compromise is delivery in hospital and discharge home after only a few hours and this is now widely practised. Hospitals should be as comfortable and homely as possible.

A major obstacle to the improvement of perinatal care is the shortage of skilled neonatal nursing and medical staff and of training posts for them to gain experience in the care of tiny and ill newborn babies. This is particularly important because of the difficulty in recognising the significance of early signs of illness in newborn babies and the rapidity with which they can become ill and die without treatment.

The lessons for perinatal care have not always been well learned in the past. In the 1950s many harmful treatments were used for new-born babies. An editorial in the *Lancet* in 1974 said 'this period must surely be regarded as the one in which modern neonatal iatrogenisis reached a peak'. For example, the widespread use of intravenous nikethamide during resuscitation was not only useless but harmful; the common use of intragastric oxygen was useless; hypoglycaemic convulsions and brain damage were common because small babies were not fed for up to five days, in order to reduce the risks of aspiration; babies were not kept warm enough; some developed kernicterus following high doses of synthetic water-soluble analo-gues of vitamin K and the indiscriminate use of sulphonamides in the newborn period; and unnecessarily high and frequent doses of chlor-amphenicol caused death due to circulatory collapse from the 'grey baby' syndrome.

The greatest harm to babies was caused by the swings in fashion in the use of oxygen therapy. Liberal amounts of oxygen in the 1940s led to many blind children with retinopathy of prematurity and, following this, the refusal to allow babies to have anything more than 40% oxygen in the 1950s led to many unnecessary deaths and much handicap from hypoxia in RDS.

The handicaps seen in the survivors of neonatal care in the 1950s led many people to feel that the intensive or special care of newborn babies would only increase the number of handicapped survivors. There is now reasonable evidence that many of the disabilities resulted from medical and nursing methods then in vogue. Improve-ment in our knowledge of the physiology of the newborn baby has increased the number of survivors; follow-up studies suggest that the prevalence of major handicaps is quite low. More than 9 out of 10 babies surviving with a birthweight of 1500 g or less are likely to be normal; this is three times more than 40 years ago. The baby who weighs less than 1000 g at birth now has more than a 50% chance of survival, as high as that for babies weighing between 1000 and 1500 g 20 years ago (Stewart *et al.*, 1981). In attempting to improve survival rates we must be careful not to introduce techniques that could damage the baby's brain or other organs. This means that in every centre which has an intensive care unit careful follow-up studies must be done to ensure that harm is not being caused. The number of children with cerebral palsy and chronic lung disease has increased recently as the techniques of intensive care are applied to smaller and smaller babies.

A major priority in an industrialized country must be to ensure a good standard of medical care throughout the whole country. This should be done carefully so that the consumer's wishes are followed. For instance, it may be necessary to arrange a regional centre for the care of women of very high risk, but this may result in long journeys during the antenatal period. Because some women need to travel to special centres, it does not follow that every woman needs such care. Attention should be paid to the convenience of individual women and their families and financial help should be given where there is need.

Adequate arrangements must be available in every country for home and hospital delivery of normal pregnant women. An obstetric and neonatal flying squad should be available where a sudden emergency occurs, so that specialist medical help is immediately available. The British Paediatric Association and the British Association for Perinatal Medicine have produced a document of categories of neonatal care (see Appendix) including a summary of the resources required for neonatal care. The English National Board has also issued guidelines for staffing units undertaking neonatal nurse training.

The following seem sensible recommendations for improving our PMR and the quality of surviving babies:

1 Special care nurseries should be available in all obstetric units. It is usually suggested that the unit should have six cots per 1000 deliveries per year. This is a high estimate as less than 10% of all newborn babies should need admission to the special care unit (see Chapter 4). A unit of 20 cots is an efficient size; this implies that obstetric units should be of a reasonable size (about 2000–3000 deliveries a year) in order to have a special care baby unit and sufficient staff. The unit should be within the maternity unit and, if possible, attached to a children's hospital or a general hospital with a paediatric unit. There should be an efficient system to allow mildly ill babies or small babies to be transported from general practitioner units or from home if they need special care and for their parents to be transferred with them.

2 There should be sufficient, adequately trained, experienced resident paediatric staff and nurses constantly available. They must be trained in special and intensive care of the newborn.

3 There should always be adequate equipment; there must be piped oxygen, air and suction and a laboratory with microtechniques to assay chemicals in blood and urine. There should be apparatus in the special care baby unit, or very near it, for measuring blood gases.

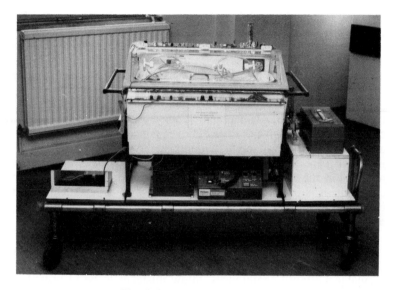

Fig. 1.7 A portable incubator

Monitoring equipment is essential and every hospital should have a technician to keep it in working order.

Every region should have at least one intensive care unit to serve a total population of about three million people. This should certainly be in a maternity hospital; two intensive care cots per 1000 deliveries are needed. Ill babies can be transported to the unit in a portable incubator by a neonatal team of doctors and nurses who can collect a baby by ambulance or helicopter (Fig. 1.7). All women in premature labour (at a gestation less than about 33 weeks) or who are likely to have a very ill baby should be advised to be transferred for delivery to a hospital with an intensive care unit. This may mean that a woman is very far from her home and family. It is important that money and transport should be provided so that members of the family, friends and, most importantly, the woman's other children can be with her and the ill newborn baby.

Every country should organise its neonatal services so that ill babies can receive skilled care. Clearly, this must be done within the resources available, which means that countries without much money and with very high mortality rates may need to pay attention to basic neonatal care before moving on to a more sophisticated system. Neonatal special and intensive care is expensive. It is particularly costly to train skilled personnel, both paediatricians and nurses, and also to buy and service elaborate equipment. But this cost is insignificant in comparison with the cost of not providing adequate perinatal care. The total expense of caring for one severely handicapped individual in Great Britain through a lifetime of 50 years is at least £$\frac{1}{2}$ million. This takes no account of the stress and suffering of the individual family concerned. It may be that neonatal intensive care is not as expensive as once believed, since babies need less space and less laundry than other patients in hospital. The cost of one intensive care cot is equivalent to an ordinary bed in a general hospital in the UK, not to the cost of a bed in an adult intensive care unit. It is important to be humane as well as technically proficient. Proper pain relief remains a challenge: severe pain may have physiological consequences as well as being very unpleasant.

It is vital that every maternity hospital should develop a team for perinatal care. There is a lot to be gained from close liaison between the obstetricians and paediatricians. Regular audit sessions, such as perinatal mortality conferences, allow mistakes to be identified and corrected. We hope that local confidential enquiries into perinatal mortality will allow maternity and neonatal services to be better planned in future.

References and Further Reading

Avery, G.B. (1987) *Neonatology: Pathophysiology and Management of the Newborn.* 3rd ed. Philadelphia: Lippincott.

British Association of Perinatal Medicine (BAPM) (1992) *Report of the working group of the BAPM and Neonatal Nurses Association on categories of babies requiring neonatal care. Arch. Dis. Child, 67,* 868–869.

Campbell, R. (1979) *Home Births Survey,* England and Wales. PhD Thesis, London University.

Chamberlain, G., Phillipp, E., Howlett, B. *et al.* (1970) *British Births Survey,* vol. 1. London: Heinemann Medical.

Department of Health (1993) Expert Maternity Group Report, *Changing Childbirth.* London: HMSO.

English National Board for Nursing, Midwifery and Health Visiting (1991) *Guidelines for Staffing of Neonatal Units Involved in ENB Courses.* Circular 1991/09/APS.

Grant, J.P. (1993) *The State of the World's Children.* Geneva: UNICEF.

Klaus, M.H. & Fanaroff, A.A. (1986) *Care of the High-risk Neonate.* 3rd ed. Philadelphia: W.B. Saunders.

Office of Population Censuses and Surveys (OPCS) (1989) *Mortality Statistics, Perinatal and Infant: Social and Biological Factors* (series DH3). London: HMSO.

OPCS (1991, 1992, 1993) *Monitor.* (series DH3) London: HMSO.

OPCS (1989) *Population Trends.* London: HMSO.

Review of the Registrar General (1993) *Births and Patterns of Family Building in England and Wales 1991.* (FMI no.20). London: HMSO.

Roberton, N.R.C. (ed.) (1992) *Textbook of Neonatology (2nd edn).* Edinburgh: Churchill Livingstone.

Sinclair, J.C. & Bracken, M.B. (eds) (1992) *Effective Care of the Newborn Infant.* Oxford: Oxford University Press.

Stewart, A.L., Reynold, E.O.R. & Lipscomb, A.P.L. (1981) Outcome for infants of very low birth weight: survey of world literature. *Lancet, i,* 1038–1041.

The National Birthday Trust (1994) 1994 Confidential Enquiry into Home Births. Information from Department of Obstetrics and Gynaecology, St George's Hospital Medical School, London SW17 0RE.

Thomas, R. & Harvey, D. (1992) *Neonatology* (Colour Guide Series). Edinburgh: Churchill Livingstone.

Trade Union Congress (1981) *The Unequal Health of the Nation.* Summary of the Black Report.

Wigglesworth, J. (ed.) (1984) *Perinatal Pathology* (Major Problems in Pathology Series). Philadelphia: W. B. Saunders.

World Health Organisation (1977) *Manual of International Statistical Classification of Diseases, Injuries and Causes of Death,* vol. 1. Geneva.

2

Prenatal Influences on the Baby

Causes of Preterm Birth

Around 70% of perinatal mortality in Britain occurs in the 7% of infants of low birthweight. Those countries with more small babies often have a higher infant mortality (Fig. 2.1): Clearly, if we are to improve survival and quality of life, we must reduce the number of babies who are born early and those who are small. We are still far from understanding the causes of preterm births in most cases. Nevertheless, if all the knowledge now available were put into practice, significant benefits would follow. Some factors we can correct; there are many that for political, social, emotional, or financial reasons are difficult to change.

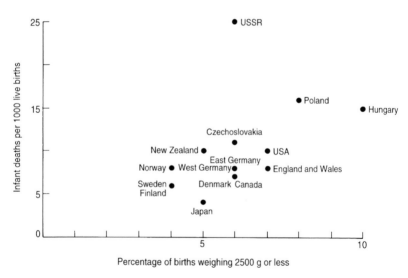

Fig. 2.1 Infant mortality rates and incidence of low birthweight for selected countries (1980–1988). (OPCS)

In an individual pregnancy, there is sometimes an obvious cause when the baby is born too small or too early. For example, the mother may have pe-eclampsia or an antepartum haemorrhage; she may have a multiple pregnancy; or the fetus may be abnormal. In most cases there is no simple explanation; it is likely that the result was the end-product of many genetic and environmental factors.

Very often, a baby is born early and is also found to be smaller than expected for gestation because growth has been too slow *in utero*. Many of the factors that are associated with preterm delivery are also associated with slow growth, so that there is much overlap between the two. It is very important that gestation should be measured as accurately as possible. Women should keep an accurate record of their menstrual history and attend an antenatal clinic early in pregnancy so that a clinical and ultrasound assessment of gestation can be made. The baby should be weighed and measured accurately shortly after birth and weight should be plotted on a birthweight/gestational age chart to show whether it is small-for-gestational-age (SFGA) (see chapter 6). Table 2.1 summarises the factors known to influence the

Table 2.1 Factors influencing the length of gestation or fetal growth.

Gestation	Fetal growth
Shortened	*Reduced*
1 Previous obstetric history	1 Maternal illness during pregnancy
2 Maternal illness during pregnancy	2 Chronic maternal disease
3 Chronic maternal disease	3 Maternal age
4 Maternal age	4 Parity
5 Fetal disease	5 Maternal height
6 Social class	6 Ethnic group
7 Multiple pregnancy	7 Genetic factors
8 Major life events	8 Birth weight of other family members
	9 Social class
Lengthened	10 Smoking
1 Drugs	11 Poor nutrition
2 Anencephaly	12 Alcohol
	13 Weight gain in pregnancy
	14 Multiple pregnancy
	15 Altitude
	16 Fetal disease
	17 Fetal abnormalities
	Increased
	1 The baby of the diabetic mother
	2 Beckwith syndrome
	3 Transposition of the great arteries

length of gestation or fetal growth which are discussed in more detail below. It is often very difficult to be certain whether a factor is associated with short gestation or produces slow fetal growth; in many cases the factors are intermingled. A baby may be born small because of short gestation, because of slow growth *in utero* or for both reasons. The care of small babies is discussed in Chapter 6.

Factors that alter the length of gestation

Short gestation

Previous obstetric history. It is common experience that women who have had mid-trimester miscarriages tend in a subsequent pregnancy to have a preterm delivery or another mid-trimester miscarriage. In some of these cases there is cervical incompetence which is often treated by cervical suture.

There has been considerable controversy about the effect of therapeutic abortion on subsequent pregnancies. Some workers have suggested that it is more likely to lead to mid-trimester miscarriage and preterm births, whereas a large study in the Far East (Chung *et al.*, 1982) suggested that it has no effect. It seems likely that the chance of a subsequent preterm birth depends on the type of operation used for therapeutic abortion. If the cervix has been greatly dilated during the operation then it is more likely to be incompetent in a later pregnancy.

Infection. There have been reports that bacterial infections of the amniotic cavity can lead to premature rupture of the membranes and preterm delivery (Chaudhrey *et al.*, 1984). In developing countries, zinc deficiency may lead to amniotic infection by reducing the antibacterial defences of the fluid.

Studies have shown that mothers with Group B streptococcal urine infection have a significantly increased risk of premature rupture of the membranes, and subsequent preterm delivery (Moller *et al.*, 1984).

Maternal illness during pregnancy. A pregnancy may have to be terminated because of serious illness in the mother: the commonest indications are the hypertensive disorders and antepartum haemorrhage from either placenta praevia or placental abruption. Very often labour is induced at term, or just before, because of only mild illness in the mother; to allow the pregnancy to continue longer might increase the risk to both mother and fetus. It is therefore common for labour to be induced at term for mild hypertensive disorders associated with other high-risk factors such as the mother's age or previous obstetric history.

Chronic diseases in the mother.   Some disorders such as chronic renal disease or essential hypertension are often complicated by pre-eclampsia during pregnancy and, therefore, a shorter gestation. It is thought that other disorders such as tuberculosis and urinary tract infection are more likely to lead to spontaneous premature labour.

Maternal age.   This appears to have very little effect on the length of gestation; the longest pregnancies occur in women during their 20s and gestation is shorter in those women over 35 or under 20 years.

Fetal diseases.   Labour may be induced when it would be dangerous to leave the fetus *in utero*, for example rhesus disease or intrauterine growth retardation.
   Congenital abnormalities are sometimes associated with short gestation, as well as with failure to grow normally *in utero*. We know that many fetuses with chromosomal abnormalities are aborted.

Major life events.   A sudden emotional upset can precipitate preterm labour (Newton and Hunt, 1984). Major life events, such as bereavement, are more common in the recent past of women in preterm labour than those at term. Certainly, our grandmothers would have believed in it.

Social class.   It is common experience that the families of babies in special care baby units have more social problems than do those of normally sized babies.
   There is a suggestion from the British Births Survey (1970) that babies born into social classes IV and V have shorter gestation than those in the middle class. The difference appears to be greater for unsupported mothers.

Multiple pregnancy.   This frequently leads to preterm labour. It is common to see twins or higher multiples in a special care baby unit. In many cases the labour occurs spontaneously and in some countries much attention has been paid to these pregnancies by using beta-mimetic drugs to delay birth. Pre-eclampsia and other disorders of pregnancy are commoner in multiple pregnancies and labour may need to be induced. Higher multiple pregnancies are much more common today as a result of treatment for infertility. The Human Fertilization and Embryology Act (1990) states that a maximum of three embryos are transplanted during *in vitro* fertlisation (IVF), but gamete intrafallopian transfer (GIFT) is not yet covered by this act.

Long gestation

Drugs. Certain drugs may prolong pregnancy. Women who take aspirin freely during pregnancy are more likely to go into spontaneous labour after term because of the drug's antiprostaglandin effect.

Congenital abnormalities. Some women bearing abnormal fetuses, for example anencephalics without pituitary glands, fail to go into labour spontaneously at the appropriate time. This is probably the result of poor fetal adrenal function.

Factors affecting fetal growth

Some of these factors appear to affect growth throughout pregnancy but most of them only have an effect towards term.

Reduced growth

Maternal illness in pregnancy. In many of the common disorders of pregnancy, such as pre-eclampsia or antepartum haemorrhage, the baby is smaller than one might expect. It is thought that maternal blood supply to the placenta is decreased in many of these disorders.

Chronic disease in the mother. Chronic hypertension and renal disease are notorious for producing very SFGA babies. Cyanotic congenital heart disease is another cause.

Maternal age. The heaviest babies are born to women in their late twenties and early thirties. There is a lower mean birthweight in babies whose mothers are under 20 or over 35. This effect is more obvious at term.

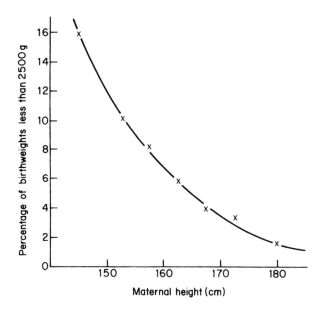

Fig. 2.2 Percentage of low birthweight babies in relation to the mother's height. From MacFarlane & Mugford (1984)

Parity. First-born babies are generally lighter than those born subsequently. Again, this effect is more obvious as term approaches.

Maternal height. Short women have smaller babies than tall women. (Fig. 2.2). The mean birthweight in the British Births Survey (1970) was 3.16 kg for women under 157 cm and 3.41 kg in those 165 cm or more.

Ethnic group. This is one of the most important factors influencing the incidence of low birthweight (Grundy *et al.*, 1978). Studies from the USA have shown that nearly 1 in 8 babies born to black mothers weighs 2500 g or less; this is about twice as many as those born to white mothers, even allowing for the positive correlation with low maternal income and poor education. Paradoxically, before 35 weeks gestation, black fetuses are heavier than white and black children are taller than their white peers at the age of 2 years. There are many studies of birthweight around the world and, in general, babies born in developing countries are lighter. This is particularly marked in babies from the Indian subcontinent; the birthweight of babies there is lower than European babies at term, but there is very little difference between the two groups before 32 weeks. It seems that the babies are SFGA because of some factor constraining growth towards the end of the pregnancy. A study in a London borough (Dawson *et al.*, 1982) showed that Indian babies were, on average, 250 g lighter than white babies and West Indian babies were intermediate. It is difficult to be certain what factor is being exerted through the mother's race. It might be a genetic factor; or a reflection of poor nutrition or short stature; it is probably a result of both.

Genetic factors.   Work before the Second World War on the size of foals at birth showed that genetic factors have an important influence on the size of the newborn animal. A pure-bred foal from a large variety is larger than a pure-bred foal from a small variety of horse. A cross breed between a large and a small horse is intermediate in size, but the size depends on whether the mare is from the large or small variety: in the horse, it is the *mother's* size that largely determines the rate of intrauterine growth in a cross between two extremes of adult size.

Birth weight of other members of the family.   The birthweight of a baby is significantly related to the birthweight of the last child born to the same mother. Some women have several children who are small at term; there is a significant correlation between the mother's own birthweight and those of her children, which is much stronger than

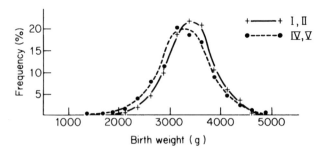

Fig. 2.3 Distribution of birthweight for social classes I, II, IV and V (singletons, LMP certain). From Chamberlain *et al.* (1975), by permission of the authors and the National Birthday Trust Fund

that between the baby's and the father's birthweights. This may be because a woman who is small at birth tends to be a small adult and therefore has a smaller uterus and placental size.

Social class.   The mean length of gestation is hardly different in the different social classes, but the mean birthweight is significantly lower in social classes IV and V when compared with social classes I and II. This indicates that there are more SFGA babies in the less advantaged. It is probable that a multitude of factors, including ethnic group, nutrition, maternal height and smoking, play an important part in influencing this. Figure 2.3 shows the distribution of birthweight in social classes I and II, compared with social classes IV and V.

Cigarette smoking.   This has been shown to be a major influence on fetal size. Figure 2.4 shows the mean birthweight for length of gestation in women who smoked in pregnancy and those who had

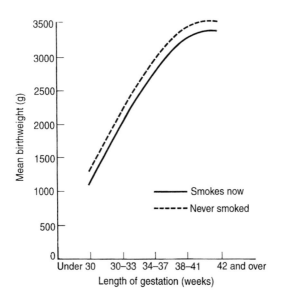

Fig. 2.4 Mean birthweight for length of gestation according to maternal smoking habits (singletons LMP certain). From Chamberlain *et al.* (1975), by permission of the authors and the National Birthday Trust Fund

never smoked. Babies are about 200 g lighter in women who smoke. There is also a lower reading age in later childhood in those children whose mothers smoked during pregnancy.

Smoking has a direct effect on the fetus and the reduced fetal growth is not simply due to smoking mothers eating less well. Women who smoke inhale nicotine and also have higher carbon monoxide levels in their blood. As a result, the fetus obtains less oxygen and grows less well. For this reason the effect on birthweight is more or less uniform at all stages of gestation (Fig. 2.4).

Recent evidence also shows a four times greater risk of sudden infant death syndrome (SIDS) from mothers smoking antenatally, and a link between passive smoking and SIDS (Mitchell *et al.*, 1993).

Nutrition during pregnancy.   It was shown in the Second World War that a period of starvation during pregnancy reduced the size of the baby at birth. This was true in Leningrad and also during a period of starvation in Holland during the winter of 1944–45 when the perinatal mortality and the incidence of low birthweight increased in women starved during the third trimester of pregnancy. Studies from Guatemala suggest that energy (calorie) supplements given to pregnant women who had chronic undernutrition in pregnancy increased the birthweight of their babies. This is very important for developing countries, as a simple energy supplement during pregnancy may improve the size of the fetus. This may cause problems at delivery because a small woman, when she moves into an area with better nutrition, may have a larger fetus and may therefore develop cephalopelvic disproportion.

Alcohol and other drugs.   Fetal alcohol syndrome has been described in babies born to chronic alcoholic women. The features of the syndrome include low birthweight and short length, microcephaly, irritability in infancy, a low IQ in later childhood and a number of minor dysmorphic features. It is not yet clear whether small quantities of alcohol taken regularly during pregnancy cause intrauterine growth retardation, but studies suggest that an intake of more than 8 units a week, (equivalent to approximately one drink per day), could damage a fetus (Forrest *et al.*, 1991). The use of narcotics or cocaine reduces the size of the baby at birth (see Chapter 6).

Multiple pregnancy.   It has long been known that this leads to SFGA babies. In general, the more babies in one pregnancy the lighter they are. The mean birthweight of twins tends to deviate from the mean for

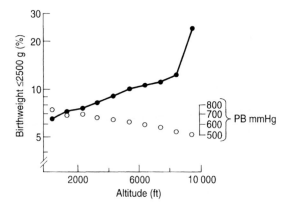

Fig. 2.5 Frequency of low birthweight related to altitude in the USA mountain states, 1952–57. Adapted from Grahn & Kratchman (1963). ●, frequency of low birthweight; ○, atmospheric pressure

singletons at about 32 weeks and that of triplets deviates at about 28 weeks.

Altitude.   This has a major effect on the growth of the fetus *in utero.* Those women who spend their pregnancies at a higher altitude have smaller babies (Fig. 2.5). Presumably this reflects the amount of oxygen that reaches the fetus, since the oxygen tension in the atmosphere is lower at high altitudes.

Fetal disease.   Congenital infection, particularly rubella, leads to slow intrauterine growth. There are usually other signs that suggest the diagnosis, such as purpura and hepatosplenomegaly.

Fetal abnormalities.   Many of these are associated with low birth-weight. This is particulary striking in chromosomal abnormalities such as the autosomal trisomies. However, many babies with other congenital abnormalities tend to be SFGA; one of the major excep-tions is transposition of the great arteries where the babies are larger than expected. It is striking that babies who are SFGA and have congenital abnormalities are symmetrically small; this means that their head circumference is small in proportion to their weight. Babies who are SFGA because of other causes of slow growth *in utero*, however, often have a relatively large head in comparison to the rest of the body (see Chapter 6).

Any of these factors may come together to influence the size of the baby. The incidence of low birthweight is a major factor in the perinatal mortality rate (PMR). Many countries with low PMRs such as the Scandinavian nations, have fewer low birthweight babies than the UK. The reasons for this are not clear, but it does seem that better social conditions and taller mothers lead to larger babies who are healthier at birth and less likely to die. Information from China is interesting because women there seem to be at low risk of having a small or preterm baby. This may account for the surprisingly low PMR in China – a developing country.

We are still ignorant of many of the factors in individual women that lead to repeated low birthweight. Clearly, we still have a long way to go before our knowledge of the various factors affecting the length of pregnancy and growth of the fetus can be used in the large-scale prevention of the birth of small babies and thus in a major improvement in perinatal mortality.

Increased growth

Factors associated with increased growth *in utero* are discussed in Chapter 15.

Antenatal Care

There are many aspects of antenatal care which are of importance to paediatricians. When assessing a baby, the paediatrician should read the antenatal notes carefully. Note the following (summarized in Table 2.2) and enter them in the baby's notes when relevant:

1 *Maternal age*
2 *Occupations of mother and father*. These will help in assessing the social class of the family and will prevent the nurse or doctor from falling into the trap of talking at too sophisticated a level for the parents, or conversely, using simplified terminology to parents, who are already well informed about medical matters – although she may have no experience of preterm or sick neonates. It is best to encourage questions to ensure that the parents have grasped the information given.
3 *Marital status*. A single mother is not necessarily unsupported; the

Table 2.2 Aspects of the antenatal history to be noted.

1 Maternal age
2 Occupations of mother and father
3 Marital status
4 Mother's medical history
5 Ethnic group
6 Family history
7 History of previous pregnancies
8 Record of antenatal care
9 Mother's menstrual history and estimate of gestation
10 Blood group and serology of mother

circumstances of each family must be individually assessed. An unsupported mother may need extra help in order to care for her baby.

4 *Mother's medical history.* In particular, note any history of tuberculosis which would mean that the baby should have BCG in the neonatal period.

5 *Ethnic group.* Certain illnesses are commoner in some groups than others. For instance, cystic fibrosis is common among the English but is rare in black people. Ashkenazy Jews have a much higher incidence of some inborn errors of metabolism, e.g. Tay–Sachs disease.

Parents who were born outside Europe and North America have a higher incidence of tuberculosis. There may therefore be a good reason for giving BCG to their babies in the neonatal period.

6 *Family history.* Note any diseases that could be inherited and any record of consanguinity, for instance cousin marriages.

7 *History of previous pregnancies.* This should be studied in great detail since there may be a recurring history of abnormalities such as preterm births or of an important inherited condition for which a special examination must be made. Any previous perinatal deaths are bound to cause anxiety at subsequent deliveries.

8 *Record of antenatal care.* Read the notes about the number of visits during pregnancy. Women should attend the antenatal clinic early in pregnancy, but it is common for some to book late; this complicates the assessment of the gestation and may mean that a number of vital tests are done late or not at all (such as serological tests for syphilis). Poor attenders at the clinic do seem to have a greater risk of perinatal death. A history of irregular attendance in the antenatal period may give a warning that there will be difficulties with the child's care. A study of the antenatal record makes certain that no abnormalities have been noted during the antenatal period, such as polyhydramnios or poor fetal growth.

9 *Mother's menstrual history and length of pregnancy.* The date of the last menstrual period is very important, but a proper assessment of gestation can be made from the date only if the mother has regular periods, with a standard cycle. Look at the history of the cycle and the last menstrual period; recalculate the estimated date of delivery. Did the obstetrician's assessment at the first visit correspond with the dates? Is there any record that the mother felt movement at the expected time (18–20 weeks for the first baby or 16–18 weeks in subsequent pregnancies)? It is very common to find that the length of gestation in the notes has been rounded up. You may well find that a baby who is only 36 weeks and five or six days gestation, has been called 37 weeks. There is an appreciable difference in mortality rate between one week of gestation and the next; weeks of gestation refer to *completed* weeks.

The dates that are obtained from the menstrual history and from clinical examination are wrong in up to 25% of cases. Some women have only a shaky memory of the date of the last menstrual period and some will be too embarrassed to mention this; they may say a date is certain when it is not. The use of the contraceptive pill has led to further confusion about dates as periods may be quite irregular after stopping the pill.

For all these reasons, careful assessment of gestation is needed during a pregnancy and ultrasound has made this much easier. An ultrasound reading of the biparietal head diameter between 10 and 20 weeks of a pregnancy, or of the crown–rump length before 10 weeks of pregnancy, gives an estimate of the expected date of delivery that is even better than the date obtained from menstrual dates. The estimate is accurate within a week either way. It seems that ultrasound is a safe method of examining the fetus although recent studies (Newnham *et al.*, 1993) suggest that five or more ultrasound and Doppler flow studies, between 18 and 38 weeks gestation, may result in intrauterine growth retardation. For gestational assessment in the newborn, see p. 437.

10 *Mother's blood group and serology.* Note the blood group of the mother, and in particular, the rhesus group. Note the results of the serological tests for syphilis: congenital syphilis should be totally prevented by careful serological testing in pregnancy. The test for rubella is especially important in assessing an SFGA infant and whether the mother needs immunization. It is becoming increasingly common to offer testing for antibodies to the human immunodeficiency virus (HIV) (see p. 367). Mothers are also screened for hepatitis B as carrier mothers could infect their infants at delivery, or the fetus transplacentally, with subsequent development of hepatitis. Sometimes other tests will have been done, such as those for toxoplasmosis.

Assessment of Fetal Growth and Wellbeing

Growth

The earlier in pregnancy ultrasound is used to determine the gestational age of the fetus, the more accurate the assessment. Serial measurements of the biparietal diameter, head circumference, abdominal circumference and femur length will show the rate of fetal growth. Plotting these recordings on intrauterine growth charts allows early recognition of growth retardation (Fig. 2.6). Most

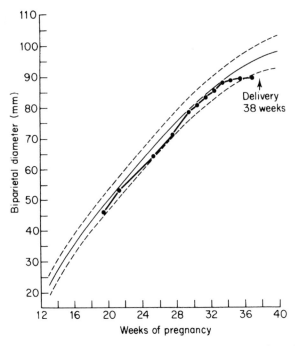

Fig 2.6 A case of intrauterine growth retardation with cessation of growth of the head late in pregnancy (see also Fig. 6.1)

SFGA babies have a relatively large head circumference compared to the other measurements, so slowing of the growth of the fetal skull indicates severe growth retardation. Interpreting the ratios of the various measurements enables the birthweight to be predicted very accurately.

A clinical assessment of fetal growth may be made from 20 to 36 weeks gestation, by measurement of the height of the fundus from the top of the symphasis pubis. At 20 weeks gestation in a normal singleton pregnancy, the fundal height is approximately 20 cm. It increases at a rate of 1 cm per week until 36 weeks when the presenting part may engage, therefore altering the measurements.

Biophysical profile

This non-invasive form of assessment was first described in 1980 (Manning *et al.*), and is now widely used. Five separate parameters are assessed using ultrasound scanning, each being given a score of 0 (when the criterion is not met) to 2 points. A total score of 8 or more, in the absence of oligohydramnios, is normal. Less than this indicates that the fetus is compromised to some degree, and further investigations may be required. Each of the five parameters are, individually, measures of fetal well being (Gabbe, 1991). The specific criteria are as follows:

1 Reactive fetal cardiotocograph.
2 One or more 30–second episodes of fetal breathing movements in 30 minutes.
3 Three or more distinct fetal body or limb movements in 30 minutes.
4 One or more episodes of extension and flexion.
5 One or more pockets of amniotic fluid measuring 2 cm or more.

Fetal cardiotocography (FCTG)

A fetus who is already compromised *in utero*, by placental insufficiency for example, may become distressed and hypoxic during labour. The fetal heart rate can be monitored intermittently using a Pinard stethoscope, or continuously using a transducer on the mother's abdomen or a fetal scalp electrode. By monitoring the fetal heart rate during uterine contractions and fetal movements, it is possible to detect early signs of hypoxia, which may indicate the need for further investigations or delivery. FCTG is discussed in more detail under Care of Labour (p. 42).

Fetal movements

Most women are aware of fetal movements by 18–20 weeks of pregnancy. A healthy fetus is active throughout the pregnancy, thus a reduction or absence of these movements may indicate intrauterine hypoxia, and fetal death may occur if no further action is taken. Ultrasound scanning allows fetal movements to be visualized. A chart designed to allow the mother to record these movements, the Cardiff 'count-to-ten' fetal activity chart, is given to all mothers at 28 weeks gestation. They record the number of movements felt in a 12-hour period, to a maximum of 10, starting from the time they wake. If there are less than 10 two days in succession, they record the actual number and are advised to contact their GP. If no movements are felt, they are told to contact the hospital immediately. Reliability of this method of assessment relies on the midwife giving clear instructions, the mother understanding the purpose of the chart, completing it and seeking advice appropriately. Findings from various studies are divided over the usefulness of these charts (Liston *et al.*, 1982; Lobb *et al.*, 1985).

Fetal breathing movements

A healthy fetus demonstrates breathing movements 80% of the time *in utero*. These can be clearly seen with ultrasound scanning. Prolonged hypoxia is necessary for breathing movements to cease completely, but the fetus should be considered at serious risk if there are prolonged apnoeic episodes.

Fetal tone

As well as demonstrating general movements, a healthy fetus can be seen stretching and relaxing limbs, during ultrasound scanning. These episodes of flexion and extension are not lost unless prolonged hypoxia has occurred.

Amniotic fluid volume

The volume of amniotic fluid is assessed by measurement in centimetres on ultrasound scan pictures. Oligohydramnios, less than 5 cm, at term is related to an increased perinatal morbidity. Severe oligo-hydramnios, less than 1 cm, has been associated with a 40–fold increase in perinatal mortality. Polyhydramnios, 20 cm or more, may be associated with congenital malformations.

Doppler studies

The blood flow from the placenta to the fetus can be visualized in wave form, using Doppler ultrasound. This technique identifies placental insufficiency very early, allowing action to be taken before the fetus is significantly compromised (Sonek *et al.*, 1990).

Detection of Abnormalities

Many parents who have a family history of congenital abnormalities or who have already suffered the tragedy of an abnormal baby do not want to have another child with such a problem. There are now a number of techniques for detecting abnormalities early enough in pregnancy for a therapeutic abortion to be performed. Unfortu-nately, most of the techniques can be used in only a small proportion of pregnancies and are unlikely to alter appreciably the number of babies born with congenital abnormalities, with the probable excep-tion of spina bifida and Down syndrome. The techniques that can be used to detect abnormalities include the following:

Chromosomal analysis (karyotype)

This is performed on cultured cells obtained by amniocentesis or chorionic villus sampling. It is used for the detection of Down syndrome (trisomy 21), which now accounts for a third of all the severely mentally handicapped persons in the UK (see also Chapter 9). There is an increased risk of Down syndrome in the babies of older women: it is about 1 in 1600 when the mother is 22 years old but 1 in 100 if she is 40 years. The abnormality is an extra chromo-some 21, so the baby has 47 chromosomes instead of the usual 46 (Fig. 2.7). This extra small chromosome usually comes from the mother, but in a third of the cases it comes from the father. There are other rarer types of Down syndrome where the extra chromosome 21 is attached to another chromosome (translocation) so that the baby has only 46 chromosomes, but has the amount of genetic material equivalent to 47 chromosomes. This can be inherited from either the

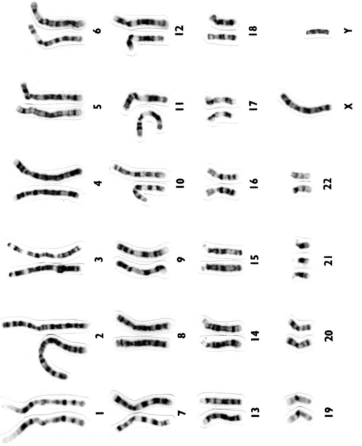

Fig. 2.7 A banded karyotype of Down syndrome (trisomy 21)

mother or the father, who can be easily identified because he or she has only 45 chromosomes but is apparently normal. Whenever a baby with Down syndrome is born, the karyotype should be examined so that these rarer types can be identified and the parents warned of the increased risk of having another child with Down syndrome. The risk in these translocations is 1 in 5 when the mother is the carrier and 1 in 100 when it is the father.

The usual practice in the UK is to offer prenatal chromosome analysis to women at increased risk of having a baby with Down syndrome, either because of a family history, or an increased risk identified on maternal serum screening or age. Fetal chromosomal analysis can be done on samples obtained from amniocentesis or chorionic villus sampling (CVS).

A decision will need to be made between the obstetrician and the parents, about whether prenatal diagnosis should be performed and which method should be used. Amniocentesis has usually been performed at 15–16 weeks, although some centres are now offering it at a much earlier gestation, 12–13 weeks. The disadvantage of amniocentesis has been that when a chromosomal or biochemical abnormality has been found, it is relatively late for termination to be performed. On the other hand the risk of miscarriage has been relatively low at 1%. There is also an increase in the number of congenital abnormalities in babies born after amniocentesis, mainly talipes equinovarus and congenital dislocation of the hip, and of respiratory distress syndrome (RDS). Sampling of the chorionic villi can be done at a much earlier stage of pregnancy, around 9–12 weeks. This allows a safer and earlier termination of pregnancy if an abnormality is found. The rate of miscarriage specifically due to the procedure is approximately 0.6% higher than from amniocentesis (National Institute of Health, 1989).

Individual parents will have their own views about whether they want amniocentesis or CVS, and some will undoubtedly be prepared to take the extra risk of miscarriage in order to avoid having a child with Down syndrome. On the other hand, many people have an objection to abortion, which is the only way of avoiding the birth of a Down syndrome baby when it has been discovered *in utero*.

It is important to recognize that about 70% of fetuses with Down syndrome occur in women aged less than 35 years. Therefore a strategy which only performs screening over a certain age, for example 37 years, would not detect a large number of abnormal fetuses. Newer screening tests involving a number of biochemical factors such as human chorionic gonadotrophin (HCG) and low alpha-fetoprotein (AFP), have been developed, and can detect approximately 60% of fetuses with Down syndrome.

Some conditions, such as haemophilia, occur only in males, and a selective abortion may be considered for male fetuses of a carrier mother – ultrasound would determine the sex of the fetus at around 16 weeks. Many people would find this objectionable and more detailed tests are now available to determine the diagnosis accurately.

Rapid advances have been made in diagnostic tests, particularly using DNA techniques, thus inborn errors of metabolism and haemoglobinopathies can be detected by CVS. Fetal blood sampling allows much more rapid karyotype examination than in the past.

Biochemical investigations on amniotic fluid or cells

Inborn metabolic errors

There are many, very rare, inborn errors of metabolism which can be diagnosed *in utero*. They are usually inherited in an autosomal recessive fashion and cause a wide variety of disorders, very often with mental handicap. Since most of them are disorders of metabolism, it is possible to detect the abnormality in the fetal cells. The absence of an enzyme can be discovered or an accumulation of metabolites shown in the cell. These cells can be obtained by amniocentesis or by CVS. An increased proportion of these diseases are now being diagnosed prenatally by the use of DNA probes, but unfortunately this is not possible in a small percentage of affected families (10–20% depending on the disease). It is essential that DNA analysis of family members should be done before a prenatal diagnosis is attempted. These disorders are very rare and the test can only be performed when there is a family history of the specific disorder; general screening is not possible. Those which can be diagnosed *in utero* now number nearly 100 and some of these are listed in Table 2.3.

Occasionally it may be possible to identify parents who could pass on the disease and are therefore heterozygous for the gene. An example is Tay–Sachs disease which is common in Ashkenazy Jews; there have been screening programmes among Jewish people in the UK and North America to identify those who might be carrying the condition and to warn them before they have children.

Autosomal recessive disorders are commoner in couples who are near relatives because they are more likely to share many genes, including a rare harmful one.

Table 2.3 Inherited metabolic diseases diagnosable prenatally.

Acatalasaemia
Acid phosphatase deficiency
Adenine phosphoribosyl transferase deficiency
Adenosine deaminase deficiency
Adrenogenital syndrome (21–hydroxylase deficiency)
Adrenoleukodystrophy (Schilder's disease)
α_1-Antitrypsin deficiency
Arginosuccinic aciduria
Aspartyl glucosaminuria
Bloom's syndrome
Carbamyl phosphate synthetase deficiency
Cerebro-hepato-renal syndrome (Zellweger's syndrome)
Chédiak–Higachi syndrome
Citrullinaemia
Cockayne's syndrome
Congenital erythropoietic porphyria
Congenital hyperammonaemia Type II
Cystathioninuria
Cystic fibrosis
Cystinosis
Cystinuria
Dihydropteridine reductase deficiency
Epidermolysis bullosa
Fabry's disease
Fanconi's anaemia
Farber's disease
Fucosidosis
Galactosaemia
Galactokinase deficiency
Galactose–4–phosphate epimerase deficiency
Gaucher's disease
Glucose–6–phosphate dehydrogenase deficiency
Glycerol kinase deficiency
Non-ketotic hyperglycinaemia
Glycogenoses (glycogen storage diseases) Type I–IV
Glutaric acidurias Types I and II
GM_1 gangliosidoses Types I and II
GM_2 gangliosidoses Type I (Tay–Sachs) Type II and III
Haemoglobinopathies
Haemophilia (A and B)
Hartnup disease
Histidinaemia
Homocystinuria
Huntington's chorea
3–hydroxy–methylglutaric aciduria
Hypercholesterolaemia
Hyperlysinaemia
Hyperoxaluria
Hypervalinaemia

Hypophosphatasia
I-cell disease
Isovaleric acidaemia
Propionic acidaemia (ketotic hyperglycinaemia)
Krabbe's leucodystrophy
Lactosyl ceramidosis
Lesch–Nyhan syndrome (hyperuricaemia)
Lysyl protocollagen hydroxylase deficiency
Mannosidosis
Maple syrup urine disease (branched chain ketoaciduria)
Menke's kinky hair disease
Metachromatic leucodystrophy
beta-Methylchrotonylglycinuria
Methylcrotonyl glycinuria
Methylmalonic acidaemia
Methyltetrahydrofolate methyl transferase deficiency
Methyltetrahydrofolate reductase deficiency
Mucolipidoses Types I–III (includes I-cell disease)
Mucopolysaccharidoses Types I–VII
Multiple carboxylase deficiency
Multiple sulphate deficiency (mucosulfatidosis)
Muscular dystrophy (Duchenne and Becker types)
Niemann–Pick disease
Ornithine-transcarbomylase deficiency
Orotic aciduria
Phenylketonuria (phenylalanine hydroxylase deficiency)
Phosphohexose isomerase deficiency
Polycystic kidney disease
Pyruvate decarboxylase deficiency
Pyruvate dehydrogenase deficiency
Refsum's (phytanic acid storage) disease
Retinoblastoma
Rhizomelic chondrodysplasia punctata
Saccharopinuria
Salla disease
Schindler disease
Severe combined immunodeficiency
Sickle cell disease
T-cell immunodificiency
Thalassaemia (alpha and beta)
Tyrosinaemia Type 1
von Willebrand's disease
Wolman's disease
Xeroderma pigmentosum
X-linked ichthyosis (steroid sulphatase deficiency)
Zellweger's syndrome

The list of disorders which can be diagnosed is growing every day and Table 2.3 should be checked against the most up-to-date list. The rapid advances in research have allowed the commonest autosomal recessive condition in Great Britain – cystic fibrosis – to be diagnosed *in utero* by the use of a gene probe.

Other inherited metabolic diseases are being investigated with a view to antenatal diagnosis. In any case of a pregnancy at risk for one of the diseases not listed, provided that the diagnosis of the previous affected child is secure, the Prenatal Diagnosis Group should be consulted for the most up-to-date information, (see Appendix).

Neural tube defects

Neural tube defects are common congenital abnormalities in Great Britain. About half are fetuses with anencephaly where the brain is exposed and the baby dies; the other half are different types of spina bifida where there is an opening over the spinal cord. The neonatal diagnosis is discussed in Chapter 10. Since severe degrees of spina bifida cause serious mental and physical handicap in later life, it is now common to make a diagnosis early in pregnancy so that the abnormal fetus may be aborted.

When the parents have had a child with anencephaly or spina bifida they have a 1 in 20 chance of having another child with a neural tube defect, although the risk is higher in Wales and Ireland (see Table 9.1) and lower where spina bifida is rare. In anencephaly and the 90% of spina bifida cases where the neural tube is exposed to amniotic fluid, body fluid from the fetus can escape into the amniotic fluid. The normal fetus produces a protein, known as alpha-fetoprotein, which is present only in fetal life and in one or two rare conditions during later life. It is present in the mother's blood in only a low concentration, but appears to peak during mid-pregnancy. If there is a possibility of a leak of body fluids from the fetus into the surroundings, the concentration of alpha-fetoprotein in amniotic fluid will be much higher than in a normal pregnancy; there will also be a greater concentration in the mother's blood. Since spina bifida produces a leak from the fetus into amniotic fluid, the discovery of this protein has permitted the early diagnosis of open neural tube defects during pregnancy. A similar leak is also found in babies with conditions such as exomphalos or congenital nephrotic syndrome, but these are much rarer.

Where there is a previous history of neural tube defect in the family, for instance where one parent has spina bifida or where the parents have had a previous child with the condition, it is important to manage the pregnancy carefully. An ultrasound examination should be done at about 16 weeks gestation, since this is the best method of diagnosing anencephaly and of confirming the gestational age. At about 16–18 weeks a sample of amniotic fluid can be taken for alpha-fetoprotein analysis. The back can also be scanned by ultrasound to detect a defect in the neural arches which would indicate spina bifida. Unfortunately, a lesion very low in the spine is difficult to diagnose by ultrasound.

The measurement of alpha-fetoprotein in the mother's plasma can be used to screen women who have no history of a baby with neural tube defect. It is best to take the sample between 16 and 18 weeks of pregnancy. At the same time it is wise to do an ultrasound examination to make certain that the gestation is correct, since the commonest cause of an apparently high plasma alpha-fetoprotein is an incorrect estimate of gestational age. At the same time the uterus can be examined by ultrasound for multiple pregnancy or missed abortion since these are other reasons for a high maternal plasma alpha-fetoprotein. If the high alpha-fetoprotein (usually over the 97th centile) is found on two occasions, amniocentesis can be offered.

The first sample of blood should be taken only from women who understand the reson for sampling and wish to be screened. Amniocentesis is done under ultrasound control and the head and back are scanned at the same time. The expertise needed for scanning the back is much greater than when ultrasound is used to assess the length of gestation and it seems that this investigation should be done only in specialist centres. It is possible to miss some cases and this causes great distress especially if a woman has been told that her baby is unlikely to have spina bifida. The sampling of blood, examination of the fetus, and amniocentesis all cause considerable anxiety to parents. This is a reason for ensuring informed consent for screening before the first blood sample is taken.

Fetoscopy

Fetoscopy involves examining the baby through a tiny fibreoptic telescope which is passed into the uterus through the abdominal and uterine walls. The first fetoscopes were fairly large and fetoscopy was often followed by miscarriage. The most recent instruments are much finer and have been used with greater success but there is a risk of miscarriage. The most obvious use of fetoscopy is to look for an external abnormality of the fetus such as a cleft lip or

Table 2.4 Indications for fetal blood sampling.

1 Bleeding disorders
2 Haemoglobinopathies
3 Karyotyping
4 Immunodeficiencies
5 Viral infections
6 Metabolic disorders
7 Non-rhesus hydrops
8 Fetal anaemia

spina bifida. It may be very difficult to use the instrument since only a small portion of the fetus can be seen at one time, and the procedure should be done in specialised centres under careful ultrasound control.

Fetal blood sampling

An even more useful technique is blood sampling under ultrasound guidance. It is possible to take a blood sample from an intrahepatic vessel, to obtain a specimen of fetal blood. The blood is examined to measure red cell size and confirm that the sample is fetal and not maternal blood. This technique can be used for the diagnosis of a growing list of conditions (Table 2.4) such as thalassaemia and sickle cell disease.

Care of Labour

Good care by experienced midwives and obstetricians is essential if a woman is to be delivered safely of a healthy normal baby. We can be particularly proud that trauma is now a very rare cause of fetal death or morbidity. The death rate from trauma in the 1970 perinatal survey was one-seventh that in the 1958 survey. This reflects the increased readiness of obstetricians to use caesarean section as the method of delivery when damage to the baby otherwise seems likely. A number of recent techniques have been added to the traditional methods of assessing the baby's health during labour. Fresh stillbirth from anoxia during labour should now be considered a preventable condition.

Diagnosis of fetal asphyxia during labour

The classic signs of intrauterine asphyxia are meconium staining of the liquor and fetal tachycardia (>180 beats/min) or bradycardia (<100 beats/min). However, clinical assessment is only crude and has therefore been refined by fetal cardiotocography (FCTG). The principle is continuous recording of the fetal heart rate and the intrauterine pressure changes, both of which are printed by the machine. The fetal heart rate can be recorded externally or directly from the scalp. There are several warning signs of asphyxia which are shown by such a record:

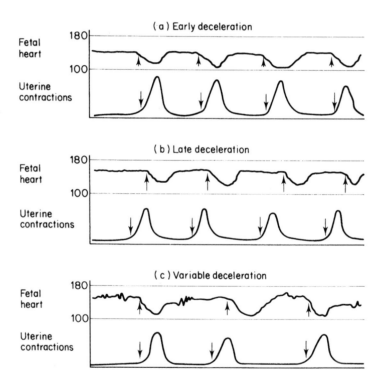

Fig. 2.8 Fetal cardiotographic tracing. (a) Type 1 or early deceleration, suggestive of head compression. (b) Type 2 or late deceleration, suggestive of uteroplacental insufficiency. (c) Variable deceleration, suggestive of cord compression. From Campbell & McIntosh (1992), with permission from the editors and Churchill Livingstone

1 *Tachycardia.* There is a normal acceleration of heart rate during contractions and fetal movements; however a rate continually above 180 beats/min is sinister.

2 *Loss of base-line variability.* The visual record normally shows an irregular line and loss of this variation occurs early in asphyxia.

3 *Bradycardia.* Continuous bradycardia is very worrying, although it is occasionally the result of complete fetal heart block.

The FCTG is mainly used to show any intermittent dips in heart rate. The dips are often divided into type I and type II (Fig. 2.8). The first occur during a contraction while the second, which are thought to indicate asphyxia, occur at the end or after a contraction. Quite often variable dips are seen. Although type I dips are usually benign, any prolonged or deep slowing of the heart rate may be a danger sign. Some obstetricians measure the area of the dip and use this as a measure of fetal distress. If there are persistent abnormalities, the fetus should be investigated further by sampling of the scalp blood for pH. Asphyxia produces a marked acidaemia; a pH below 7.25 is usually considered to be sign of hypoxia.

Preterm labour

A baby who is born early has a much greater chance of dying than one born at term. If one could prevent preterm delivery one could greatly reduce perinatal mortality. The methods of stopping preterm labour are still not very successful. Where there is clear cervical incompetence, possibly from a previous termination of pregnancy, cervical suturing may prevent premature dilation of the cervix and therefore preterm delivery. Some success has been claimed with the use of betasympathomimetic drugs, such as ritodrine for reducing uterine contractions (Leveno *et al.*, 1986).

Even when labour cannot be postponed until term, it may be useful to put off preterm labour for several days in order to allow steroids such as betamethasone to have an effect on lung surfactant production (see Chapter 8). Controlled trials (Collaborative Groups, 1981) suggest that where betamethasone has been given to the mother more than 24 hours before delivery, the incidence of respiratory distress syndrome in the baby is less.

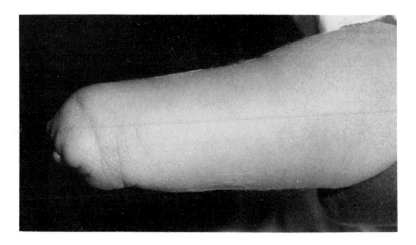

Fig. 2.9 The results of thalidomide: there is no hand on this arm

Drugs in Pregnancy

A number of different drugs and classes of drugs have been shown to be associated with an increased risk of fetal abnormalities when taken by the pregnant mother. The best know example is, of course, thalidomide (Fig. 2.9). The striking and severe abnormalities produced by this drug led to its early incrimination and withdrawal. Great care will need to be taken to ensure that it is not used during pregnancy again, now that it has been reintroduced on to the market. Most drugs have much subtler adverse effects and it is important during pregnancy to avoid using newer drugs, except in exceptional circumstances.

In all cases the value of a drug to the mother must be weighed against possible risks to the fetus. Thus it is reasonable to use high-dose quinine to treat chloroquine-resistant malaria, but not for malaria prophylaxis as it increases the risk of abortion. Similarly, one may use frusemide to treat heart disease in pregnancy, but not for physiological ankle oedema as there is a risk of reducing maternal intravascular volume and placental perfusion. As a general rule, all drugs should be avoided during pregnancy unless they are essential.

Table 2.5 Drugs that may affect the fetus if given during the first trimester of pregnancy.

Drugs	Use	Proved or suspected abnormalities
19–nor–progestagens (such as norethisterone and norethynodrel	For treatment of recurrent abortion	Masculinisation of female fetus
Isotretinoin (and related drugs)	Acne	Abortion and central nervous system defects
Etretinate	Acne	Pregnancy should be avoided for two years after stopping Etretinate and four weeks after stopping Isotretinoin
Lithium	Mania	Cardiovascular malformations
Phenytoin	Anticonvulsant	Folic acid antagonist producing cleft lip, finger and toe abnormalities, diaphragmatic hernia. There is increased risk if toxic levels are present and blood levels should be monitored throughout pregnancy
Trimethoprim (in co-trimoxazole)	Urinary tract infection	Folic acid antagonist producing congenital malformations; probably a theoretical risk, but folic acid supplements should be given
Warfarin	Anticoagulant	Nasal bone hypoplasia, bony defects in limbs, and punctate epiphyses
Sodium valproate	Anticonvulsant	Increased risk of neural tube defects (screening advised)
Carbemazepine	Anticonvulsant	Slight increased risk of neural tube defects (screening advised)

Table 2.6 Drugs that may affect the fetus if given during the second and third trimester of pregnancy.

Drugs	Effects on fetus or newborn
Antibiotics and related agents	
Tetracyclines	Chelate with calcium and therefore are deposited in tissues undergoing mineralisation. Produce yellow teeth and reduce bone growth
Sulphonamides and co-trimoxazole	If given shortly before delivery they might possibly displace bilirubin from protein binding sites, leading to neonatal kernicterus
Streptomycin	Poorly excreted by the newborn kidney and toxic to the eighth cranial nerve
Aminoglycosides	May cause auditory or vestibular nerve damage. Deafness has been reported with Streptomycin. Risk with gentamicin and tobramycin is probably small
Nitrofurantoin	May produce haemolysis if used at term in G–6–PD deficient babies
Rifampicin	Risk of neonatal bleeding may be increased due to vitamin K deficiency
Drugs acting on the central nervous system	
Hypnotics and sedatives	All can depress neonatal respiration
Narcotics Opioid Analgesics	Respiratory depression, poor feeding, withdrawal fits (see Chapter 14)
Barbiturates	Produce deficiency of vitamin K dependent liver clotting factors leading to haemorrhagic disease. In anticonvulsant doses they may also produce withdrawal fits or apnoeic attacks
Diazepam Benzodiazepines	Hypothermia, hypotonia, poor sucking, jaundice, withdrawal fits and apnoeic attacks
Tricyclic antidepressants	Neonatal tachycardia, irritability, tremor, muscle spasms have been reported
Lithium	May produce neonatal goitre. Neonatal lithium toxicity produces hypotonia and cyanosis

Table 2.6 Drugs that may affect the fetus if given during the second and third trimester of pregnancy (*Contd*).

Drugs	Effects on fetus or newborn
Alcohol	Growth retardation and neonatal withdrawal syndrome in babies of alcoholic mothers
NSAIDs (non-steroidal anti-inflammatory drugs)	A possible risk of premature closure of the ductus arteriosus, pulmonary hypertension and periventrical haemorrhage
Antihypertensives Reserpine	Bradycardia, poor temperature control, nasal obstruction, lethargy and respiratory depression
Ganglion blockers	Hypotension and paralytic ileus
Thiazide diuretics	A very small risk of thrombocytopenic purpura
Betablockers e.g. Atenolol, Propranolol	May cause intrauterine growth retardation (IUGR) if prolonged use. Fetal and neonatal bradycardia may occur
Endocrine system Radioactive iodine	Permanent hypothyroidism
Sulphonylureas Chlorpropamide Tolbutamide	Neonatal hypoglycaemia may occur
Carbimazole or thiouracil Propylthiouracil	Goitre, hypothyroidism
Iodides (e.g. in cough mixtures or contrast media used in radiography)	Goitre, hypothyroidism
Anticoagulants Coumarins (e.g. Warfarin)	Fetal or neonatal haemorrhage due to prolonged prothrombin time. Heparin which does not cross the placenta should be substituted for these oral drugs about one month before the expected date of delivery
Corticosteroids	Possible increased risk of intrauterine growth retardation and long-term effect on subsequent growth
Antidiabetic drugs Chlorpropamide	Possibility of neonatal hypoglycaemia

The first trimester

If dangerous and possibly teratogenic drugs are to be avoided in early pregnancy, it is important for the doctor to assume, when prescribing, that any woman of child-bearing age is pregnant unless she can give specific assurances that she is not. If this rule is not followed, teratogenic drugs may be given inadvertently before either the family doctor or the woman herself knows that she is pregnant.

X-rays should be avoided in pregnancy. Small doses (e.g. for a chest radiograph) are probably not harmful, but larger doses may cause fetal death or abnormalities such as microcephaly or, possibly, childhood leukaemia.

Some drugs which may affect the fetus if given during the first trimester of pregnancy are listed in Table 2.5. It must be emphasised that with all these drugs there is only a small increase in the risk of the specific abnormalities mentioned when compared with the general population.

Second and third trimesters

Substances with molecular weights of less than about 600 cross the placenta easily. Most drugs come into this category, and they are often more toxic to the fetus than to the mother (Table 2.6). This may be because drugs such as barbiturates can enter the brain more easily, or because drugs are less well excreted by the fetal kidneys or liver, for example chloramphenicol, sulphonamides and phenytoin. The persistence of maternally derived drugs in the newborn baby must be considered when prescribing safely in late pregnancy or during labour. In addition many drugs are excreted in breast milk (see Chapter 7).

References and Further Reading

Anthony, A.N. (1947) Children born during the seige of Leningrad in 1942. *Journal of Pediatrics*, *30*, 250.

Campbell, A. and McIntosh, C. (eds) (1992) *Forfar and Arneil's Textbook of Paediatrics* 4th ed. Edinburgh: Churchill Livingstone.

Chamberlain, R., Chamberlain, G., Hewlett, B. *et al.* (1975) *British Births 1970.* London: Heinemann Medical.

Chaudhrey, H., Nergesh, T., Uma, L.V. *et al.* (1984) Silent chorioamnionitis as a cause of preterm labour to tocolytic therapy. *Am. J. Obstet. Gynecol. 149*, 726–730.

Chung, C.S., Smith, R.G., Steinhoff, P.G. *et al* (1982) Induced abortion and spontaneous fetal loss in subsequent pregnancies. *Am. J. Public Health*, **72**, 548–554.

Collaborative Groups in Antenatal Steroid Therapy (1981) Effect of antenatal dexamethasone administration on the prevention of respiratory distress syndrome. *Am. J. Obstet. Gynecol. 141*, 276–287.

Dawson, I., Golder, R.Y. & Jonas, E.G. (1982) Birthweight by gestational age and its effect on perinatal mortality in white and in Punjabi births: experience at a district general hospital in West London 1976–75. *Br. J. Obstet. Gynaecol. 1*, *89*, 896–899.

Forrest, F., Florey, C du V., Taylor, D. *et al* (1991) Reported social alcohol consumption during pregnancy and infants development at 18 months. *BMJ*, *303*, 22–26.

Gabbe, S. (1991) Antepartum fetal evaluation. In *Obstetrics: Normal and Problem Pregancies*, 2nd ed., eds S. Gabbe, J. Niebyl & J. Simpson, pp. 377–424. New York: Churchill Livingstone.

Grahn, D. & Kratchman, J. (1963) Variations in neonatal death rate and birth rate in the US and possible relations to environmental radiation, geology and altitude. *Am. Journal of Human Genetics*, *15*, 329.

Grundy, M.F.B., Hood, J. & Newman, G.B. (1978) Birthweight standards in a community of mixed racial origin. *Br. J. Obstet. Gynaecol.*, *85*, 481–486.

Leveno, K.J., Klein, V.R., Gusick, D.S. *et al.* (1986) Single centre randomised trial of ritodrine hydrochloride for preterm labour. *Lancet*, *i*, 1293–1295.

Liston, R.M., Cohen, A.W., Mennuti, M.T. *et al.* (1982) Antepartum fetal evaluation of maternal perception of fetal movement. *Obstet. Gynecol.*, *60*, 424–426.

Lobb, M.O., Beazley, J.M. & Haddad, N.G. (1985) A controlled study of daily fetal movement counts in the prevention of stillbirths. *J. Obstet. Gynaecol. 6*, 87–91.

MacFarlane, A. & Mugford, M. (1984) *Birth Counts (Statistics of Pregnancy and Childbirth)* London: HMSO.

Manning, F., Platt, L. & Sipos, L. (1980) Antepartum fetal evaluation: Development of a fetal biophysical profile. *Am. J. Obstet Gynecol.*, *136*(6), 787–795.

Mitchell, E.A., Ford, R.P.K., Stewart, A.W. *et al.* (1993) Smoking and the sudden infant death syndrome. *Pediatrics*, *91*(5), 893–896.

Moller, M., Thompson, A.C., Borch, K. *et al.* (1984) Rupture of fetal membranes and prematurity associated with group B streptococci in urine of pregnant women. *Lancet*, *ii*, 69.

National Institute of Health Chorionic Villi Sampling Study Group (1989) The safety and efficacy of chorionic villi sampling compared to amniocentesis for prenatal diagnosis. *New Eng. J. Med*, *320*(10), 609–617.

Newnham, J.P., Evans, S.F. & Michael, C.A. (1993) Effects of frequent ultrasound during pregnancy: a randomised controlled trial. *Lancet*, *342*, 887–891.

Newton, R.W. & Hunt, L.P. (1984) Psychosocial stress in pregnancy and its relation to low birthweight. *BMJ*, *288*, 1191–1194.

Sonek, J., Reiss, R. & Gabbe, S. (1990) Antenatal fetal assessment. In *Manual of Obstetrics and Gynecology*, 2nd ed., eds Z. Zuspan E. Quilligan, pp. 57–95. St Louis: Mosby.

Whittle, M.J. & Connor, J.M. (1990) *Prenatal Diagnosis in Obstetric Practice*. Oxford: Blackwell Scientific.

3

Resuscitation and Care of the Baby at Delivery

The use of mouth-to-mouth resuscitation dates from antiquity. Benjamin Pugh in 1754 said: 'If the child does not breathe immediately upon delivery . . . wipe its mouth and press your mouth to the child's, at the same time pinching the nose with your thumb and finger to prevent air escaping; inflate the lungs'. Intubation and ventilation using oxygen was described in 1780 by Chaussier in Dijon; it is very surprising that so many useless methods of treating asphyxia have been used since.

The newborn baby is better able to survive a period of asphyxia than an adult. There are several reasons for this: they include the relatively immature brain with its reduced metabolic requirements; the ability to utilize substrates other than glucose for metabolism, for example glycerol, free fatty acids and ketone bodies; and the ability to metabolize glucose anaerobically.

None the less, a baby who is apnoeic with a slow or falling heart rate represents an extreme emergency. In such a situation, treatment, if it is to be effective, must be applied rationally. Many techniques have been developed over the last century which are irrational. These included intragastric oxygen, analeptic drugs, hyperbaric oxygen or electrical stimulation of the phrenic nerve.

The physiological changes underlying the initiation of respiration are described below. Once they are understood the reasons for active resuscitation can be easily appreciated. There are a number of situations in which problems may be predicted before birth so that a paediatrician may be called in good time to attend the delivery and before an emergency arises. These include:

1 Premature onset of labour (35 weeks or less of gestation).
2 Abnormalities found at rupture of membranes, for example polyhydramnios, oligohydramnios or meconium-stained liquor.
3 Breech presentation or other malpresentation.
4 Caesarean section under general anaesthesia.
5 Evidence of intrapartum asphyxia shown by type II dips on the cardiotocograph, a large dip area, irregular fetal heart rate, fetal

tachycardia, fetal bradychardia, or low fetal blood pH on scalp sampling.

6 Antepartum haemorrhage.

7 Prolapsed cord.

8 Severe pre-eclampsia or chronic hypertension.

9 Maternal diabetes.

10 Rhesus isoimmunization.

11 Heavy maternal sedation.

12 History of previous neonatal death or of major congenital abnormalities.

The British Birth Survey 1970 showed how common apnoea is after abnormal delivery. Of the 16 000 babies in the survey 4.7% had not breathed by three minutes, but nearly a quarter of babies born by the breech or caesarean section had not breathed by that time. The recent changes in maternal anaesthesia have altered the incidence of apnoea. Thus, it is now uncommon to see apnoea in a baby whose mother has an elective caesarean section at term after an uncomplicated pregnancy. It is not necessary to send a paediatrician to such a delivery; the doctors may be better employed in the neonatal intensive care unit.

In an emergency, the resuscitator must be able to rely on the equipment. Therefore before *every* delivery:

1 Check the resuscitation table and its equipment:

(a) laryngoscope of the appropriate size with bright light, spare batteries and bulb (we find the small curved Penlon 'O' and straight Penlon 'WIS' 'O' most useful);

(b) range of endotracheal tubes and standard connectors (2.5 mm for small babies, 3 mm for most babies; 3.5 mm tubes are particularly useful for large mature babies who have aspirated meconium). Some paediatricians and midwives like to have an endotracheal tube introducer available;

(c) manometer at 30 cm of water, or some other method of limiting the volume used such as an inflating bag. It is common to use an Ambu or Laerdal bag. A range of round masks for inflation without an endotracheal tube is necessary;

(d) source of suction which is working and has no loose connections;

(e) range of suction catheters (5,6 and 8 FG);

(f) oxygen [check the cylinder (and that a cylinder spanner is available) if piped oxygen is not available];

(g) mucus extractors;

(h) clock;

(i) umbilical venous catheters (8 and 5 FG);
(j) stethoscope;
(k) scissors;
(l) equipment for securing an endotracheal tube, so that a preterm baby can be transferred to the neonatal unit on mechanical ventilation.
2 Check drugs:
(a) dextrose 5% and 10%;
(b) sodium bicarbonate 4.2%;
(c) naloxone;
(d) normal saline;
(e) adrenalin 1:10000;
(f) syringes and needles in a range of sizes.
3 Check that the labour ward temperature is adequate. Close the windows. Turn on the overhead heater. We suggest a labour ward temperature of about 26°C, but at least 20°C. A fan heater could be used to boost the temperature of the room at the time of delivery.
4 Check that the portable incubator is warm.
5 Check the obstetric notes for problems that may be expected.
6 Check that someone has put on sterile gloves and has a sterile towel to receive the baby from the midwife or obstetrician. Warm towels must be available.

At birth

1 Turn on the clock.
2 Place the baby on the already warm resuscitation table. Have the head towards you. (Some doctors believe that it is harmful to have the head lower than the feet because pressure on the diaphragm from the liver and other organs could hinder breathing.) Gently apply suction to oropharynx and nostrils.
3 Quickly dry the baby by wiping off vernix and amniotic fluid and wrap in a dry, warm towel so as to reduce heat loss by evaporation.

By one minute after birth, an assessment of the baby's condition must be made. Subsequent management will vary according to whether asphyxia is present and, if so, whether the baby has primary or terminal apnoea (see Table 3.1).

Asphyxia

A baby with too little oxygen in the blood (hypoxaemia) and an accumulation of carbon dioxide and lactic acid (acidaemia) is said

Table 3.1 Differential diagnosis of asphyxia livida and asphyxia pallida.

Primary apnoea (asphyxia livida)	Terminal apnoea (asphyxia pallida)
Apnoea or gasping	No respiratory effect
Cyanosed	Pale and grey
Muscle tone normal or increased	Reduced muscle tone
Heart rate greater than 100/min or less than 100 but rising	Heart rate less than 100/min
Reflex grimacing on stimulation	No response to stimulation
The stage of primary apnoea lasts longer if the mother is given narcotic or anaesthetic drugs. It is shorter if gentle peripheral stimulation or pharyngeal suction is given. This stage is followed by either (*a*) onset of regular respiration or (*b*) more severe asphyxia (terminal apnoea)	If unduly prolonged, may produce brain damage followed *inevitably by death* unless: *intervention* by endotracheal (ET) intubation and intermittent positive pressure ventilation (IPPV)

to be asphyxiated. Failure to breathe is a consequence of asphyxia and of course will itself lead to further hypoxaemia, hypercapnia and asphyxia.

A baby may be born in either primary or terminal apnoea (Fig. 3.1). This terminology has come from experimental asphyxia in animals. There are four characteristic phases of respiration when any newborn mammal is made anoxic: a period of hyperventilation; a period of apnoea usually called primary or preterminal apnoea; gasping; and finally terminal or secondary apnoea. In the period of primary apnoea the animal will survive if it has air to breathe. In terminal apnoea, it dies unless the lungs are ventilated, with cardiac massage and the reversal of acidaemia with alkalis if necessary. Narcotic drugs such as pethidine will greatly prolong the period of primary apnoea, but this can be reversed by naloxone. Brain damage occurs only during terminal asphyxia as a result of prolonged cardiac arrest.

A baby in terminal apnoea will have passed through the stage of primary apnoea and the last spontaneous gasp by the time of birth. As the management of these two types of asphyxia is quite different, it is important to be able to recognise them clinically. The tems of asphyxia livida (blue) and asphyxia pallida (white) have been out of fashion for some time but are useful when a shocked baby needs active resuscitation. In general, asphyxia pallida is the same as terminal apnoea when the heart rate is very slow and the baby is

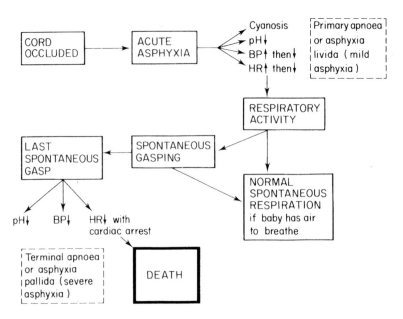

Fig. 3.1 The sequence of events following umbilical cord occlusion

shocked. The differentiation of these conditions is summarised in Table 3.1, and the causes of neonatal asphyxia are shown in Table 3.2.

The assessment of the baby's condition was formalised by Dr Virginia Apgar in 1953 by assigning a score of 0 to 2 for each of five facets of the baby's state (Table 3.3). The assessment at one minute is important for the further management of resuscitation. However, it has been shown that an assessment at five minutes is much more reliable as a predictor of the risk of death during the first 28 days of life and of the child's neurological state and risk of major handicap at the age of one year (Nelson & Ellenberg, 1981; Rehnke *et al.*, 1987). It is therefore customary to do both one-minute and five-minute Apgar scores. The five signs are not equally important – heart rate and respiratory effort are crucial – but each factor is relevant in the differentiation of mild from severe asphyxia. The score identifies high-risk infants in both the short and the long term. The higher the score the better; if the five-minute score is 7 or less it should be repeated at 10 minutes (Table 3.3).

Table 3.2 Causes of neonatal asphyxia

Immaturity

Respiratory
Obstruction, such as mucus or choanal atresia
Aspiration of blood or meconium
Pneumothorax, usually produced by overenthusiastic resuscitation
Congenital pneumonia
Hypoplastic lungs, as in renal agenesis
Surfactant deficiency, which will later lead to hyaline membrane disease
Diaphragmatic hernia

Metabolic
Acidaemia from antenatal hypoxia
Hypoglycaemia

Cerebral
Congenital cerebral abnormalities
Drugs, such as those given to the mother for sedation
Reflex apnoea, often caused by deep suction of the pharynx
Shock caused by serious blood loss
Severe infection such as group B streptococcal septicaemia
Traumatic birth

Table 3.3 Apgar Scoring (modified after Apgar, 1966).

	Score		
	0	1	2
Heart rate	Absent	Less than 100/min	More than 100/min
Respiratory effort	Absent	Gasping or irregular	Crying or rhythmic breathing
Muscle tone	Flaccid	Some flexor tone	Good with movement
Response to stimulation	None	Poor (with a facial grimace)	Good (with a cry)
Colour of tongue or abdominal skin	Pallor	Cyanosis	Pink

Some obstetricians and paediatricians now believe that cord blood should be taken from the placenta after every delivery. This will give an indication of any asphyxia which may have taken place.

Immediate check

Normal baby: spontaneous respiration established

1 Dry the baby and wrap warmly.
2 Check for obvious abnormalities such as spina bifida or imperforate anus; abrasions, fractures, or haemorrhage due to trauma; listen to the heart and lungs; palpate the abdomen for masses or enlarged viscera; examine the genitalia.
3 Put on an umbilical cord clamp about 3 cm from the umbilicus and cut off the rest of the cord. Check for the presence of two arteries (small, thick-walled) and one vein (large, thin-walled).
4 Give the baby to the mother. It is nice for the baby to be in skin-to-skin contact with her (Fig. 3.2) with the blanket to cover both of them. The baby can then take the first feed.
5 Transfer mother and baby together to the postnatal ward.

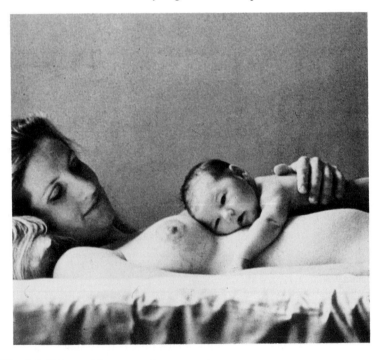

Fig. 3.2 Skin-to-skin contact in a warm labour ward. By courtesy of Professor J. Hedgecoe

The infant with primary apnoea

Action can be taken in the following order:

1 Gentle pharyngeal suction. This provides reflex stimulation of the posterior phyaryngeal wall and produces a powerful stimulus for respiration.
2 Blow oxygen over the face (too fast a jet merely cools the baby).
3 Flick the feet – lightly!
4 Ventilation by bag and mask if the baby has not breathed by about two minutes.

If the heart rate falls or the baby remains unresponsive, proceed with the schedule for terminal apnoea.

The infant with terminal apnoea

1 Inspect the vocal cords with a laryngoscope; aspirate any liquid under direct vision.
2 Intubate with the largest possible endotracheal tube (ET) (3 mm diameter for the average baby); do not advance more than 1–1.5 cm beyond the glottis (for technique see below).
3 The endotracheal tube should already have a connector attached to it; this can then be fitted on to an inflating bag. The alternative technique is to attach the side limb of a Y connector down which oxygen can flow at approximately 2 1/min.
4 In general the pressure should not exceed 30–35 cm of water (a pressure valve may need setting manually or a water manometer may provide automatic blow-off). However, it is important to achieve adequate ventilation and movement of the chest wall gives a good guide to this. In some cases the pressure may need to be quite high in order to inflate the lungs (Milner, 1991). When a bag is used it is safe to use higher pressures since the volume is controlled.
5 Occlude the open end of the Y connector with your thumb and release rhythmically at about 30 times per minute or inflate with the bag; ensure that all connections are tight.
6 Check that both sides of the chest move and there are breath sounds on both sides; the heart rate should gradually increase to normal, and the baby should become pink. If this does not happen consider the problems described on pp. 65–68.
7 Maintain artificial respiration until the baby has started breathing spontaneously and this has become well established (for several minutes).

8 Extubate the baby.

9 Give the baby to the parents.

10 Do *not* transfer to the special care baby unit unless there are other indications (see Chapter 4). Routine observations can be carried out on the postnatal ward.

NB. If the baby is obviously in terminal apnoea, do not wait for 1 min before starting resuscitation. A preterm baby should be intubated if he is in any respiratory difficulty, and it is common to use routine intubation for babies under 30 weeks gestation.

If in doubt as to whether apnoea is primary or terminal, proceed as for terminal apnoea – intubate.

Management of cardiac arrest

Press the upper sternum sharply but gently downwards with two fingers once per second (preferably get an assistant to do this); intubate and ventilate as above; if single-handed give five beats of external cardiac massage before intubating; check efficacy of massage by feeling femoral pulses; discontinue massage when the heartbeat is established; too heavy a pressure or pressure too low down on the sternum may rupture the liver with possible fatal haemorrhage. Cardiac massage is often useful if the heart rate is very slow (< 60/min).

Use of drugs in apnoea

The use of drugs, even when indicated, should never delay intubation and artificial ventilation if this is necessary. It is possible to use:

1 *Alkali.* A baby who has been apnoeic for some time develops metabolic acidaemia. The best way to correct this is to treat the hypoxia which causes it – by intubation and ventilation with added oxygen. In the most severely affected babies alkali may be given. It must be given *slowly* and *sparingly* as 8.4% sodium bicarbonate (which contains 1 mmol in 1 ml) diluted in an equal volume of 10% dextrose or as 4.2% $NaHCO_3$. Not more than 3 mmol/kg body weight should be given at a rate of not more than 1 mmol/min. A useful rule is to give sodium bicarbonate if the baby has not breathed spontaneously by five minutes. It can be given through a needle into the umbilical vein at the base of the cord, but some paediatricians feel happier to give it through an umbilical venous catheter.

2 *Naloxone.* If the mother has been given pethidine or morphine within a few hours of delivery *and* the baby is slow the breathe adequately after resuscitation, naloxone may be given intravenously, 0.01 mg/kg once only to counteract the respiratory depression that they cause. Naloxone has the advantage over previously used narcotic antagonists that it has no respiratory depressant action of its own. It can be given intramuscularly, but this is less satisfactory as the sole route of administration. However, it may be useful to give an additional 0.01 mg/kg intramuscularly because it will have a longerlasting effect.

3 *Analeptics* (e.g. nikethamide). These drugs should *not* be used: they are unnecessary in primary apnoea and dangerous in terminal apnoea as they will not effect respiration and may cause fits and hypotension.

Some techniques used in resuscitation

Laryngoscopy and endotracheal intubation (Fig 3.3)

1 Lay the baby on its back.

2 Hold head with right hand so as to keep the neck slightly flexed and the head extended on the neck.

3 Hold laryngoscope in the left hand and pass the blade along the groove on the right of the laryngoscope, displacing the tongue to the left.

4 Advance blade until it rests in the vallecula between the epiglottis and base of tongue.

5 Tilt tip of blade slightly upwards so as to bring the glottis (top of trachea) into view.

6 If necessary, pressure on the cricoid cartilage in the throat with another finger of the left hand will produce a better view.

7 The glottis may be obscured by fluid. If so, a fine suction catheter is used to reveal it as a black slit with the vocal cords on each side.

8 An appropriate size of endotracheal tube is taken in the right hand and passed through the glottis under direct vision.

9 It should go no further than 1–1.5 cm beyond the glottis otherwise one main bronchus will be entered, so occluding the other and causing collapse of that lung.

10 Check the position by auscultation over both lungs and the stomach.

11 Air entry should be equal on both sides of the chest. The first breath should be quite prolonged (about five seconds) to ensure expansion of the lungs. Subsequent breaths should be approximately

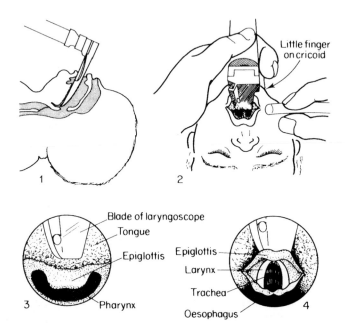

Fig. 3.3 How to intubate. 1, Lie the baby on its back if possible, with the head tilted slightly downwards. Extend the neck so that the chin points upwards. 2, Take the infant laryngoscope with a straight blade and insert the blade into the infant's mouth, gently lifting the tongue. 3, The epiglottis can be seen at the base of the tongue; it hangs down obscuring the entrance to the larynx. 4, Slide the laryngoscope to the base of the epiglottis and tilt the tip of the blade upward. At the same time press gently on the cricoid cartilage with the little finger. The entrance to the larynx will then come into view. An endotracheal tube can then be guided carefully into the trachea. From S. Wallis & D. Harvey (1979), by permission of the authors and editors

one second. The pressure may need to be increased if there is no movement of the chest wall.

Mask and bag ventilation (Fig. 3.4)

For new medical staff, or nurses and midwives who are inexperienced in resuscitation, and when no immediate skilled help is available, this is probably a safer method of resuscitating an asphyxiated baby than unskilled endotracheal intubation. Bags used for neonatal resuscita-

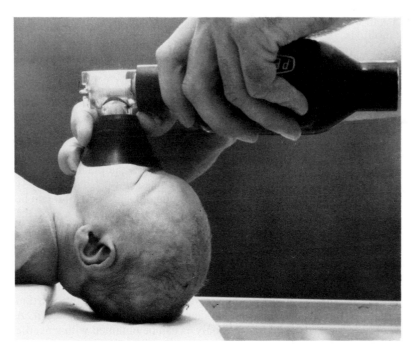

Fig. 3.4 The Cardiff infant inflating bag and mask. (By courtesy of Penlon Ltd)

tion have a valve that ensures that it is impossible to maintain inappropriately high pressure for more than a fraction of a second. Twenty to thirty breaths per minute should be given.

Chest movement should be the method of judging the efficacy of resuscitation. Make sure that the baby is on its back with the neck slightly flexed and the head extended. The neonatal face-mask should be positioned so as to produce a good seal over the mouth and nose.

Insertion of umbilical venous catheter

This is the most reliable way of administering drugs.

1 Fill a 8 or 5 FG polyvinyl catheter with normal saline via a three-way tap.
2 Close the tap so that no air may get to the baby on insertion.

3 Cut cord with sterile scissors or scalpel blade to about 2 cm from umbilicus.
4 Grip cut end with forceps and insert the catheter under sterile conditions 5–10 cm into umbilical vein (the large, single, thin-walled vessel).
5 Drugs may be given through the side limb of the three-way tap.
6 *Never* open the umbilical venous catheter to air.

Obtaining cord blood

It has been common to allow blood to drip from the placental end of the cord, but the blood is easily contaminated with Wharton's jelly and it is better to collect the blood with a needle and syringe. It can be taken from a vein on the cord itself or on the fetal surface of the placenta.

It has now been shown that arterial pH at birth is a better measure of recent asphyxia than the Apgar score. (Goldenberg *et al.*, 1984; Vintzileos *et al.*, 1987). There is some controversy over its sensitivity as a predictor of neurological impairment (Nelson & Ellenberg, 1981). In any birth where this is necessary, such as intrapartum hypoxia or preterm delivery, two clamps can be put on the cord. A sample of arterial blood for gas analysis can be obtained with a needle and syringe.

Complications of endotracheal intubation

Unskilled resuscitation may be dangerous. Errors usually stem from lack of experience and lack of understanding of the physiological mechanisms underlying the onset of respiration. Examples include:

1 Advancing the laryngoscope blade too far, obscuring the glottis and revealing the oesophagus which may be intubated in error. In this situation withdraw the blade slowly and point the tip slightly upwards. The glottis will then come into view.
2 Overextension of the baby's head: this precludes a good view. The neck should be slightly flexed and the head extended (see Fig. 3.4)
3 Insertion of the endotracheal tube too far beyond the glottis (see above).
4 Overenthusiastic use of drugs: the establishment of respiration by artificial ventilation must precede the use of alkali or naloxone. In addition, alkali should not be given unless there is adequate circulation as it will remain in the liver and not progress further.

5 Pneumothorax (see p. 68 and 182).

The techniques of resuscitation cannot be learnt from a book. It is useful to practise on models but there is no substitute for constant practice in the company of someone experienced in these techniques. The most important rule is that you must see the larynx before you intubate. It is easy to become agitated and to push the tube down into the oesophagus.

Examination of the Placenta

The placenta should be examined after every delivery because of its relevance to fetal growth. Conditions in which this is particularly useful include ascertaining the zygocity of twins, fetal haemorrhage, intrauterine infection with chorioamnionitis, birth asphyxia with retroplacental clots and placental infarcts, and intrauterine growth retardation (associated with a small placenta). Any abnormal placenta, including those from multiple pregnancies, should be sent to the pathologist for an opinion.

Indications for Transfer to Special or Intermediate Care Baby Unit

These indications are listed fully in Chapter 4. In summary, babies who have been born by caesarean section or forceps delivery or those who have minor abnormalities should *not* be routinely transferred to the special baby care unit. It is much more difficult for parents to form an attachment to their baby there and also more difficult to establish breast feeding.

Other Emergencies

There are a number of conditions which require urgent treatment in the labour ward.

Meconium aspiration

This condition is commonly seen in term babies, particularly those who are SFGA or who have had acute intrapartum asphyxia. It is rare in the preterm. It is also discussed in Chapters 6 and 8. If meconium is inhaled a chemical pneumonitis ensues. This may often be complicated by secondary bacterial pneumonia or pneumothorax.

The most important prophylactic procedure is to aspirate the mouth and pharynx thoroughly as soon as the head is born. Although it is no longer considered good practice to aspirate the pharynx deeply in a normal delivery, it is essential when there is thick meconium in the amniotic fluid. Some units have a policy of holding the chest firmly to stop the first breath but this is very difficult to do, of doubtful benefit, and may even be dangerous. It seems more practical to do the aspiration while the body is still inside the birth canal.

If thick meconium is aspirated from the mouth, it is essential to inspect the larynx with a laryngoscope. If meconium is seen on the larynx itself, an attempt should be made to aspirate the trachea. This can be done either by passing a suction catheter through the glottis, or by passing an endotracheal tube and passing the catheter through that. (Linder *et al.*, 1988). Of course, it is necessary to start ventilation when the suction has been performed. It is not helpful to perform bronchial lavage.

If meconium is aspirated into the lungs, the baby develops respiratory distress because of pneumonitis and plugging of the bronchioles with skin debris, mucus and meconium. Affected babies show signs of respiratory distress with tachypnoea, recession and sometimes cyanosis. A chest radiograph (Fig 6.9) at this time is characteristic, showing irregular areas of subsegmental atalectasis with associated hyperaeration. Such babies may need increased inspired oxygen concentrations to maintain normal arterial oxygen tensions. Arterial oxygen levels should be monitored and inspired oxygen concentrations adjusted appropriately. Such babies should also be screened for infection and started on antibiotics because of the high incidence of secondary bacterial pneumonia.

Diaphragmatic hernia

Embryologically, the diaphragm develops from several tissues. Sometimes there are defects where these tissues have not properly fused. Most commonly there is persistence of the left pleuroperitoneal canal through which bowel herniates. This produces an acute emergency as the lung is unable to expand. Air entering the bowel following delivery causes increasing dyspnoea and cyanosis and displacement of the heart to the right. Other signs include bowel sounds audible in the chest and a scaphoid abdomen due to absence of bowel. Treatment is by endotraceal intubation and intermittent positive pressure ventilation (IPPV) until surgery can be arranged to replace the bowel in the abdomen and repair the diaphragmatic defect. It is useful to sedate the baby heavily with an opiate to suppress respiration and to use a paralysing agent, thus allowing adequate mechanical ventilation. Many surgeons now feel it is better

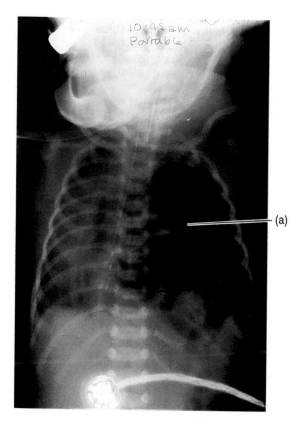

Fig 3.5 X-ray showing diaphragmatic hernia; note bowel in the chest (a)

to delay operation for a day or two. Ventilation should never be by face-mask as air will be swallowed causing the bowel to distend and increasing the dyspnoea. For this reason, it is useful to pass a gastric tube and empty the stomach of air with a syringe. Associated abnormalities are common, and the prognosis is only fair because there is usually pulmonary hypoplasia. This is another reason why it is difficult to expand the lungs (Fig. 3.5).

Pneumothorax

Pneumothorax (see also Chapter 8) is a common complication in the newborn, particularly following meconium aspiration, ventilator therapy, or staphylococcal pneumonia. It may complicate overenthusiastic resuscitation in the labour ward. If a tension pneumothorax develops, the situation may be extremely dangerous. The diagnosis should be considered in any baby who suddenly deteriorates or in whom resuscitation proves particularly difficult. In this situation, there is usually no time for radiographic confirmation (Fig. 3.6). Action should be taken on the basis of clinical signs, but these may be very difficult to detect and so transillumination has proved very valuable. It is necessary to use a very strong fibreoptic source of light. The chest glows brilliantly when a pneumothorax is present, but the investigation is not so useful for babies over 34 weeks gestation as the chest wall is thicker.

Emergency treatment is by aspiration of the pleural air. This is conveniently done by using a 21 gauge butterfly needle filled with sterile water. The free end of the tubing is placed a few centimetres under the surface of sterile water in a sterile container. The needle is inserted at the fourth intercostal space in the anterior axillary line. If there is a pneumothorax on that side, air will be seen to bubble out from the tubing under the surface of the water on aspiration.

Hydrops fetalis

The signs of hydrops include severe anaemia with a greyish pallor or cyanosis, ascites and generalized oedema and hepatosplenomegaly. The commonest cause of hydrops fetalis in the UK is still severe haemolytic disease of the newborn associated with rhesus alloimmunization although it is much less common than it was; anti-D immunoglobulin has prevented many cases (see p. 297), and fetal transfusions ensure that the babies are born in better condition. The birth of so severely affected an infant should normally be anticipated

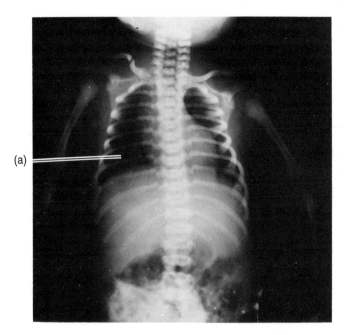

Fig. 3.6 Right-sided pneumothorax (a)

before delivery. Treatment is urgent. Clamp the cord immediately: adequate respiration must be established; laryngeal oedema may be very severe, so do not take the endotracheal tube out too early. Paracentesis to reduce respiratory embarrassment should be performed through the left iliac fossa to avoid an enlarged liver; it is probably easiest to use a polyvinyl intravenous cannula. Heart failure should be treated by giving intravenous frusemide 2 mg/kg, and if necessary by venesection (10–20 ml of blood removed from the umbilical vein) and digitalization (see p. 274). Ventilation is very useful in treating pulmonary oedema, but drains may be required for pleural effusions. A partial exchange transfusion is then carried out using Group O rhesus-negative packed cells up to a total of 100 ml. Sometimes peritoneal dialysis is required.

Fetal haemorrhage

Fetal haemorrhage may complicate twin delivery (bleeding into the other twin), antepartum haemorrhage, or accidental incision of the placenta by the obstetrician at caesarean section. The baby looks very pale and has tachypnoea and tachycardia. The cord should be tied late and as much blood as possible transferred to the baby before this is done. A transfusion of 20 ml/kg should be given as an emergency. This may be given as Group O rhesus-negative blood; a bottle of blood of this group should always be available in the labour ward for this purpose.

Choanal atresia

The newborn baby is able to breathe mainly through the nose. Any nasal obstruction therefore causes extreme respiratory embarrassment. In choanal atresia, the nasal airway is blocked by a bony or membranous septum across the posterior nasopharynx. This condition should be suspected if there is persistent respiratory difficulty or cyanosis from birth. It is relieved by crying, as it is only in this situation that the baby can inspire through the mouth. The diagnosis is made by inability to pass a feeding catheter down either nostril. Immediate treatment is by inserting an infant oral airway. Elective surgery may then be carried out at a later date.

Exomphalos and gastroschisis (see also chapter 9)

Exomphalos occurs in about 1 in 10 000 births. The abdominal contents have herniated through the umbilicus into a sac made up of peritoneum and amnion. There are commonly associated abnormalities of the heart, intestines or genitourinary system. Sometimes the sac has perforated before birth.

In gastroschisis there is a defect in the whole thickness of the anterior abdominal wall, usually just to the right of the umbilicus. A large proportion of the gastrointestinal tract including stomach may prolapse through this defect and there is no covering sac. Both conservative and surgical treatment have been advocated; in each the immediate management in the labour ward is identical:

1 Cover the sac or bowel with saline-soaked gauze or silastic sheeting in the form of a bag.
2 Pass a nasogastric tube and aspirate stomach contents at frequent intervals to prevent intestinal distension.
3 Consult a surgeon. (Details about the preparation of babies for transfer to a regional neonatal surgical unit, and for surgery are given in Chapter 9.)

Babies Who Need Transfer to a Regional Centre for Intensive Neonatal Care

Ideally, if problems can be anticipated, a baby should be transferred *in utero*. This is not always possible – serious unpredicted problems can arise after delivery which necessitate transfer to a regional centre for intensive neonatal care for specialist management. It is important for the referring hospital staff to maintain the baby in as stable and satisfactory a condition as possible until the transfer. It is better to arrange with the obstetric staff for the mother to go with the baby if at all possible; but in any event the parents should be given an instant photograph of their baby – preferably before too many tubes and monitors are attached. The referring hospital should consider having the following specimens ready to accompany the baby or have arranged for them to be processed: (a) maternal high vaginal swab and clotted blood sample, (b) placenta (in sealed bag), (c) cord blood, and (d) (from the baby) surface swabs (ear, nose, throat, umbilical, rectal), blood cultures and gastric aspirate – all should be obtained before antibiotic treatment is started.

The team who collect the baby must check that they have all the appropriate equipment. This would include:

1 Portable heated incubator with working ventilator and circuit.
2 Full oxygen and air cylinders and spare full cylinders with spanners.
3 Portable heart-rate monitor, and transcutaneous Po_2 monitor and syringe pump.
4 Gamgee, blankets and bubble sheeting.
5 Other equipment including mucus extractors, ambu bag, torch, suction catheters, intubating equipment with assorted endotracheal tubes and connectors, electrodes and cream, artery forceps, oxygen tubing.
6 Drugs.
7 Instant camera and flash.

A check list must be kept with the transport incubator and equipment used must be replaced immediately on return. All equipment must be checked daily and kept in optimum working order ready for a flying squad call at any time.

The flying squad team, on arrival at the referring hospital, should be prepared to spend time getting the baby into optimal condition for the journey. For example, the baby may require warming if cold, blood gases should be checked as acidosis or hypoxaemia may need correction and intubation and mechanical ventilation may be needed if there are signs of respiratory distress. It may be helpful to pass an arterial umbilical catheter.

When the baby is warm and stable, prepare for the journey:

1 Make sure incubator and wrappings are warmed.
2 Check oxygen and ventilation settings.
3 Place cardiac electrodes and transcutaneous Po_2 probe on baby.
4 Place baby in incubator and wrap in prewarmed gamgee and insulating bubble sheet.
5 Connect baby to ventilator; check ventilator settings, oxygen concentration and air entry.
6 Connect baby to appropriate monitors.
7 Make sure baby is comfortable and well padded for journey – in case of emergency stops.
8 Check records and if necessary obtain photocopies of notes relating to delivery and early neonatal care.
9 Check specimens are obtained and consent form completed if appropriate.
10 Check baby is wearing two namebands

Before departure make sure that the parents have seen the baby. Remember to keep the parents and referring staff fully informed of how the baby is progressing.

References and Further Reading

Apgar, V. (1953) Proposal for new method of evaluation of newborn infant. *Anaesthesia and Analgesia, 32*, 260–267.

Apgar, V. (1966) The newborn scoring system. *Pediatric Clinics of North America, 13*(3), 645–650.

Goldenberg, R.L., Huddleston, J.F. & Nelson, K.G. (1984) Apgar scores and umbilical arterial pH in preterm newborn infants. *Am. J. Obstet. Gynecol., 149*, 651–654.

Linder, N., Aranda, J.V., Tsur, M. *et al.* (1988) Need for endotracheal intubation and suction in meconium-stained infants. *J. Pediatr., 112*, 613.

Milner, A.D. (1986) ABC of resuscitation: resuscitation at birth. *BMJ, 292*, 1657–1659.

Milner, A.D. (1991) *Arch. Dis. Child, 66*, 66.

Moore, K.L. (1988) The Developing Human Clinically Orientated Embryology. 4th ed. Philadelphia: W.B. Saunders.

Nelson, K.B. & Ellenberg, J.H. (1981) Apgar scores as predictors of chronic neurologic disability. *Pediatrics, 68*, 36–44.

Rehnke, M., Carter, R.L., Hardt, N.S. *et al.* (1987) The relationship of Apgar scores, gestational age and birthweight to survival of low-birthweight infants. *Am. J. Perinatol.*, *4*, 121–124.

Vintzileos, A. *et al.* (1987) The relationships among the fetal biophysical profile, umbilical cord pH and Apgar scores. *Am. J. Obstet. Gynecol. 157*, 627–631.

4

Care of the Normal Newborn Baby

The First Routine Examination

It is usually possible to carry out a quick examination of the baby while still in the labour ward. This may be done by the midwife or doctor and is mainly concerned with the detection of serious abnormalities, for example cleft lip and palate or spina bifida. It is a mistake to attempt a full examination at that time, as the baby may become very cold.

Within the first 24 hours a full examination must be carried out by the doctor. This is best done by the mother's bedside so that she can watch: in this way she is able to ask questions as the examination proceeds and the doctor is able to provide specific reassurances for any worries that she may have. It is an advantage for the examining doctor already to be aware of any unusual circumstances in the family, social, obstetric or paediatric history. Parents may be very anxious about what, to the doctor, seems to be a trivial blemish on the baby, e.g. stork bite marks, crumpled ears or milia. The parents' anxieties must always be taken seriously and full explanation given. An over-glib response will only increase their anxiety. Always ask about family illnesses, any abnormalities of pregnancy, the gestation and any family history of tuberculosis.

1 Take a good history. Before the routine examination mother's notes must be read carefully for important clues (see Chapter 2).
2 Emergency conditions should have been excluded by the quick examination at birth, but it is surprising how many conditions can be missed – for example a cleft palate is easily overlooked. For this reason a routine examination should be very thorough.
3 Develop a routine method of examining the baby. There are several schemes for this, but it is probably easiest to examine the baby methodically from fontanelle to toe so that no important points are missed. It may be useful to have a printed examination chart to be filled in for every baby.

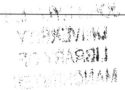

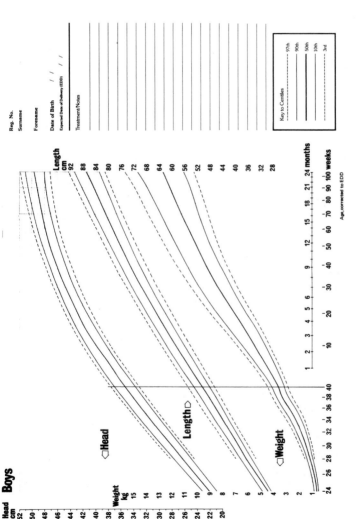

Fig. 4.1 Pearson–Gairdner Chart. This is the 1988 edition extended from Gairdner, D. and Pearson, J. (1985) *Archives of Disease in Childhood* **60**, 1202. Reproduced with permission from Castlemead Publications. Reference GPB3 boys.

Head and skull

The baby may have a large or small skull circumference, or it may be within the normal range but out of proportion to the rest of the body. The occipitofrontal circumference at birth may be misleading because the head can change shape quite markedly within the first three days. A baby born by the vertex usually has an elongated head from moulding and this turns to a round shape within a day or so. The doctor should, therefore, always measure the head. It is useful to plot the result on a Pearson and Gairdner chart (Fig. 4.1), although this chart may not be appropriate for babies of certain ethnic groups such as those from the Indian subcontinent. The baby's head size can be compared with weight and length. Length is impossible to measure accurately in the newborn period with a tape measure. Inexpensive portable equipment is now available, for example neonatal mat as well as the neonatometer. Centile charts for non-caucasian babies are becoming available and will be particularly useful to units serving populations with a high proportion of immigrants.

The fontanelle and sutures should be examined carefully. A small-for-gestational-age (SFGA) baby has a relatively large anterior

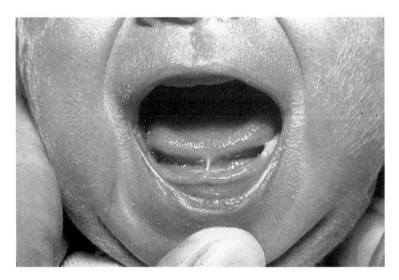

Fig. 4.2 Tongue-tie

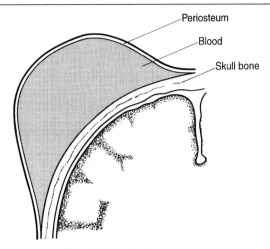

Periosteum

Blood

Skull bone

Fig. 4.3 Cephalhaematoma

fontanelle. If there is any suggestion that the fontanelle is very large or that the sutures are markedly separated, serial measurements of the occipitofrontal circumference should be made, in case the baby is developing hydrocephalus. A third fontanelle between the anterior and posterior fontanelles is one of the supporting signs of Down syndrome, but it is very inconstant and should not be relied on.

The scalp should be examined carefully because a fetal scalp electrode may have been overlooked. Some babies have marked oedema over the presenting area or bruising where a ventouse cup was applied, known as caput succadaneum. Cephalhaematoma (Fig. 4.3), a collection of blood between the periosteum of one of the skull bones and the bone itself, is very common (see Chapter 5). It should not be confused with the rare and dangerous subaponeurotic haemorrhage (see Chapter 5) in which the head circumference rapidly enlarges and there is a boggy feel to the whole of the scalp. A baby with this condition needs urgent transfusion to prevent exsanguination.

Microcephaly is an inappropriately small head circumference. One should take care before informing the parents about any abnormality of the head circumference because the *rate* of growth of the head is more important than a single circumference reading.

Eyes

Both eyes should be carefully examined. Any discharge or inflammation in the first 24 hours should be investigated urgently as it may indicate gonococcal infection. Ophthalmia neonatorum is a notifiable condition. The baby's eyes are usually open for the first few hours after birth, but it is common for the lids to become very swollen during the next two days and it may be difficult to see the eye itself. The swelling is more common after a difficult delivery. The lids should be carefully separated to reveal the eyeball to make certain that it is present. If the eye itself can be seen the cornea should be observed for size and clarity. A congenital glaucoma causes a cornea which is more than 11 mm in diameter and is cloudy.

There is often a subconjunctival haemorrhage. This disappears within 10 days and is of no significance except that it is upsetting to the parents. It usually appears as a tiny bright red crescent-shaped mark in the white of the eye.

If it is easy to inspect the eye itself it is useful to shine a light or an ophthalmoscope through the pupil. On looking through an ophthalmoscope, the retina appears red and this is called the red reflex. In this way a cataract may be found. However, the commonest abnormalities of the retina are haemorrhages which again disappear without causing any problem.

Babies often seem to have difficulty in coordinating their eyes during the early weeks of life. They may therefore appear to squint and their gaze sometimes wanders. It should be explained to parents that this is a normal appearance at this age. Babies can see very well at birth, and are thought to see things clearly in focus about 25 cm away – about the distance of the breast from a mother's face. It is important to remember this when examining babies as they will enjoy looking at a face; you should be certain that you are the right distance away and are clearly visible.

Ears

The ears should be inspected to ensure that they are not very low set on the head or sticking out abnormally and, most importantly, that there is an auditory meatus. Ears should be considered low set when the helix meets the cranium at a level below that of a horizontal plane with the corner of the orbit. Small lumps of cartilage, usually called accessory auricles, are often found just in front of the ear and may need to be removed if they are very obvious. Some tiny skin tags can be tied off, but larger blemishes should be referred to a plastic surgeon to ensure that all the cartilage is removed.

Marks on the face

A birthmark on the face is usually very obvious, and most of them are entirely benign. The commonest is the simple naevus or 'stork bite mark'. This is usually present as a V-shape mark on the forehead or eyelids (hence the name stork bite since this is supposed to represent the mark of the stork's beak when he carried the baby).

Nose

A baby's nose often appears squashed if there was oligohydramnios. This usually corrects itself within a few days. If the baby has any respiratory difficulty it may be necessary to pass a catheter down each nostril to make certain that there is no choanal atresia (see Chapter 3).

Mouth

A cleft lip is obvious but a cleft palate is not. To be certain that a cleft palate has been excluded, it is necessary both to look at the palate and to feel it. The tongue can be depressed with a wooden spatula to reveal the whole length of the palate; it is possible to have a cleft of the soft palate which cannot be seen without depressing the tongue. A submucosal cleft of the hard palate can be missed by inspection alone. It will become obvious when felt. Other abnormalities in the mouth are usually obvious, such as incisor teeth present at birth, a very enlarged tongue or cysts of the gum.

Some minor abnormalities of the mouth may cause concern to the parents. It is common to see tiny white cysts along the midline of the palate or in the gums. These are often called Epstein's pearls and disappear without any problem.

Skin of the face

There are a number of common minor abnormalities of the skin. A baby may have tiny blister-like lesions over the face at birth. These are called miliaria crystallina; they burst and disappear spontaneously although it is usually wise to take a swab to ensure that there is no infection.

Tiny white spots on the nose are known as milia (milk spots) and are due to sebaceous gland enlargement. Tiny white cysts are often seen on the face. They are often given long names which are not of great importance.

Neck

It is usually obvious if the neck is abnormally short, but the neck must be palpated to ensure that there are no cysts, webbing or an enlarged thyroid. Occasionally sinuses discharging from the neck can be seen.

Arms

Look at the arms to see if they are the same length. It may be obvious that the baby is moving only one arm, in which case the commonest reasons are brachial plexus palsy (Erb's palsy) (see Chapter 5) or a fractured clavicle or humerus (see Chapter 5). It is easy to miss such common abnormalities as syndactyly or an absent or extra finger; count the fingers on each hand and examine the hand carefully. A single palmar crease is a common physical sign of Down syndrome. Do not make this diagnosis on the basis of a single palmar crease alone as it occurs in 1% of the normal population.

Heart

Some doctors start the examination with the heart because it is easier to listen to it before the baby starts to cry. Look for central cyanosis by inspecting the tongue and look for any breathlessness. Many newborn babies have various soft systolic murmurs but a loud systolic murmur or any diastolic murmur is a reason for immediate cardiac investigation. The femoral pulses should be palpated, but this is usually done later in the examination.

Chest

Look for tachypnoea or retraction of the intercostal spaces or of the ribs or subcostal area. Auscultation of the chest is not very useful but is traditional. It is also useful for junior doctors and midwives to be familiar with normal breath sounds in the newborn so that an emergency (for example an endotracheal tube slipping into the right main bronchus) can be recognised.

Breasts

Assessment of breast size is important as part of the gestational assessment of the baby (see below). Breast engorgement is not usually obvious at the first examination.

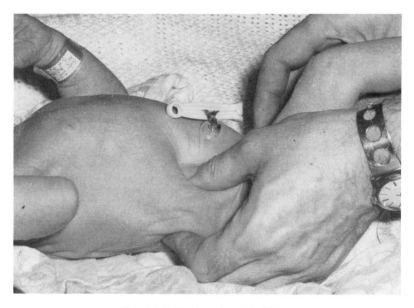

Fig. 4.4 Palpating the right kidney

Abdomen

Look for marked distension; this may indicate ascites which often occurs in a baby with hydrops. The liver, spleen and kidneys should be felt for. The spleen may normally be palpable just below the costal margin, but it is greatly enlarged in rhesus disease. The liver is most easily felt in the epigastrium; it is usually about half way between the umbilicus and the xiphisternum. A liver edge at or below the umbilicus is abnormal. The kidneys can be palpated by bimanual examination or by using one hand with the thumb in front of the abdomen and the fingers behind the loin (Fig. 4.4). Pelvic enlargement of the kidneys is now usually diagnosed by ultrasound before birth.

Umbilicus

Even though the cord has been clamped at birth, it is possible to see whether there are three vessels in the cord. It is common for the skin of the abdomen to encroach on the base of the cord and this may suggest that an umbilical hernia will develop later. The base of the cord should be examined carefully for minor degrees of exomphalos which are easily missed; this is a hernia containing gut with a transparent membrane. Inflammation of the umbilicus is unusual in the first 24 hours.

Femoral pulses

The hips should be abducted into a frog position; the femoral pulses can be felt in the midpoint of the groin. They are sometimes rather difficult to find; it is important to wait for the baby to stop crying. If the pulses cannot be found, coarctation of the aorta may be present; but the usual reason is that they were not very obvious and they are easily palpable later in the first week. Coarctation may be present with normal femoral pulses because the ductus arteriosus can supply the aorta. It is, therefore, possible to find them on the first day, but they then disappear several days later when the ductus closes. Any baby with a suspected cardiac abnormality should have the femoral pulses examined repeatedly.

Hips

A careful examination for congenital dislocation of the hips is essential; it is described in detail on p. 231. The important findings are limited abduction and the sudden jump when the hip is dislocated or reduced.

Genitalia

Boys

The first week of life is the most important time to establish whether the testes have descended. A careful record that the testes have descended ensures that there is no later worry about whether testes are undescended or merely retractile. Each of the testes should be present in the scrotum after 36 weeks gestation (Fig. 4.5). If the testes have not descended, an appointment should be made to see the baby in three months time because they often descend meanwhile. After three months the testes are unlikely to descend, unless the baby was very premature.

The penis should be examined carefully. The foreskin cannot be retracted at birth and the meatus may look very small, but this is not an indication for circumcision. Some boys have hypospadias: the

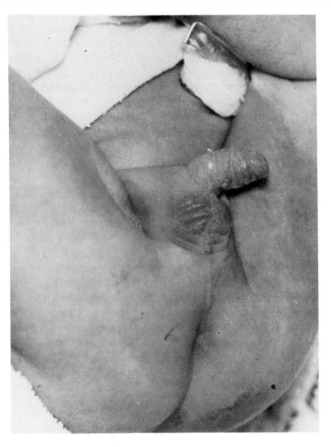

Fig. 4.5 Undescended testes in a baby of 35 weeks gestation

urethral meatus is not on the tip of the penis but on the ventral surface somewhere between the tip and the scrotum. In this condition the foreskin is cleft on the ventral surface (Fig. 4.6) and is often called hooded. The baby looks as if he has been circumcised naturally. A careful search for the meatus should be made, as there is often a small dimple on the tip of the penis which is thought to be the meatus when in fact the urine emerges further down the penis. If there is any doubt, the mother should be asked to watch micturition to see where the urine emerges and that the baby produces a good stream. A dribble rather than a good stream is an important physical sign and should always be recorded because urethral valves may be present which could lead to permanent renal damage unless they are resected (see Chapter 10). A boy with hypospadias should not be circumcised because some of the skin may be needed for repair of the urethra. If circumcision is needed for religious reasons, it is possible to take a tiny piece of skin and leave plenty for the plastic surgeon. The parents are often concerned about the boy's future sexual function and fertility. These will not be problems and this should be explained.

A very small penis (micropenis) may be a sign of hypopituitarism, particularly if there is associated hypoglycaemia.

The scrotum is often pigmented and the usual reason for this is racial. However, do not forget adrenal hyperplasia which can produce the same appearance (see p. 239).

Girls

The labia minora and the clitoris look surprisingly large in the newborn, particularly if the baby is preterm. If there is any doubt about the size of the clitoris a senior opinion should be obtained because some forms of adrenal hyperplasia may cause masculinization and need urgent treatment. Separate the labia majora; the vaginal

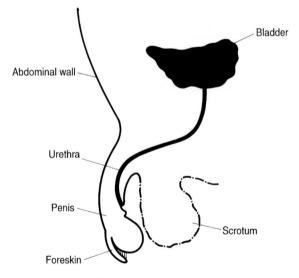

Fig. 4.6 Hypospadias

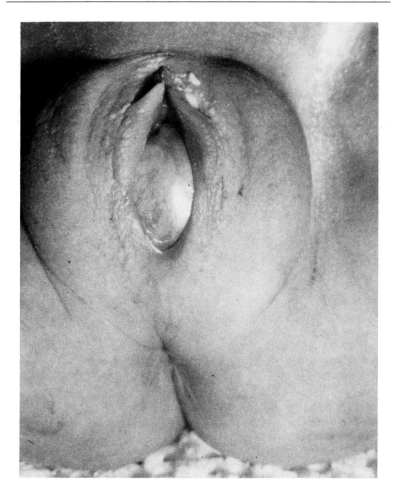

Fig. 4.7 Hydrocolpos (imperforate hymen)

opening should be obvious. If it is not, probe very gently because it is important not to miss an absent vagina. Discharge of meconium through the vagina indicates a fistula from the bowel.

There are often small tags around the vagina or even small cysts. Most of these disappear within a few weeks. If the hymen is completely sealed over it may be bulging from retained secretions and will need operation by a paediatric gynaecologist (Fig. 4.7).

Anus

The baby's bottom is often covered with meconium. Be careful to wipe it all away because a number of minor abnormalities of the anus still allow the baby to pass meconium. There should be a reasonable gap between the posterior part of the scrotum or vulva and the anus. Meconium may not be passed for the first 24 hours after birth. If there is any further delay, a gentle rectal examination should be done. If any obstruction is found, no force should be used otherwise the rectum could be ruptured. The commonest abnormality is atresia of the anus, but it is sometimes merely covered by a triangular flap of skin.

Legs

Straighten the legs to see if they are the same length. They are normally bowed outwards. The knees occasionally show dislocation with the tibia dislocated forwards on the femur.

Feet

Abnormalities of the feet are very common; the parents are often worried about club feet. The commonest variety is talipes equino-varus (TEV) in which the foot is adducted and plantar flexed. This is described in the section on congenital abnormalities. The most important procedure during examination is to see how far one can reduce the abnormality by pressure on the sole of the foot; TEV which is completely reducible is often called positional talipes and has an excellent prognosis (Fig. 4.8). Talipes calcaneovalgus is shown by a foot in eversion and dorsiflexion; this also has a good prognosis if the deformity can be completely reduced. Count the toes to look for any abnormalities such as extra toes or syndactyly.

Back

There is sometimes a pit in the lumbosacral region. If it is possible to see the bottom of the pit, no action need be taken, but if there seems to be a track passing inwards, the baby should be referred to a paediatric neurosurgeon as infection may spread to the central nervous system causing meningitis. Run a finger up the back to ensure that there are no swellings. It is particularly easy to miss a small encephalocele covered by skin and hair on the back of the head

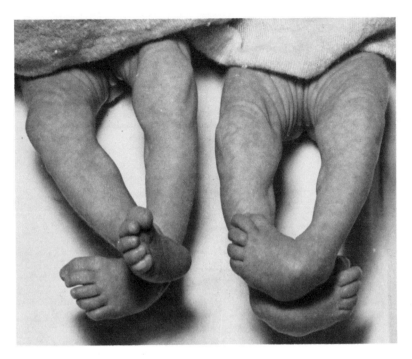

Fig. 4.8 Twins with talipes equinovarus. The one on the right has severe irreducible talipes and that on the left reducible (positional) talipes

(Fig. 4.9). Mongolian blue spots are large areas, usually over the sacrum or buttocks, which look rather like bruises. They are found in black or oriental babies and it is important that they should not be confused with bruising due to non-accidental injury (Plate I). A simple capillary naevus is very common over the cervical and lower lumbar spine.

Neurological examination

During the examination, it should be possible to test the baby's responses. A normal newborn baby has a number of simple reflexes which show that the skin is sensitive and that the central nervous system, nerves and muscles are working (Dubowitz & Dubowitz, 1981). The grasp reflexes are the easiest to demonstrate; a baby will clench a hand or foot in response to pressure on the palm or

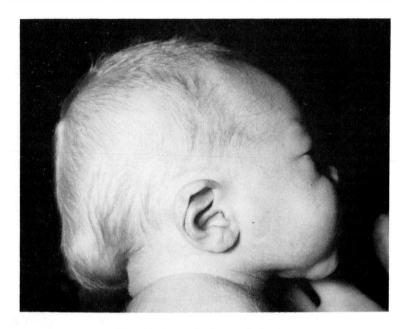

Fig. 4.9 A cervical encephalocele

sole. When doing the palmar grasp it is usual to pull the baby forward to see whether there is a response of lifting the head slightly or pulling with the arms. A baby whose head flops helplessly backwards has abnormally low tone. The Galant reflex is shown when the baby has been turned over: a finger touches the loin and the baby swings the bottom over to that side.

The Moro response is the most famous primitive response; if the cot is tapped on either side of the baby, or the baby's bottom is lifted and allowed to fall gently onto the cot, or if the baby's head is lifted off the cot and allowed to fall back a few degrees on to the hand, a characteristic response follows – the baby flings the arms sideways, spreads the fingers and then adducts the arms as if in an embrace. During this the legs also extend. The baby looks startled and often cries. If it is felt necessary to elicit this response, it should be done very gently indeed as babies do not like it. It can, however, be useful when looking for a difference between the two sides in a baby who has brachial plexus palsy or a fractured clavicle. It is possible to make a formal score from the neurological examination but this is not necessary for a routine examination.

The primitive responses which are usually described might suggest that newborn babies are capable only of very simple neurological responses. In fact, they are much more alert to their surroundings than we used to think. There is a period of an hour or two shortly after birth when babies are particularly alert and look around (Klaus, 1970; Klaus *et al.*, 1976). They will usually look at a face intently and are not so interested in non-human objects; they will also respond to being talked to. It is important to explain this to the parents who may have been told by others that a baby cannot see or hear at birth.

Babies are sensitive. It is a misconception to think that they do not feel pain. Studies have shown that their palms sweat when a heel prick is done (Harpin & Rutter, 1982); a circumcision without an anaesthetic must be extremely painful.

At the end of the examination, it is nice to place the baby in the arms of one of the parents, so that they can explore and get to know their child fully. They may need encouragement to undress the baby. The room should be kept reasonably warm so that the cold does not inhibit getting to know one another. It is also an ideal time to put the baby to the breast – early feeding is known to help in establishing breast feeding (Taylor *et al.*, 1986).

The Discharge Examination

A baby needs several examinations during the first week if there are any worrying signs. However, every baby should be examined again before going home, and in many units this is now done by a midwife. This is just one of the regular examinations which should be done throughout childhood to ensure that an infant is progressing steadily and normally. The purpose of the discharge examination is to make sure that a baby has not developed an infection or other serious condition which could not be managed at home and has no congenital abnormality which has been missed. It is common for cardiac abnormalities to show no abnormal signs during the newborn period – a murmur may appear later. The examination can follow the same plan as the first examination, but there are a number of specific checks to be made:

1 *Jaundice*. A baby who is jaundiced at discharge will need further checks from the midwife at home and the health visitor or general practitioner may carry out a later check to ensure the jaundice has disappeared by two weeks of age (see Chapter 12).

2 *Heart.* Another complete examination of the cardiovascular system is needed in case any physical signs have appeared during the first week.

3 *Hips.* A further check is needed since it is very easy to miss a congenital dislocation.

4 *Umbilicus.* This is a common site of infection. A note should be made about whether the umbilical cord has separated. The parents should be given information about cord care. Studies (Lawrence, 1982; Barr, 1984) have shown no increase in infection when cords are treated with antibacterial powder alone or not treated at all, and separation occurs by the seventh day.

5 *Breast engorgement.* (Fig. 4.10). This may occur around seven to ten days of age in both sexes due to a surge of prolactin and oestrogen secretion; it normally subsides without treatment. Warn the parents not to try and express milk from them as this may lead to infection. Rarely, breast abscess may result (see Chapter 16).

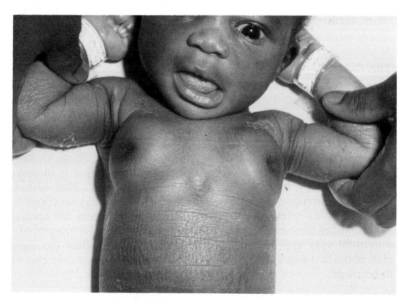

Fig. 4.10 Breast engorgement

Follow-up

When a baby is discharged from hospital it has been common to give the parents an appointment to come back to the follow-up clinic. However, it is important not to duplicate services which are available in the community, since this may give the parents many unnecessary journeys to the hospital and it is likely that this will be much less convenient for them than calling at the local clinic to see the health visitor and community paediatrician. It is extremely important to communicate information about the baby to them and the general practitioner. Modern methods of communication will make this easier. Fax, electronic mail and computer networking will become increasingly important.

In general, there are two good reasons for follow-up. The first is that the baby has a high risk of disability, because of the birth history or other abnormalities. Follow-up is necessary for coordination of care and for detection of other developmental abnormalities; the baby should be discharged to the care of the community services as soon as there is no longer any need for hospital services, such as neurological investigations. The second is that every neonatal unit running a special or intensive care service should monitor the number and types of abnormalities in the babies who have passed through the unit. Constructive changes in neonatal paediatrics can be made only by finding out whether babies survive and whether they survive without abnormalities. The following are suggested reasons for follow-up at the hospital:

1 *Birthweight under 1000 g.*
2 *Major congenital abnormalities* (although it may be better to refer the baby to an appropriate specialist and to leave the coordination of care to the general practitioner and consultant community paediatrician).
3 *Urinary tract infections*, because of the risk of ureteric reflux and other abnormalities of the urinary tract.
4 *Jaundice* with a peak bilirubin over 380 µmol/l in term babies, but lower in those of low birth weight.
5 *Severe asphyxia.* We suggest that an Apgar score of less than 4 at five minutes would be a reasonable criterion.
6 *Major neurological abnormality* in the neonatal period such as convulsions during the first 48 hours of life, or definite subarachnoid haemorrhage.
7 *Symptomatic hypoglycaemia.*

8 *Neonatal abnormalities* such as Erb's palsy which are likely to resolve fairly quickly and which are therefore more easily managed by a few visits to the outpatient department than by referral to another centre. Any long-lasting problems are not best managed from a maternity hospital.

9 Less than 32 weeks gestation.

This list, of course, does not include particular problems which are the special interest of an individual hospital.

Intermediate or Transitional Care Unit

To some extent the criteria for admission to special care nurseries have varied with the availability of paediatric and nursing expertise in the postnatal wards. In many units, babies who were born by forceps delivery, for example, were routinely admitted to a special care nursery, often even without consultation with the paediatric staff. The percentage of babies admitted to special care baby units has often fluctuated. It became popular in the 1970s to admit many babies for observation and to receive the skilled attention of the doctors and nurses in the unit. In some units this even reached 40% of all births, whereas an admission rate of 6% was common in the early 1960s. We now know that it was a mistake to have a high admission rate because many babies were separated from their mothers unnecessarily; it also reduced the skills of the nurses in the postnatal wards. The dangers of admitting well babies to special care nurseries are now appreciated: separation from the mother produces anxiety which may lead to impaired lactation or even cessation of breast feeding and a disordered relationship between the mother and her baby, sometimes called poor bonding. There is an increased risk of healthy babies acquiring an infection if they are transferred to a unit in which there are already ill babies; pathogenic and resistant bacterial strains are commoner in a special care nursery. The easy availability of phototherapy or a lower threshold for the use of antibiotics and other drugs may increase the risk of iatrogenic illness in such units.

It is now common for a maternity hospital to have an intermediate or transitional care unit. This can be a section of a postnatal ward where babies needing special care can be nursed with their mothers. The midwifery staff in this area need special training and there should be a higher ratio of staff to babies than in an ordinary postnatal ward, because the babies need frequent feeding, weighing and observations. The babies can be assessed by a paediatrician in the labour ward using the following admission criteria:

1 Well babies of *low birthweight*.
2 *Rhesus disease* which does not require an immediate exchange transfusion.
3 *Infants of insulin-dependent diabetics.* These have usually been observed in the special care baby unit for 24 hours, but in well-staffed hospitals they could easily be managed on a postnatal ward. Large babies or babies of mothers who have had an abnormal glucose tolerance test in pregnancy should be on a postnatal ward.
4 Babies requiring *short-term tube feeding* before discharge.
5 Suspected *meconium aspiration* with no respiratory problems.
6 *Phototherapy* if it cannot be done on an ordinary postnatal ward.

Such a unit is not suitable for infected babies.

Transfer to Special Care Unit

The following are reasonable indications justifying transfer to a special care baby unit:

1 *Birth weight* under 1700 g or gestational age less than 32 weeks.
2 *Birth asphyxia* with persistent central nervous system or respiratory signs or symptoms. Mild birth asphyxia (Apgar 5 or more at five minutes) with no subsequent problems is not an indication for transfer.
3 *Aspiration* including meconium aspiration with respiratory symptoms and signs. Meconium staining of the skin with no evidence of aspiration is not an indication for transfer.
4 *Rhesus haemolytic disease.* A rhesus-negative mother or a rhesus-positive mother with antibodies is not an indication for transfer; some mild cases do not need admission if they can be carefully observed on a postnatal ward or in intermediate care.
5 *Respiratory* signs such as transient tachypnoea or respiratory distress syndrome. This would include such complications as pneumothorax or recurrent apnoeic attacks, as well as other causes of respiratory distress.
6 *Congenital malformation* with symptoms such as congenital heart diseases.
7 *Convulsions.*

8 *Major infection*, for example meningitis, pneumonia or septicaemia. Other infections such as those of the urinary tract or staphylococcal infections of the skin do not indicate a need for transfer, but some may need isolation only.

9 *Persistent vomiting*. This does not include minor feeding problems, 'mucusy' babies or babies with regurgitations or occasional vomits. A baby who is persistently feeding poorly may need transfer.

10 *Jaundice* requiring exchange transfusion. Phototherapy for full-term well babies should be given at the mother's bedside on the postnatal ward.

11 *Fetal haemorrhage* or haemorrhage from the cord.

It is worth re-emphasising those circumstances in which babies should *not* be routinely transferred. In addition to those already mentioned these include:

1 *Abnormal delivery* including forceps, ventouse and caesarean section.

2 *Malpresentation*.

3 *Mild hypothermia*.

4 The babies of a *multiple pregnancy*.

5 *Previous adverse history* for example, obstetric, neonatal death or stillbirth.

6 The *jittery baby*.

7 *Maternal illness* or *therapy*.

8 *Traumatic cyanosis*.

9 *Malformations* which do not threaten life such as Down syndrome, cleft lip or talipes equinovarus.

10 *Infant of a mother with well-controlled diabetes mellitus.*

Reasons for Isolating Babies

The usual reason that a baby needs isolation is because of actual or potential infection, which would be a risk to other infants:

1 Admission from outside the hospital.

2 Staphylococcal skin lesions.

3 Gastroenteritis.

4 Severe ophthalmia.

5 Group B β-haemolytic streptococcal infection.

6 Necrotizing enterocolitis.

7 Colonization with a potentially dangerous organism.

There is a need for an isolation unit for infected term babies and also for a small isolation area within the neonatal intensive care unit because some of these babies are very ill.

Quite often a baby needs isolation because the mother is infected. Examples of such conditions are maternal tuberculosis, genital herpes and hepatitis B.

Rooming-in

This means that the mother has her baby in the cot beside her for most of the 24 hours. The advantages are that mother and baby are able to get to know one another earlier, and that breast feeding is more easily established. It is most successful in single rooms or in units containing up to four beds, otherwise there may be too much disturbance to mothers from babies other than their own. None the less, even in many larger wards, rooming-in has been satisfactorily established.

Weighing

A normal newborn baby may lose up to 10% of the birth weight during the first week and not regain it until two weeks of age. Babies normally gain weight thereafter at a rate of about 200 g per week. There is no question that adequate gain in weight and length is crucial during the early months of life. This is the time when brain growth is at its greatest and any shortfall during this time may not be made up afterwards. It is adequate to weigh a well newborn baby on alternate days whilst in hospital. In this way, day-to-day variation due to such things as a feed or a bowel action will not give rise to needless anxiety on the part of the mother or attendants. An ill or small baby, of course, requires more frequent weighing. Test weighing of breast-fed babies should not be done because it reduces the chance of successful breast feeding by making the mother worry about how much she should be producing. The quality of the breast milk is equally as important as the quantity. Weight is best plotted graphically, as inadequate weight gain is then more obvious.

Temperature

The baby's temperature is taken on admission. Some check the temperature daily thereafter, but this is probably unnecessary in a well baby. Routine taking of the temperature rectally is undesirable as it may rarely cause rectal perforation. Axillary temperatures are satisfactory, but a figure below 36°C or an ill baby should be checked with a rectal reading. A low-reading thermometer should always be used.

Passage of Meconium and Urine

Failure to pass either meconium or urine within the first 24 hours should be reported to the paediatrician who should examine the baby carefully. Remember that less than 1 in 100 babies will not have passed urine by 48 hours of age. Check for abdominal or bladder distension which might suggest urethral obstruction (much commoner in males and due to urethral valves; Fig. 10.25). Look for the position of the urethral orifice but do not attempt to retract the foreskin or to probe with a catheter. Ensure that the external genitalia are normal.

The passage of meconium during delivery should be recorded. Not doing this is a common reason for believing that the baby has not passed meconium in the first 24 hours. Low birthweight, preterm or ill babies may have delayed passage of meconium, but always check for abdominal distension or vomiting indicating intestinal obstruction (see Chapter 11). If in doubt take an erect plain abdominal radiograph. Hirschsprung's disease, cystic fibrosis and imperforate anus are all causes of failure to pass meconium.

Baths

Early and frequent baths are unnecessary and may lead to hypothermia. A full bath should never be done in the first 24 hours. The baby's face can be cleaned shortly after birth and any very soiled areas can be cleaned. One unit in India greatly reduced the neonatal mortality rate by cutting out a bath shortly after birth.

BCG

Tuberculosis still occurs in Britain. It has a high prevalence among immigrants from outside Europe, North America and Australasia; in certain inner-city areas it is safest to immunise all babies against the disease shortly after birth. This is done by giving an injection of BCG before the baby leaves the maternity unit; 0.05 ml is given intradermally. There is a problem about giving it over the deltoid because of keloid formation. Some use the scapula or the upper buttock. BCG usually provides long-lasting protection against contracting tuberculosis.

If the mother is being treated for tuberculosis there is no need to separate her from the baby or stop her breast feeding. The baby can be immunized with special isoniazid-resistant BCG and treated with a course of isoniazid. In this way one can be doubly sure that the baby does not get tuberculosis.

Guthrie Test

The Guthrie test is a simple blood test for abnormal amounts of phenylalanine, an essential amino acid converted in the liver to tyrosine. In those suffering from phenylketonuria (PKU), there is a lack of the liver enzyme which carries out this conversion. The enzyme is known as phenylalanine hydroxylase. In such babies the blood phenylalanine level becomes very high and causes brain damage, leading to severe mental retardation. The condition can be successfully treated from birth with a low phenylalanine diet.

Before birth, phenylalanine does not accumulate in the fetus because it can pass across the placenta into the mother. After birth, the newborn baby with PKU has a steadily rising phenylalanine level after milk feeds are started. Thus infants with PKU are not brain damaged at birth; they only become so once they have started ingesting phenylalanine in milk. The disease is uncommon; it occurs in about 1 in 7000–10 000 births in this country, but varies. However, once the parents have had one affected baby, there is a 1 in 4 chance of their having another infant with PKU because it is inherited as an autosomal recessive disorder. It is therefore sensible to have a universal screening test which can be used to detect the condition.

The test is carried out as follows: on about the sixth day of life the baby has a simple blood test. This is done by pricking the baby's heel and collecting four drops of blood on a piece of absorbent paper (Fig.

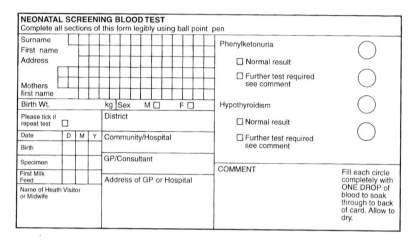

Fig. 4.11 The Guthrie test card

4.11). The test cannot be carried out earlier, because there has to be time for phenylalanine to be taken in by the baby as milk before abnormally large amounts can be detected in his blood. The paper is sent to a laboratory, where the blood spots are punched out and placed on an agar plate. This contains the phenylalanine antagonist beta-thionylalanine which inhibits the growth of a phenylalanine-dependent strain of *Bacillus subtilis*. If the level of phenylalanine in the blood sample is high, this inhibition is overcome and the bacteria are able to grow. This provides a simple and semiquantitative screen for raised levels of phenylalanine. Thus if, following overnight incubation, a turbid zone of growth is found around the test disc, this indicates a positive result. A rough serum phenylalanine level is determined by comparison with control discs. A value of 4 mg/100 ml (240 µmol/l) or more is presumed to be positive for phenylketonuria, but before diagnosis is firmly established a full investigation must be carried out.

The test should be explained to parents before it is done and they must be warned that it is occasionally necessary to repeat the test, without this necessarily implying there is anything wrong with the baby. The commonest reason for repeating the test is that there was not enough blood to cover the circled areas on the card completely. The repeat test is nearly always satisfactory.

Modifications of the Guthrie test using agar media impregnated with other *B. subtilis* inhibitors can be used to detect a variety of other inborn errors of metabolism. Some centres do the screening by a plasma amino acid chromatogram.

Tests for Cystic Fibrosis (CF)

Screening tests for this disease would be important because it is common and affects about 1 in 2000 babies. The most reliable test so far uses blood immunoreactive trypsin. A positive test is a reason for a definitive sweat test. There is increasing evidence that very early diagnosis of cystic fibrosis improves the prognosis, and allows early genetic counselling.

The only effective way of reducing the birth prevalence of cystic fibrosis will be by *prenatal* screening. The gene for CF has now been sequenced; there appear to be a number of different abnormal genes. Prenatal diagnosis using this technique is now possible in 90% of cases, although screening is still not possible.

Screening Tests for Hypothyroidism

Congenital hypothyroidism is commoner than PKU; it affects about 1 in 4000 infants. If detected early, it can be treated with thyroxine, preventing mental handicap and ensuring normal growth. Obvious physical signs – including prolonged jaundice, cretinous facies, big tongue, coarse cry and umbilical hernia – are often not present in affected newborn babies and, therefore, a screening test is particularly useful. It is now carried out on all babies born in the UK, using blood from the Guthrie test card. It is possible to measure either T_4 or thyroid-stimulating hormone (TSH). Ideally both should be measured, if no cases are to be missed, but TSH alone seems to be satisfactory and is measured in the UK. The rare pituitary and hypothalamic causes of congenital hypothyroidism are not detected. This is not a major disadvantage as the hypothyroidism in these circumstances is less severe (so treatment is less urgent) and is usually part of a broader spectrum of hypothalamopituitary disease (so the problem may be suspected for other reasons, such as hypoglycaemia or micropenis).

In as many as 1 in 8000–10 000 normal babies there is a temporary rise of TSH. It is very important to start treatment early, but also to check thyroid function fully before treatment with thyroxine is started

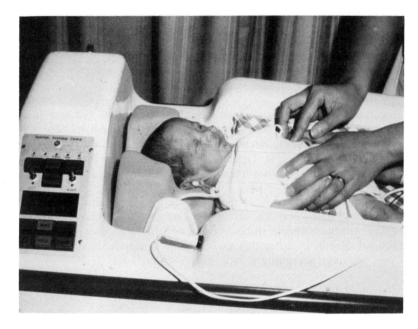

Fig. 4.12 The auditory response cradle

to ensure that the problem is persisting. If it is not, treatment should be stopped as soon as the definitive results become available.

The presence or absence of any functioning thyroid tissue can be assessed by scanning following the injection of radioactive iodide (^{123}I) or technetium-99m pertechnetate. This may help to identify some inborn errors of thyroxine metabolism which have an autosomal recessive inheritance. Their final identification may require further special diagnostic procedures.

The initial dose of thyroxine replacement is around 10 µg/kg/day. The dose per kilogram falls with increasing age but remains around 100 µg/m²/day. The aim of treatment is to achieve normal growth and development. TSH levels may take many months to fall on treatment and provided T_4 levels are in the upper half of the normal range and growth is normal this is not an indication for increasing the dose of thyroxine.

Vision and Hearing Tests

Parents often ask if their babies can see and hear normally (Dubowitz *et al.*, 1980). It is easy to demonstrate sight, as the baby will blink in response to a bright light. It is also possible to show the parents that the baby will gaze at a smiling face with great interest. More sophisticated tests will be done during developmental checks later in the first year.

Tests of hearing are becoming more sophisticated. A baby will quieten at the ring of a bell in the first week and most parents will be certain in the first few months that their baby can hear something. All babies should be tested at eight months using a very soft rattle and other sounds at no more than 40 decibels. The baby turns the head towards a sound. More sensitive hearing tests for screening the newborn are being developed.

Tests for brain stem evoked responses are now more widely available and can be used to evaluate the hearing of even very preterm infants (Lary *et al.*, 1985).

References and Further Reading

Barr, R.J. (1984) The umbilical cord: to treat or not to treat? *Midwives Chronicle Nursing Notes, July*, 224–226.

Clarke, A. (1978) *Culture, Childbearing, Health Professionals*. Philadelphia: Davis.

Dubowitz, L. & Dubowitz, V. (1981) *The Neurological Assessment of the Preterm and Full Term Newborn Infant. Clin. Dev. Med., 79*. SIMP/ Heinemann: London.

Dubowitz, L.M.S., Dubowitz, V., Morante, A. *et al.* (1980) Visual function in the premature and full term newborn infant. *Dev. Med. Child Neurol, 22*, 465–475.

Harpin, V.A. & Rutter, N. (1982) Development of emotional sweating in the newborn infant. *Arch. Dis. Child, 57*, 691–695.

Klaus, M.H. (1970) Human maternal behavior at first contact with her young. *Pediatrics, 46*, 187.

Klaus, M.H. & Kennell, J.H. (1976) Maternal–infant bonding. St Louis: Mosby.

Lary, S., Briassoulis, G., de Vries, L. *et al.* (1985) Hearing threshold in preterm and term infants by auditory brainstem response. *J. Pediatr., 107*, 593–599.

Lawrence, C.R. (1982) Effect of two different methods of umbilical cord care on its separation time. *Midwives Chronicle Nursing Notes, June*, 204–205.

Perry, D. (1982) The umbilical cord: Transcultural care and customs. *Journal of Nurse-Midwifery*, *27*(4), 25–30.

Taylor, P., Maloni, J. & Brown, D. (1986) Early suckling and prolonged breastfeeding. *Am. J. Dis. Child*, *140*, 151–154.

Vulliamy, D.G. & Johnston, P.B. (1987) *The Newborn Child*, 6th ed. Edinburgh: Churchill Livingstone.

—5

Birth Trauma

Severe birth trauma is now a rare complication in normal obstetric practice. However, minor trauma associated, for example, with rotational forceps, ventouse extraction, shoulder dystocia or breech delivery is still a problem (Effer *et al.*, 1983). Preterm babies are at particular risk (Liu & Fairweather, 1984). Because of their small size they pass rapidly through the pelvis with little time for the skull to mould; the brain is only semi-solid and easily contused, with tearing of its septa such as the falx cerebri or tentorium cerebelli and

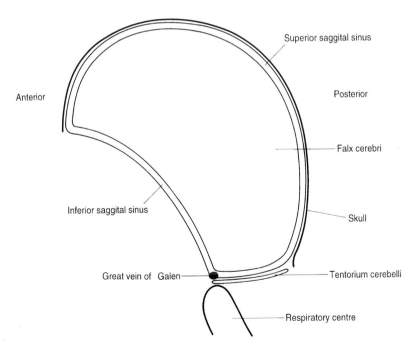

Fig. 5.1 LS of fetal skull showing internal anatomy

resultant haemorrhage (Fig. 5.1). The preterm baby's blood vessels are also friable and easily torn. There is no evidence that the prophylactic use of forceps for very preterm or low birth weight babies is of any benefit.

Bleeding may also result from hypoxia during delivery. Both trauma and hypoxia frequently coexist in a difficult labour. Venous distension or high blood pressure due to anoxia may be sufficient in itself to cause haemorrhage. There are often petechial haemorrhages throughout the brain or periventricular haemorrhage.

Traumatic Cyanosis

Cyanosis is seen following difficult delivery, especially if the cord is tightly round the baby's neck. The appearance can be frightening. The baby's face is bright blue or reddish-blue with petechial haemorrhages and ecchymoses. At first glance, the baby may be thought to have cyanotic congenital heart disease, but closer inspection reveals no cyanosis below the neck and a pink tongue. Examination is otherwise normal. If you press on the face, the cyanosis does not fade. Parents need strong reassurance about the appearance of the baby and must be told that the bruising may take up to a few weeks to disappear completely. A watch should be kept for the development of jaundice as blood is reabsorbed.

Occasionally these babies develop respiratory obstruction due to associated oedema and need careful observation in the first 24 hours. If the lips are very swollen tube-feeding may be necessary for a short period.

Fat Necrosis

These areas of hard thickening occur under parts of the baby's skin that have had pressure applied during delivery. They may occur over the mandible, in front of the ears, on the elbows or in the parietal regions (Plate II). Thus fat necrosis often results from a forceps delivery, but may follow a normal delivery. Sometimes widespread fat necrosis is seen all down the extensor surfaces after perinatal asphyxia. Usually no treatment is necessary and explanation is all that is required. If large areas are involved they may become secondarily infected, requiring antibiotics. Occasionally, parietal fat necrosis may ulcerate.

Cephalhaematoma

Bleeding between a skull bone and its outer covering (periosteum) is common even following normal delivery, and is due to mild shearing trauma (Fig. 5.2, see also Fig. 4.3). Most commonly one, or sometimes both, parietal bones are affected, rarely the frontal or occipital. The swelling is sharply limited by the suture lines which the blood is unable to cross. The swelling becomes visible as the moulding subsides and can be a great source of worry to the parents, who should be reassured that the baby's head will be a normal shape. No attempt should be made to aspirate the haematoma because of the risk of introducing infection; it may take several weeks or even months to disappear and will meanwhile calcify hardening from the edge inwards, thus feeling like a depressed skull fracture after one to two weeks. The baby may become significantly jaundiced as blood is reabsorbed.

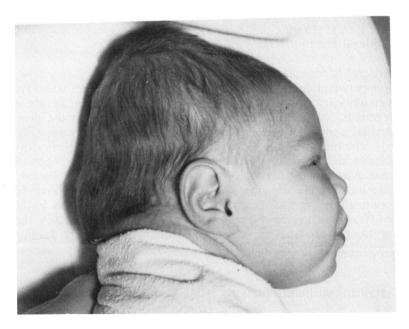

Fig. 5.2 Occipital and parietal cephalhaematoma

Subaponeurotic Haemorrhage

Unlike cephalhaematoma, which is common, subperiosteal and benign, subaponeurotic haemorrhage is rare, dangerous and extends widely into the areolar tissues of the scalp under the epicranial aponeurosis. Babies particularly at risk include those born by ventouse extraction and African babies born by any means. It is possibly a manifestation of haemorrhagic disease of the newborn (see Chapter 13) but tends to occur earlier. Affected babies develop a boggy swelling of the scalp during the first two days of life with rapid onset of pallor, shock and subsequently, jaundice. The baby may lose a large proportion of the blood volume in this way. Treatment is by emergency blood transfusion (fresh frozen plasma may need to be given in the first instance) and intramuscular injection of 1 mg of vitamin K_1 to prevent further bleeding (vitamin K dependent clotting factors II, VII, IX, X are low). The condition may be largely prevented by giving vitamin K_1 at birth to all babies following forceps or ventouse deliveries and all non-Caucasian babies. Many paediatricians routinely give all infants vitamin K_1 at birth (see Chapter 13).

Subdural Haemorrhage

Subdural haemorrhage is due to trauma and must be distinguished from periventricular haemorrhage found in preterm babies who have been hypoxic. Subdural haemorrhage arises from a tear in the falx or tentorium, leading to rupture of and haemorrhage from the great cerebral vein (of Galen) or one of the other cerebral veins (Fig. 5.1). The infant is often lethargic with apnoeic attacks, occasionally irritable and convulsing. The anterior fontanelle may be boggy or tense. Management is conservative with minimal handling, warmth, tube feeding and sedation if appropriate. The diagnosis may be confirmed by subdural tapping but often the haemorrhage is in the posterior fossa and may be missed. The prognosis in those babies who survive the neonatal period is good, although some may develop convulsions or be left with mental handicap.

Nerve Injuries and Fractures

Depressed *skull fractures* are uncommon and are usually managed conservatively. Rarely, especially in breech delivery, there is associated intracranial bleeding with usually fatal results. Spinal cord injury is also uncommon.

Facial palsy (Fig. 5.3) is nearly always unilateral and may follow either forceps or, perhaps surprisingly, normal delivery. When the baby cries the asymmetry becomes more obvious, with only the unaffected side showing any movement or expression. Often the lower lip alone is paralysed on one side. Sometimes, in addition, the baby may be unable to close the affected eye. In nearly all cases recovery is complete.

Brachial plexus nerve injuries are often associated with a fracture of the clavicle, but may occur independently. An upper plexus lesion (Erb's palsy, Fig. 5.4) follows severe traction on the shoulders during breech delivery or may occur with shoulder dystocia; it results in an arm that hangs limply in pronation (waiter's tip position) and does not take part in the Moro reflex. Treatment is often unnecessary. It is not a good idea to pin the arm with the hand in supination alongside the infant's head because it is easy for someone to pick the baby up, forgetting the arm is pinned, and cause severe damage. Recovery usually takes place within a few weeks. Occasionally the phrenic nerve is damaged, producing unilateral diaphragmatic paralysis with dyspnoea and cyanosis.

Uncommonly, a lower brachial plexus lesion occurs (Klumpke's paralysis) with paralysis of the small hand muscles. It may be difficult to detect: there is loss of sensation on the inner forearm and medial three and a half fingers. Eventually there may be muscle wasting in the hand. It may be associated with damage to the cervical sympathetic nerves and Horner's syndrome (ipsilateral ptosis, enophthalmos and meiosis). The hand and forearm should be splintered in a cock-up position.

Radial nerve palsy may occur due to pressure on the nerve as it winds round the outer aspect of the elbow. An area of fat necrosis may overlie the nerve where it was compressed. Wrist drop may result and treatment is again by cock-up splint.

In the event of *fractures of the humerus or clavicle*, the baby does not move the affected arm and has an absent Moro reflex on that side. Crepitus may be felt over the bone. However, in many cases the result of the fracture is noticed only as a bump due to exuberant callus formation after a couple of weeks. Brachial plexus lesions may be associated. Usually no treatment is necessary, but splinting the arm with a tongue depressor sometimes relieves pain.

Fracture of the femur occurs rarely. Treatment is by gallows skin traction: suspending the baby's legs with strapping around the legs and ankles so that the buttocks are held just above the bed.

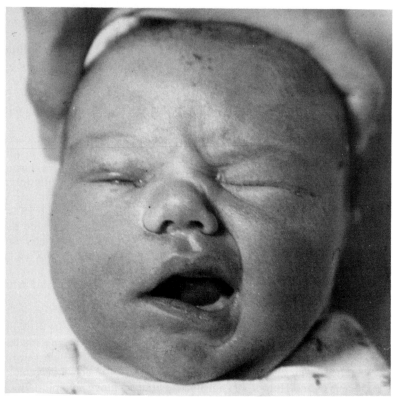

Fig. 5.3 Right facial palsy.

Sternomastoid Tumour

Occasionally a painless firm lump is noticed in the sternomastoid muscle on one or other side within a week or two of birth. No treatment is necessary, other than reassurance for the parents. Torticollis is said to occur subsequently, but this is rare. For this reason physiotherapy is sometimes given. The aetiology of the condition is unclear. However, it seems not to be due to traumatic haemorrhage as was once supposed.

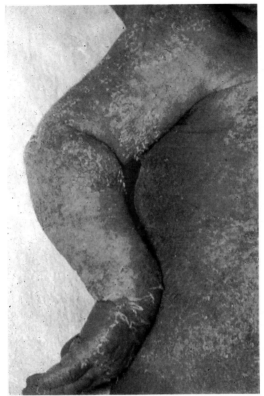

Fig. 5.4 Erb's palsy

References and Further Reading

Avery, G.B. (1987) *Neonatology: Pathophysiology and Management of the Newborn*, 3rd ed. Philadelphia: Lippincott.

Campbell, A. & McIntosh, C. (eds) (1992) *Forfar & Arneil's Textbook of Paediatrics*, 4th edn. Edinburgh: Churchill Livingstone.

Effer, S.B., Sangal, S., Raud, C. *et al.* (1983) Effect of delivery method on outcomes in the very low birth weight breech infant: is the improved survival related to caesarian section or other perinatal case manoeuvres? *Am. J. Obstet. Gynecol.*, *145*, 123–128.

Liu, D.T.Y. & Fairweather, D.V.I. (1984) The management of preterm labour. In *Preterm Labour*, eds M.G. Elder & C.H. Hendricks, pp. 231–259. London: Butterworths.

Sinclair, J.C. & Bracken, M.B. (eds) (1992) Effective Care of the Newborn Infant. Oxford: Oxford University Press.

—6

Care of the Low Birthweight Baby

Babies may be small at birth for two main reasons: because they are born early (preterm babies), or because they have not grown adequately *in utero* (small-for-gestational-age (SFGA) babies). It is important to decide to which category a baby belongs, as each group has particular problems in the perinatal period. Some babies who weigh less than they should for their gestational age *and* are born early are doubly at risk.

It is best not to use the term 'premature' because it was used in the past for any baby of 2500 g or less. A preterm baby is born before the end of the 37th week from the beginning of the last menstrual period; a SFGA baby weighs less than would be predicted from the gestational age, either two standard deviations below the mean (defining some 3.5% of all babies), or below the 10th centile. It is more useful to use the 10th centile as it will identify all babies who may be at risk of hypoglycaemia (see below). It does mean, however, that 1 in 10 babies is classed as SFGA. The baby must first be weighed and measured accurately (see Chapter 4). The results are then plotted on a growth chart.

These have been derived by plotting the birthweights of a large population of newborn babies against their gestational ages. Lines are drawn which divide that population into centiles: 10th, 50th, 90th, etc. A baby whose weight is just above the 90th centile for his gestational age is heavier than 90 out of every 100 babies in that normal population. A chart is reproduced in Chapter 4. It should be noted that these may not be appropriate for certain ethnic groups.

Before a baby's weight can be plotted on the graph, the gestational age must be known (see Chapter 2). After birth the gestational age may be estimated by observing a number of physical characteristics and neurological responses (Dubowitz *et al.*, 1970). The baby is scored on certain key features and the score enables the baby's gestational age to be read from a chart. The score is probably accurate within two weeks either way, providing that the baby is aged between 4 and 48 hours when assessed, and is not ill. It is more accurate in babies weighing more than 1000 g, (see Appendix under Gestational Assessment). The baby's gestational age may then be plotted against the birthweight and the infant defined as large-for-gestational-age (LFGA), appropriate-for-gestational-age (AFGA) or small-for-gestational-age (SFGA).

An AFGA infant has probably grown at a normal rate *in utero* and may be born before term, at term or after term. A SFGA baby has grown at a slower rate *in utero*, whether born before, at or after term. The commonest infant to be LFGA is the baby of a diabetic or prediabetic mother; those babies have their own special problems (See Chapter 15).

If the baby is SFGA, this may be because the growth rate was slow throughout pregnancy, or growth may have slowed only late in pregnancy (Fig. 6.1; and see Fig. 2.6). These types may be distinguished by serial ultrasound measurements of biparietal diameter and abdominal circumference during pregnancy. The prognosis for

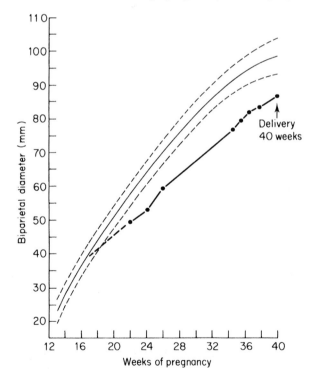

Fig. 6.1 Prolonged intrauterine growth retardation

growth and development varies with the time of the start of slow growth. Malnutrition during the period of most rapid brain growth (the middle and third trimesters of intrauterine life and the early months after birth) may reduce the number of brain cells produced and may permanently impair the baby's future intellectual development potential. Babies who grow slowly before about the 37th week may be short and light at birth, feed poorly as infants and show a number of dysmorphic features in childhood, such as asymmetry between the sides of the body, clinodactyly (short incurving little fingers) and short stature – the Russell–Silver syndrome. Some SFGA babies have an obvious reason for slow growth *in utero*; these include those with congenital rubella, chromosome disorders or major congenital abnormalities. Many such pregnancies end in spontaneous miscarriage.

Intrauterine growth retardation is now thought to be important not just in the short term (e.g. neonatal hypoglycaemia), or medium term (e.g. feeding difficulties in infancy and poor growth), but also because of possible long-term consequences in adulthood. Epidemiological evidence suggests that small fetuses are more likely to develop hypertension, other cardiovascular diseases and type 2 diabetes mellitus (Barker *et al.*, 1990, 1993; Barker, 1992; Law *et al.*, 1993; Osmond *et al.*, 1993). There is also epidemiological evidence that babies most at risk of subsequent hypertension are those who are born small with large placentae (Barker *et al.*, 1990). It is unclear whether 'normal' birthweight babies who are in fact lighter than they should have been for their parents (and thus also starved *in utero*) are at risk in any way.

There has been speculation that fetal adrenal steroiogenic patterns, which could reflect placental and fetal growth, might provide a link with the eventual development of adult hypertension (Benediktsson *et al.*, 1993; Edwards *et al.*, 1993).

The Preterm Baby (Fig. 6.2)

If preterm labour could be prevented, the perinatal mortality would fall considerably as preterm babies are particularly at risk. Unfortunately, except in certain specific cases (for example, mid-trimester abortions which may be prevented by cervical suturing), preterm delivery cannot be reliably predicted or prevented in an individual patient.

There are a number of predisposing factors (risk factors). They are

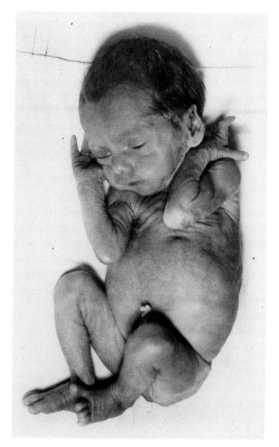

Fig. 6.2 A preterm baby born in 1954 at 28 weeks gestation and weighing 1.1 kg. He was discharged in good health after 11 weeks in hospital

discussed fully in Chapter 2. Many women suffer from a combination of risk factors. For instance, there is an association between low social class, short stature, non-attendance for antenatal care, malnutrition, previous termination and so on. It is to these women that resources of money and manpower must be preferentially directed if perinatal mortality is to be further reduced.

Some immigrant groups have a particularly high perinatal mortality rate (Young & Clarke, 1987) and the women may not attend for antenatal care. The Asian Mother and Baby Campaign (Rocheron & Dickinson, 1990) is an example of the sort of action that needs to be taken (Evans *et al.*, 1985). There should be literature in the appropriate language and interpreters to give health education and assistance in health centres and hospitals.

The lower the gestational age, the greater the risk of perinatal problems: less mature lungs suffer respiratory distress syndrome, fragile capillaries in the brain rupture easily following trauma or hypoxia, infections are poorly resisted and anaemia may develop.

Feeding

The preterm baby of less than about 34 weeks gestation often has physical difficulty in taking, digesting and absorbing feed. Sucking, swallowing and cough reflexes are particularly poorly developed before 34 weeks so feeds may be taken slowly or be aspirated into the trachea. Aspiration into the lungs may also occur if the baby should regurgitate or vomit because of slow stomach emptying. For these reasons, early feeds may have to be given through a tube passed into the stomach (nasogastric/orogastric tube), or occasionally the jejunum (nasojejunal/orojejunal tube). In the smallest babies (usually less than 32 weeks gestation), feeds are often given intravenously using a combination of special preparations (for details see Chapter 7). Preterm babies require a high energy intake (500 kJ/kg/day or about 120–150 kcal/kg/day) (or even higher) to grow adequately.

There is still no ideal milk for very immature babies; expressed mature breast milk is not entirely satisfactory because of its low protein and fat content. Nevertheless, freshly expressed breast milk is still superior to any currently available artificial milk in preventing infection, particularly necrotizing enterocolitis (Lucas & Cole, 1990); it is also well tolerated. New artificial milks have been developed for low birthweight babies; they contain more protein and sodium than the ordinary baby milks. When enteral feeding is possible, feeds should be started early so as to avoid hypoglycaemia and this is one reason for putting the baby to the breast in the labour ward when possible. A 2 kg infant at 35 weeks gestation may not need special care and might be completely breast-fed fairly soon, although theoretically preterm and low birthweight. Many preterm babies require more than 200 ml/kg/day of milk to grow adequately. Babies weighing less than 1300 g need sodium supplements (3 mmol/kg/day or more) (see Chapter 7 for details).

Jaundice

Neonatal jaundice has many causes and is discussed in Chapter 12. Preterm babies are particularly at risk of developing jaundice leading to bilirubin encephalopathy (kernicterus). There are several reasons for this:

1 Their immature enzyme systems (especially liver glucuronyl transferase).
2 The low blood levels of 'Y' and 'Z' carrier proteins which facilitate entry of bilirubin into liver cells.
3 Relative hypoalbuminaemia (bilirubin is bound to albumin in the blood during transport to the liver for conjugation).
4 The greater risk of hypoxia and hypoglycaemia which can alter the blood–brain barrier.

A high unconjugated bilirubin level is dangerous, whatever the cause, because of the risk of kernicterus. Preterm babies may be damaged at lower bilirubin levels than mature babies, and this should always be remembered when assessing the significance of a bilirubin estimation.

Jaundice appearing within the first 24 hours of life needs immediate investigation and is never physiological or due to prematurity alone.

Hyaline membrane disease

This very important disorder is discussed in Chapter 8.

Hypothermia

The preterm baby has difficulty maintaining body temperature and easily becomes cold. This results from small size and a high surface-area to body–weight ratio, so heat is lost rapidly. There is an inability to produce heat by shivering, and deposits of brown fat are also smaller. Brown fat is situated in the neck and abdomen (Findlay, 1984) (Fig. 6.3); it warms blood flowing through it and enables a mature infant to resist, to some degree, the stress of a low environmental temperature. The smaller preterm babies can lose a lot of water through the skin and therefore lose heat by evaporation.

Labour rooms are frequently cool, providing comfort for mother, midwife and obstetrician but danger for the baby. A small, naked wet baby loses heat very rapidly so the resuscitation table heater must be switched on before delivery. The baby should be dried quickly. Warm

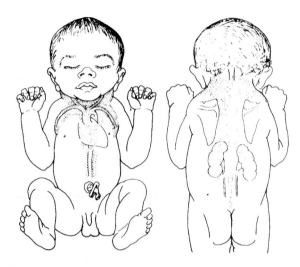

Fig. 6.3 The areas where brown fat is found. From Wallis & Harvey (1979), by permission of the authors and editor

towels are also valuable. Special care must be taken during baths, radiographic procedures, clinical examinations, surgery, and when babies are naked in incubators. Hypothermic babies are more likely to die or to develop a serious illness, such as respiratory distress syndrome. This has been known since the end of the nineteenth century (Fig. 6.4).

For each baby there is an ideal range of environmental temperature. If nursed within this range the least possible oxygen and energy are used to keep the body temperature normal. This temperature range is known as the neutral thermal environment and for a small naked baby is very narrow. In practice, special care nursery temperatures should be maintained between 26°C and 28°C, and incubator temperatures between 34°C and 37°C (Table 6.1). Perspex heat shields (simply and cheaply made in most workshops) or plastic bubble sheeting, are useful for reducing radiant heat loss without impeding a clear view of the baby (Fig. 6.5). One end of the Perspex shield should be closed to prevent its acting as a wind tunnel and cooling the baby. The head accounts for a large proportion of the preterm baby's total surface area; a scalp cap lined with gamgee will cut down heat loss significantly and clothes are often advisable, even when the baby is in an incubator. The aim should be to maintain the skin at 36.5 ± 0.3°C

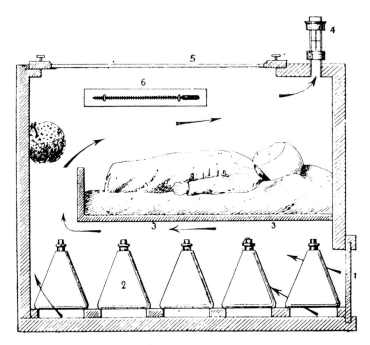

Fig. 6.4 An incubator used in Paris at the end of the nineteenth century. At the time it was shown clearly that cold babies were more likely to die

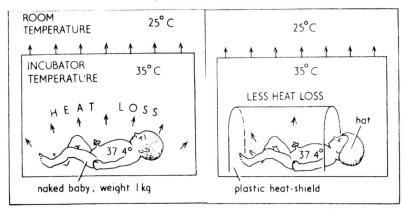

Fig. 6.5 How heat loss can be reduced by dressing the baby and using a plastic heat shield. From Wallis & Harvey (1979) by permission of the authors and editor

Table 6.1 Suggested initial temperatures for nursing babies.

Weight (kg)	Incubator* (°C)	Cot† (°C)
1	36	31
2	35	28
3	34	26

* Baby nursed naked with a Perspex heat shield
† Baby dressed

Table 6.2 Normal temperature ranges.

Rectal	36.6–37.5°C
Axillary	36.5–37°C
Anterior abdominal wall skin	36.2–36.8°C

(Table 6.2). The probe is often placed on the proximal part of a limb and it is sometimes useful to connect it to the servocontrol of the incubator. In this way the incubator heater automatically increases or reduces the heat produced to maintain the baby's temperature. This is convenient, but a disadvantage is that pyrexia may pass unnoticed and there may be swings of temperature in the incubator. When the servocontrol is not in use the baby's axillary temperature should be taken regularly and checked by rectal temperature when necessary. Low-reading thermometers are essential.

Infections

Newborn babies have a number of specific and non-specific mechanisms for dealing with infection. In the preterm baby many of them are less well developed. In particular, IgG levels are low because less has been transferred from the mother across the placenta, making the baby vulnerable to many common bacterial and viral infections. IgM production is low, leading to particular susceptibility to Gram-negative infections. Cellular immunity is also poorly developed. For a general discussion of infection in the newborn see Chapter 16.

Neurological disability

The preterm baby has a soft brain with fragile vessels. Damage, with tearing of blood vessels and of supporting structures such as the falx

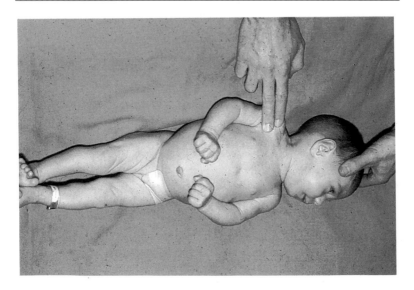

Fig. 6.6 Hypertonic baby with cerebral palsy

cerebri or tentorium cerebelli (Fig. 5.1), is easily caused by trauma during delivery, but this is now less common. Until about 1960 the incidence of mental retardation, cerebral palsy (Fig. 6.6), convulsions, deafness and blindness was very high in these babies; but now, in the best centres, the incidence of mental retardation or major handicap has dropped to less than 10%, even though many more are surviving. Now that many babies weighing less than 750 g are surviving, the number of survivors with neurological disabilities may be rising a little.

The improved outlook is associated not only with good paediatric care, but also with active obstetric intervention to prevent perinatal asphyxia, the gentle delivery of preterm babies with generous episiotomies or even less traumatically by lower-segment caesarean section. The elective use of caesarian section to deliver the preterm baby is therefore becoming commoner and is being encouraged, especially for breech presentation.

Many preterm babies under 34 weeks have periventricular haemorrhages which usually begin in the anterolateral walls of the lateral ventricles of the brain. Up to 30% of preterm babies have been shown by ultrasound (Fig. 6.7) to have such haemorrhages but most absorb without ill effects. Permanent damage may occur from

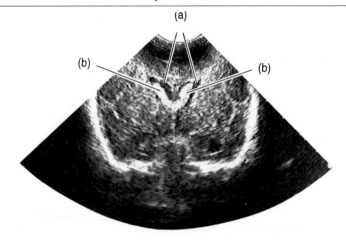

Fig. 6.7 Coronial cranial ultrasound scan showing intraventricular haemorrhages (b) in dilated lateral ventricles (a).

post-haemorrhagic hydrocephalus or porencephalic cysts from hae-morrhage ploughing into the parenchyma of the brain (Stewart *et al.*, 1983). The technique of real-time ultrasound has shown other abnormalities in the brain, including periventricular leucomalacia which is associated with a poor outcome (de Vries *et al.*, 1985; Cooke, 1987) (see Chapter 14).

Sudden infant death syndrome (SIDS)

This condition occurs in 0.2–0.3% of live births but low birthweight infants are probably at much greater risk – perhaps 10 times as great. One study showed that 10% of postneonatal deaths (between 28 days and 1 year) in infants nursed initially on a neonatal unit were due to SIDS. Near-miss SIDS also occurs more frequently in low birthweight survivors.

Anaemias

Milk is a poor source of iron. The full-term baby has sufficient iron stores acquired *in utero* to last about four to six months. A reason for introducing mixing feeding at about this time is to provide an increased dietary intake of this essential element. Preterm babies do not gain much of the iron which they would have stored if they had not been born too soon. Thus unless prophylactic iron supplements are given these babies will develop an iron-deficiency (hypochromic) anaemia. This anaemia, which would develop at around the age of six months, should be prevented by giving iron. Many centres give ferrous sulphate 30 mg twice daily from the third week of life for six months. Not only may babies suffer from anaemia, but there is now evidence that neurological development is delayed in iron deficiency.

Anaemia after six months should be contrasted with the early anaemia of preterm infants. There are several reasons for the early drop in haemoglobin:

1 For adequate tissue oxygenation the fetus and neonate require about 11 g/dl of haemoglobin. As the placenta is only about 65% efficient at oxygenating haemoglobin, the total haemoglobin level *in utero* must be about 19 g/dl which is the level at birth. After birth, the lungs oxygenate haemoglobin about 96% effectively and therefore the total haemoglobin can be allowed to fall to about 12 g/dl; the bone marrow goes into a resting phase and is restimulated as the level of oxyhaemoglobin tends to fall below 11 g/dl. The preterm baby's bone marrow is often slow to respond to such stimulation and thus anaemia may develop during the second month of life. All preterm babies are usually given supplements of 50 μg folic acid daily for six months.
2 At the same time, there is an extremely rapid rate of growth in the preterm baby leading to a rapid increase in circulating blood volume; the bone marrow is unable to respond adequately.

This early anaemia is normochromic and, if treatment is necessary, it should be by simple top-up transfusion. Transfusion is not indicated in most preterm babies because it tends to suppress bone marrow haemopoiesis further. Clear indications for transfusions are signs or symptoms of cardiac failure (such as shortness of breath on feeding, tachycardia or hepatomegaly). In addition, it is probably wise to transfuse those babies with a haemoglobin below 8 g/dl even if they appear well. The aim is to raise the haemoglobin level to about 12 g/dl. It is, however, common practice to transfuse any ill newborn baby with a haemoglobin below 14 g/dl, particularly if there is a respiratory disorder. Blood is best given slowly and partially packed so as to reduce risks of circulatory overload. It is useful to remember that a transfusion of 20 ml/kg (equivalent to 16 ml/kg of packed cells) raises the haemoglobin level by 25%. Alternatively, the volume required may be calculated from the formula:

$V = W \times$ number of g/dl by which the haemoglobin is to be raised $\times$ 6

where V is the volume of whole blood to be transfused (ml), and W is the baby's weight (kg).

A very few preterm babies (less than 1500 g birth weight) may show peripheral oedema due to a third and distinct type of anaemia. The blood film shows haemolysis with a high reticulocyte and platelet count and low packed cell volume. Vitamin E levels are low and the anaemia responds to treatment with this vitamin (15 mg/day). Some even doubt the existence of such a condition – certainly the cause is not fully understood – but giving iron supplements in the newborn period has been shown to interfere with vitamin E absorption.

Vitamins

Recommended vitamin intakes for newborn babies are:

Vitamin A 1500 iu daily
Vitamin C 15–30 mg daily
Vitamin D 400 international iu daily

Supplements are usually recommended for breast-fed babies in the form of proprietary vitamin drops. Artificial milks have added vitamins, but in inadequate amounts, so that drops are still necessary, although in smaller doses.

The enteral vitamin needs for preterm infants may not be satisfied by human milk (see also Chapter 7). The vitamin intakes from commercial formulae specifically designed for preterm infants by and large meet the minimum requirements for ascorbic acid, B_1, B_2, B_6 and niacin but there is considerable variation between different formulae. Folate supplements should be given (50–100 μg/day) to all babies under 1500 g birthweight.

In our present state of knowledge it is reasonable to suggest a vitamin B_{12} intake of 0.15 mg/100 kcal per day in formula-fed preterm infants. Infants born of vegetarian mothers should be particularly carefully monitored with regard to their vitamin B_{12} metabolism.

Early hypocalcaemia

Some preterm babies are found to have low levels of calcium and sometimes magnesium during the first three days of life. They respond to calcium or magnesium supplements or both (calcium gluconate 10% 0.5–1 ml orally with each feed, or magnesium sulphate 50% 0.5 ml orally with each feed). The mechanism of the hypocalcaemia may simply be immaturity of the parathyroid glands (magnesium is necessary for parathyroid hormone release). In many hospitals serving immigrant populations, however, a common cause of neonatal hypocalcaemia is osteomalacia (vitamin D deficiency) in the mother, who should be investigated.

Rickets

Rickets seems to be common in very immature infants, whether they are breast or artificially fed. Even large doses of vitamin D (up to 2000 iu per day) will not prevent it (de Curtis et al., 1986). Babies of birthweight less than 1500 g should be regularly monitored for rickets with alkaline phosphatase measurements. If very high levels are found (over 1000 iu/l) an X-ray examination should be made of the long bones. If rickets is then confirmed it should be treated with alfacalcidol 0.1 µg/kg/day and phosphorus supplements of 0.5 mmol/100 ml (Bishop, 1989). The rate of bone-mineralization is accelerated at approximately 42–43 weeks post-conceptual age (Congdon et al., 1990).

Patent ductus arteriosus

This is discussed in connection with hyaline membrane disease (Chapters 8 and 11).

Hypertyrosinaemia

Immaturity of liver enzymes causes hypertyrosinaemia in about 1 in 10 preterm babies, particularly those having a high protein intake or vitamin C deficiency. Blood levels of phenylalanine also rise and therefore these babies may have false-positive Guthrie tests (see Chapter 4). Normal tyrosine levels in neonatal blood are between 0.7 and 5.6 mg/dl (40–310 µmol/l). The condition probably has no long-term effects and plasma levels usually return to normal by three months. It can be corrected by lowering the protein intake or giving a course of vitamin C (100 mg daily for several days).

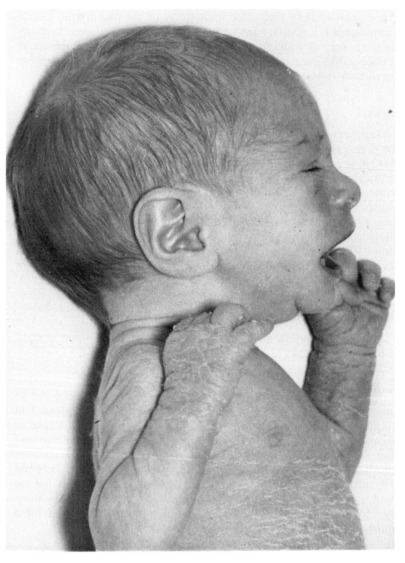

Fig. 6.8 The small-for-gestatational-age (SFGA or dysmature) baby

The Small-for-Gestational-Age (SFGA) Baby

SFGA babies (Fig. 6.8) show the results of their impaired intrauterine growth: there is little subcutaneous fat, loose dry skin, muscle wasting, especially over buttocks and cheeks, scaphoid abdomen and thin umbilical cord. Scalp hair is sparse. They are often long and thin, as longitudinal growth is not as retarded as subcutaneous fat is diminished; only the most chronically and severely affected babies have head circumference and length, as well as weight, below the 10th centile. The babies are usually active and vigorous, but they are vulnerable to particular illnesses in the newborn period and differ in their susceptibilities from the preterm baby who may weigh the same at birth.

Perinatal asphyxia

SFGA babies have frequently been chronically hypoxic during the last part of pregnancy. Not surprisingly, they are poor at withstanding the stresses of normal labour and may require active resuscitation. They need very careful monitoring in labour. Their chronic intrauterine distress may cause the passage of meconium into the amniotic fluid with gasping *in utero*. Thus before and during delivery these babies may aspirate meconium-stained liquor into the oropharynx, trachea and large bronchi. The first few breaths suck the meconium into the terminal bronchioles and alveoli (Fig. 6.9). If a SFGA baby is expected because of the presence of any predisposing factors (listed in Chapter 2) or there is evidence of poor fetal growth, a paediatrician should be present at the delivery. One should also be present if meconium-stained liquor is found when membranes rupture or are ruptured. The management of these babies is urgent and is described in Chapter 3.

Hypoglycaemia

Hypoglycaemia is common among SFGA babies because of their large, metabolically active brains which need a lot of glucose and their small livers with poor glycogen stores (Barber, 1987). There is controversy as to whether asymptomatic hypoglycaemia causes brain damage in newborn babies. It is possible that the newborn's brain can utilise other substances, such as lactic acid, as energy sources. There is no doubt that symptomatic hypoglycaemia can cause brain damage and levels below 1.4 mmol/l (25 mg/dl) are undesirable. Symptoms

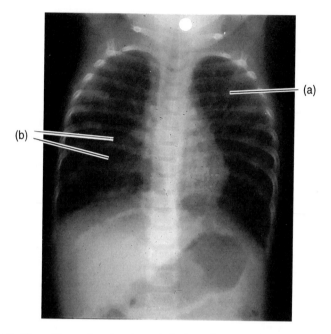

Fig. 6.9 Chest X-ray showing hyperinflation of lungs (b) and patchy shadowing (a) in meconium aspiration syndrome.

are largely non-specific – limpness, apathy, poor feeding, apnoeic attacks – and therefore all babies at risk (those below the 10th centile for weight for their gestational age) should be screened routinely and regularly using blood glucose monitoring strips. Estimations should be done every four to eight hours for 24 hours unless there are low levels, when they should be done more often. They may subsequently be checked less frequently. A reading below 1.4 mmol/l should be checked by blood glucose estimation (although this should not delay treatment if the baby has symptoms). Asymptomatic hypoglycaemia should be treated (and can almost always be prevented) by early and frequent feeding. If symptoms are present, glucose (dextrose) must be given intravenously; 10 ml of 20% glucose can be used as an emergency measure followed by 5% or 10% dextrose by intravenous infusion. Large amounts of dextrose or continuous dextrose infusions should be avoided, if possible, as they stimulate the baby's own insulin production and may lead to sudden hypoglycaemia when treatment is stopped.

Heat loss

Like the preterm baby, the SFGA baby easily becomes cold because of its high surface area and poor supply of subcutaneous fat.

Pulmonary haemorrhage

Pulmonary haemorrhage is an uncommon complication in SFGA babies and its aetiology is not fully understood, but it is thought to be haemorrhagic pulmonary oedema from heart failure. It develops suddenly in the first few days of life and presents with blood welling up the trachea. It is commoner in babies who are also ill (for example hypoglycaemic or hypothermic). Some babies do survive and require mechanical ventilation. It may now be much less common because SFGA babies are fed much earlier, kept warmer and are not allowed to become or remain hypoglycaemic.

Transient neonatal diabetes mellitus

This is a rare complication. The babies present with rapid weight loss and severe dehydration. They also have thirst and polyuria but for obvious reasons these are not usually noticed in a newborn baby. They look pale and lively in contrast to babies unwell with most other causes of dehydration, for example gastroenteritis. On testing, the urine contains sugar but no ketones, while despite high blood sugar levels they are not acidotic. Insulin levels are usually in the high normal range. On diagnosis babies should be treated with insulin to which they are very sensitive. For this reason it is best to start with 0.1 iu/kg/h as a continuous infusion. Normal saline is used initially and changed to a glucose solution when the blood glucose falls below 10 mmol/l. Potassium supplements are needed, so long as the baby is passing urine. Careful monitoring of ECG, blood glucose and plasma potassium is essential to prevent complications. This condition emphasizes the importance of screening SFGA babies with blood glucose monitoring strips and testing their urine for glucose.

Skin infections

The dry, cracked, peeling skin provides a ready port of entry for organisms such as staphylococci which are widely present on attendants, linen and in dust. The ways in which such infections can be largely prevented are discussed in Chapter 16. In general, babies with infective skin lesions should be isolated and topical treatment is usually adequate. The main dangers are either that the infection will spread systemically (when parenteral antibiotics should be given) or that other babies will be infected, with potentially serious results.

Poor feeding and poor growth

As indicated at the beginning of this chapter, some SFGA babies have grown slowly throughout pregnancy while in others there has been slow growth only at the end of pregnancy (see Figs. 2.6 and 6.1). The latter group feed avidly from the first days after birth. Instead of losing weight initially and regaining their birth weight only by about the 10th day, they immediately gain weight and grow rapidly as if making up for lost time. In contrast, those babies who have grown slowly throughout pregnancy seem programmed for extrauterine slow growth also, however intensively they are fed. They have a retarded bone-age and, therefore, their epiphyses fuse late so that some catch-up growth may take place, but short stature may persist into adult life.

High packed cell volume with increased blood viscosity

Many SFGA babies have haemoglobin levels over 20 g/dl and correspondingly high packed cell volumes (PCV, also called haematocrit) which is the proportion of the baby's blood volume made up of red cells. As the PCV increases above 65% the blood viscosity increases very rapidly and this leads to a number of complications. These babies look plethoric and lethargic and are cyanosed because there is more than 5 g of reduced haemoglobin present even with normal amounts of oxyhaemoglobin. They may become jaundiced, hyperexcitable or even develop respiratory distress or convulsions. It is customary to give additional fluid, orally if feeds are being absorbed, but this is not of proven benefit. The introduction of oral feeds is often delayed, due to the associated increased risk of necrotizing enterocolitis. If symptoms develop, exchange transfusion with 20–30 ml/kg plasma may be necessary. In practice, this is rarely required.

The fetal alcohol syndrome (FAS)

At one time, alcohol was felt to be safe in pregnancy. There is now increasing evidence that the drug has a serious effect on the growing fetus. The fetal alcohol syndrome was first recognised in the babies of chronic alcoholic mothers. It now seems that even a moderate intake may inhibit intrauterine growth, with a weekly intake of more than eight units (equivalent to one drink daily) thought to be deleterious.

Affected babies are SFGA and may have a number of dysmorphic features: microcephaly, a long phittrum to the upper lip, short palpebral fissures, maxillary hypoplasia and abnormal palmar creases. Ultimately, they may show developmental delay and mental retardation.

The incidence of FAS is approximately 1–2 per 1000 live births. There is a less serious diagnosis of fetal alcohol effects which occurs in approximately 3–5 per 1000 live births (Abel, 1983; Spohr *et al.*, 1993).

It is often useful to have problem sheets or even problem-orientated case notes for small and sick, or potentially sick babies. Their management may be made easier because problems are less likely to be overlooked.

References and Further Reading

Abel, E.L. (1983) *Fetal Alcohol Syndrome and Fetal Alcohol Effects*. New York: Plenum.

Barber, G.D. (1987) Hypoglycaemia of the newborn. *Midwives Chronicle and Nursing Notes, Feb.*, 46–49.

Barker, D.J.P. (1992) *Fetal and Infant Origins of Adult Disease*. London: BMJ Publishing Group.

Barker, D.J.P., Bull, A.R., Osmond, C. *et al.* (1990) Fetal and placental size and risk of hypertension. *BMJ*; *301*, 259–262.

Barker, D.J.P., Martyn, C.N., Osmond, C. *et al.* (1993) Growth *in utero* and serum cholesterol concentrations in adult life. *BMJ*, *307*, 1524–1527.

Benediktsson, R., Lindsay, R., Noble, J. *et al.* (1993) Glucocorticoid exposure *in utero*: a new model for adult hypertension. *Lancet*, *341*, 339–341.

Bishop, N. (1989) Bone disease in preterm infants. *Arch. Dis. Child*, *64*, 1403–1409.

Congdon, P.J., Horsman, A., Ryan, S.W. *et al.* (1990) Bone mineral repletion in preterm infants after 40 weeks post-conception. *Arch. Dis. Child*, 65, 1038–1042.

Cooke, R.W.I. (1987) Early and late ultrasonographic appearances and outcome in very low birthweight infants. *Arch. Dis. Child*, *62*, 931–937.

de Curtis, M., Nicholson, S., Fenton, T. *et al.* (1986) Failure of mineral supplementation to reduce the incidence of rickets of prematurity in infants weighing less than 1000 g at birth. *Pediatr. Res.*, *20*, 98.

de Vries, L.S., Dubowitz, L.M.S., Dubowitz, V. *et al.* (1985) Predictive value of cranial ultrasound in the newborn baby: a reappraisal. *Lancet*, *ii*, 137–140.

Dubowitz, L.M.S., Dubowitz, V. & Goldberg, C. (1970) Clinical assessment of gestational age in the newborn infant. *J. Pediatr.*, *77*, 1–10.

Edwards, C.R.W., Benediktsson, R., Lindsay, R. *et al.* (1993) Dysfunction of the placental glucocorticoid barrier: link between fetal environment and adult hypertension. *Lancet*, *341*, 355–357.

Evans, R., Pearson, M. & Ahmed, A. (eds) (1985) *Multiracial Initiatives in Maternity Care: a Directory of Projects for Black and Minority Ethnic Women*. London: Maternity Alliance.

Findlay, A. (1984) *Reproduction and the Fetus*. London: Edward Arnold.

Harvey, D., Cooke, R.W.I. & Levitt, G.A. (1989) *The Baby under 1000 g*. London: Wright.

Law, C.M., de Swiet, M., Osmond, C. *et al.* (1993) Initiation of hypertension *in utero* and its amplification throughout life. *BMJ*, *306*, 24–27.

Levine, M.I., Williams, J.L. & Fawer, C-L. (1985) *Ultrasound of the Infant Brain. Spastics Medical Publications*, *92*. Oxford: Blackwell Scientific Publications.

Lucas, A. & Cole, T.J. (1990) Breastmilk and neonatal necrotising enterocolitis. *Lancet*, *336*, 1519–1523.

Osmond, C., Barker, D.J.P., Winter, P.D. *et al.* (1993) Early growth and death from cardiovascular disease in women. *BMJ*, *307*, 1519–1524.

Rocheron, Y. & Dickinson, R. (1990) The Asian mother and baby campaign: a way forward in health promotion for Asian women? *Health Education Journal*, *49*(3), 128–133.

Rocheron, Y., Dickinson, R. & Khan, S. (1989) *Evaluation of the Asian Mother and Baby Campaign*. Centre for Mass Communication Research.

Spohr, H-L., Willms, J. & Steinhausen, H-C. (1993) Prenatal alcohol exposure and long-term developmental consequences. *Lancet*, *341*, 907–910.

Stewart, A.L., Thornburn, R.J., Hope, P.L. *et al.* (1983) Ultrasound appearances of the brain in very preterm infants and neurodevelopmental outcome at 18 months of age. *Arch. Dis. Child.*, *58*, 598–604.

Young, I.D. & Clarke, M. (1987) Foetal malformations and perinatal mortality: A ten year review with comparison of ethnic differences. *BMJ*, *295*(6590), 89–91.

7

Nutrition

Small babies have poor energy reserves (Table 7.1). Adequate nutrition and fluid intakes are essential for their survival. Despite the risks, intravenous alimentation may be life saving and promotes optimal brain growth during a crucial period.

Breastfeeding

Breastfeeding is the normal and natural way of feeding a newborn baby. It is only in very recent times, mainly during the last two centuries, that our industrial society has turned to the superficial attractions and convenience of bottle feeding. There are a number of artificial milk preparations derived from cow's milk which are more or less adapted for human needs. Earlier in the century, bottle feeding was used largely by the upper social classes whilst working class women were more likely to breastfeed. Until a few years ago there had been a continuing increase in the number of women who bottle fed their babies. Following an improvement in breastfeeding initiation and continuation rates between 1975 and 1980, the situation has changed little in the past decade.

It seems likely that infant feeding habits have been largely socially determined. Unlike 50 years ago, breastfeeding is now particularly popular amongst the more affluent. It is the women in social classes IV and V who are less likely to breastfeed now. In these days of smaller families, many young mothers have never even seen a baby

Table 7.1 Representation of energy reserves in babies of different birthweights.

Weight at birth of neonates (g)	Carbohydrate (g)	Fat (g)	kcal	Reserves (calculated in days)
1000	0	10	90	1
2000	9	100	936	5
3000	34	560	5176	18

being breastfed; they do not look upon it as natural. In addition, many mothers now wish or need to go out to work after the baby has been born in order to supplement or provide the family's income. There is also no doubt that even the most friendly maternity ward is less relaxing for the new mother than her own familiar surroundings at home. Some of the suggestions made by maternity hospitals may seem more like rules to some mothers and may even hinder breastfeeding; anxiety easily inhibits the natural development of lactation and can cause a woman to give up breastfeeding. It takes at least six weeks to fully establish breastfeeding and most mothers are discharged home long before this. Unfortunately some medical and midwifery advice in the past has been to feed babies on a fixed routine of feeding schedules, rather than to allow the mother to feed on demand, which is the natural way to breastfeed a baby.

To encourage the initiation of breastfeeding in hospital, the attitude of midwives, obstetricians and paediatricians is of crucial importance. The UNICEF Baby Friendly Hospital Initiative aims to promote beneficial breastfeeding practices and discourage detrimental ones. To facilitate this WHO/UNICEF have published 'Ten Steps to Successful Breastfeeding' (1989). Women who have some doubt about the value of breastfeeding should be encouraged to breastfeed. Restricting the time of the baby on the breast by a schedule such as allowing the baby to feed only for three minutes the first day, five the second and seven the third has been shown to decrease the success rate of breastfeeding when compared with a schedule that allows the mother to do what she and the baby want.

The time to teach the importance of breastfeeding is in school. It should form part of the national curriculum, like sex education, and both boys and girls should understand the vital importance of nutrition for a young baby. A breastfeeding mother could be invited to the school. Although it is less usual to persuade the mother to change her mind once the baby has been born, the advice and example of other mothers may be extremely helpful and breastfeeding mothers can be invited to antenatal classes. When there is a high rate of breastfeeding within a maternity ward, undecided mothers are more likely to breastfeed. The subject should be clearly discussed during the antenatal period, but one difficulty is that the mother who is less likely to breastfeed is also less likely to attend for antenatal care.

The long-term establishment of breastfeeding is greatly helped by putting the baby to the breast in the labour ward immediately after delivery. More mothers continue to breastfeed after discharge from hospital if this has been done. The establishment of breastfeeding does take time and trouble. Some hospitals employ a lactation mid-wife or infant-feeding sister, who spends the entire day giving individual help to feeding mothers and educating the staff in feeding techniques and practices.

Newborn babies may take many feeds each day. A baby who is allowed to feed completely on demand may at times feed for a very short duration as often as twice an hour. The arbitrary stipulation that babies should be fed at regular intervals, and have a certain length of time on the breast, makes it very difficult to establish natural breastfeeding. Babies should be fed on demand and, contrary to popular belief, such babies have been shown to settle down to a routine more quickly than babies who are forced to fit into a rigid timetable. The use of dummies and artificial teats should be avoided for breastfed babies. Their use will interfere with natural breastfeeding and may cause nipple–teat confusion (Mathur et al., 1990; Cesar et al., 1993).

The practice of 'rooming-in', where babies stay in cots with their mothers during the night, is also important for establishing breastfeeding. In the past night staff have kept many breastfed babies in the nursery, giving bottles of artificial milk at feed times, in order to allow the mother to rest. Far from helping, this practice makes it more difficult to establish lactation successfully, and it is now known that even one bottle of artificial feed may be sufficient to cause cow's milk allergy in a susceptible infant. Forty-five per cent of breastfed babies were given at least one bottle of artificial milk whilst in hospital, according to the 1990 OPCS survey into infant feeding.

Advantages

It is worthwhile taking trouble to establish breastfeeding because the breastfed baby has a number of potential advantages over a bottle fed peer. These advantages are worth considering in some detail.

Emotional relationships with the mother

Observation of infants in many different societies suggests that care of young infants is very different in modern industrialized societies from that in most parts of the world. In developing countries, and presumably in all countries in the past, a baby is carried around in close contact with the mother, is fed frequently on demand, is pacified immediately when miserable and sleeps in the parents' bed. In contrast, a baby in an industrial society is more likely to be fed

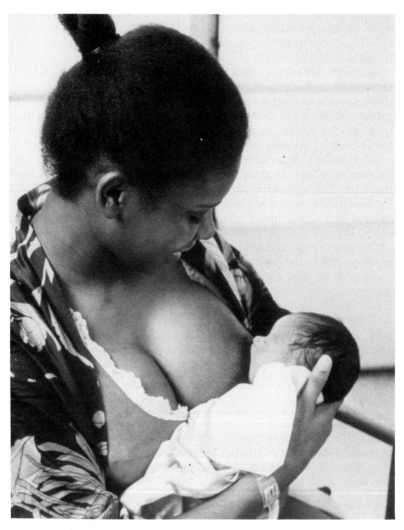

Fig. 7.1 Breastfeeding

less frequently, is allowed to cry when miserable, is rarely carried around and has much less bodily contact with an adult. The early part of infancy is a period of great need for emotional warmth and love manifested as close and regular body contact. Thus the baby who is breastfed is satisfying not only nutritional needs but also emotional needs (Fig. 7.1). There is good evidence that a baby at the breast takes in most fluid and energy requirements during the first few minutes of suckling. Much of the remainder of the time on the breast serves for oral pleasure and close body contact.

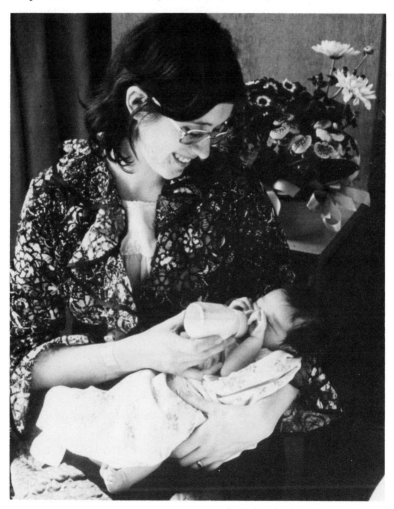

Fig. 7.2 Bottle feeding

The bottle fed baby is much more likely to be fed by other people than the mother. Feeding is more likely to be done in public and the baby may be deprived of the very close contact typical of breastfeeding. Of course, many mothers who bottle feed their babies do establish a warm and loving relationship with them (Fig. 7.2) but one sometimes sees the baby being bottle fed at arm's length while the adult is engrossed in the television or newspaper. A bottle-feeding mother may have to make a real effort to provide the emotional satisfaction that the breastfeeding mother does more naturally. We do not want this to sound too much like a sermon but there do seem to be very clear advantages to breastfeeding.

Decreased likelihood of infection

The widespread morbidity and mortality among newborn babies in developing countries in recent years has partly stemmed both from mothers' lack of knowledge of the rudiments of sterilization of bottles and feeds and from poverty. Epidemics of infantile gastroenteritis have been the result. Even in the UK many mothers in socially deprived areas have neither the facilities nor the ability to produce properly sterilized artificial feeds. There are, however, specific factors present in breast milk, and not in artificially prepared cow's milk feeds, which protect the newborn baby from infection (Howie *et al.*, 1990; Table 7.2). An immunoglobulin, IgA, is secreted in high concentration in breast milk, and, more particularly, in colostrum

Table 7.2 Composition of human and cow's milk.

Milk Composition per 100 ml	Mature breast milk	Cow & Gate low birthweight	Cow & Gate premium	Cow & Gate plus	Cow & Gate soya
Energy (kj)	270–315	336	275	274	274
Protein (g)	1.2–1.4	2.2	1.4	1.9	1.8
Fat (g)	3.7–4.8	4.4	3.6	3.4	3.6
Carbohydrate (g)	7.1–7.8	8.5	7.5	7.3	7.1
Calcium (mg)	32–36	108	54	85	54
Phosphorus (mg)	14–15	54	27	55	27
Calcium: phosphorus	2.3:1	2:1	2:1	1.5:1	2:1
Sodium (mg)	11–20	32	18	25	18
Potassium (mg)	57–62	71	65	100	65
Chloride (mg)	35–55	45	40	60	40
Iron (µg)	62–93	900	500	500	500

during the first few days of life. This substance lines the breastfed baby's gut and, in conjunction with lactoferrin also present in colostrum, helps establish a bacterial flora of non-pathogenic lactobacilli, while suppressing the growth of potentially pathogenic strains of *E. coli*. The bottle fed baby's bowel flora is predominantly *E. coli*. Even in Britain gastroenteritis is more common in bottle fed babies. Breast milk contains live cells which may have immunological properties.

Reduced incidence of eczema and other forms of atopy

It is becoming clear that the incidence of eczema is greater in babies who have had even one or two artificial feeds during the early weeks or months of life. There is a substance in the protein fraction of cow's milk which sensitizes many babies. This manifests itself as eczema during infancy and may be associated with the subsequent development of such diseases as asthma, urticaria, hay fever and allergic rhinitis. It is of particular importance that the breastfed baby is not given any artificial cow's milk complement, and if these are avoided the risk of atopy is significantly reduced (Lucas *et al.*, 1990).

Some babies can be very demanding in the first few days when the mother's milk is just coming in. In these circumstances it is particularly important to avoid the use of any supplements, either milk-based or clear fluids, as they will interfere with establishing lactation, not help. This advice applies to all breastfed babies, and a mother's lactation is best promoted by feeding the baby on demand, with no fixed guidelines over the length or frequency of feeds.

There has been a recent suggestion, based on epidemiological evidence, that breastfeeding may help to protect an infant from the later development of diabetes mellitus. If this is true the mechanism would presumably be immunological.

Reduced likelihood of biochemical upset

The composition of unmodified cow's milk and human milk is shown in Tables 7.2 and 7.3. The predominant protein in human milk (lactalbumin) is much more digestible than that in cow's milk (casein); there is more carbohydrate, but also the fat content, being much more evenly distributed throughout the milk, is more easily digestible. In addition there are significant biochemical differences. For example, cow's milk contains some three to four times as much calcium as human milk but about seven times as much phosphate. It contains four times as much sodium and its osmolality is three times

Table 7.3 Composition of breast milk, and some examples of artificial formulae and cow's milk.

Composition	Breast milk	SMA (S26)	Cow's milk
Carbohydrate*	6.8	7.2	4.9
Fat*	4.5	3.6	3.7
Protein*	1.1	1.5	3.5
Sodium (mmol/l)	7	7	22
Phosphorus (mg/l)	140	330	920
Calcium (mg/l)	340	445	1170

* grams per 100 ml of formula.

that of human milk. Until some years ago, the artificial milks available also contained too much phosphate. Many babies fed on these preparations developed hypocalcaemic fits during the second or third week of life. This is because there is an inverse relationship between calcium and phosphate in the body and ingesting too much phosphate tends to make the blood calcium concentrations low. In the last decade artificial milk preparations have reduced the phosphate load in the milk, thus making this problem much rarer.

An analogous problem has been the high sodium content of artificial milks. The newborn baby's kidney is not very efficient by the standards of older children. When a bottle-fed baby is well, there is just sufficient reserve to enable the kidney to fulfil the demands made on it. If such a baby develops diarrhoea, for example, this precarious balance is lost and severe biochemical disturbances can follow. Each baby milk preparation comes with its individual scoop. These are not interchangeable from make to make and failure to appreciate this may lead to feeds being made up in the wrong strength. If baby milk powder is packed into the scoop or it is not levelled off, over-concentrated feeds are given to the baby. Similarly, if the powder is put into the bottles before the water, and the volume then made up to the gram mark, the feed will be too concentrated. This may be very dangerous in itself, but if the baby is already unwell with gastroenteritis and crying for more feed because of thirst, an over-concentrated feed will make this plight worse. It used to be common for such babies to be brought into hospital casualty departments with dehydration and associated plasma sodium levels of over 160 mmol/l. There was considerable mortality amongst such babies and convulsions and brain damage were common in those who survived.

Reduced incidence of cot deaths (sudden infant death syndrome, SIDS)

There is a lower incidence of cot deaths amongst breastfed babies (Mitchell *et al.*, 1991). The reasons for this are not altogether clear; cot death is probably not one condition but has a multitude of different causes. Many of these deaths may be related to some of the factors already described, which are more likely in the bottle fed baby. In addition, the bottle feeding mother is less likely to have come for antenatal care and cot deaths amongst the infants of such mothers are commoner (see also p. 390).

Less likelihood of obesity

The fluid intake of the healthy baby amounts to 150–200 ml/kg/day. This is equivalent to 450–600 kJ daily (about 110–150 cal/kg); some preterm babies may need even more if they are to thrive. This is a rough guide as no two babies are alike. The natural way of feeding is to demand feed. With rare exceptions, a healthy baby will regulate intake in a satisfactory manner. Attempting to enforce an arbitrary feeding regimen is neither desirable nor recommended. There is a natural tendency among some bottle feeding mothers to overfeed their babies. This is because of the mistaken idea that fat babies are healthy babies, and because a baby who is feeding a lot and over-weight tends to be a placid individual. A fat baby does not necessarily develop into a fat child or adult. Nevertheless, an obese baby is not a healthy one and is more susceptible to respiratory infection.

Contraindications

There are few contraindications to breastfeeding. One recently recog-nised one in a developed country, is if the mother has HIV infection. This is discussed further in Chapter 16 (Thiry *et al.*, 1985; Van de Perre *et al.*, 1991).

The usual reason for not breastfeeding is the mother's reluctance to do so. It is not likely that you will succeed in persuading her once her mind is made up; this will only be counter-productive by suggesting that she is a less than adequate or conscientious mother for not wishing to breastfeed.

Only rarely is breastfeeding contraindicated because of drugs (e.g. lithium) that the mother it taking. In untreated tuberculosis, the mother who is already established on treatment may be allowed to

Table 7.4 Excretion methods which allow drugs to appear in the milk.

1 Water-soluble substances with a molecular weight of 200 or less, e.g. ethanol or urea, diffuse through pores and may achieve the same concentration in milk as in plasma

2 Active excretion, e.g. thiouracil

3 Most drugs are weak acids or weak bases and enter milk in their non-protein-bound, unionized forms to reach concentrations that depend on the pH difference between plasma (pH 7.4) and milk (pH 7.0), and on the degree of ionization of the drug at physiological pH, its protein-binding capacity and its lipid solubility. Weak acids reach *lower* concentrations in milk than in plasma, while weak bases reach concentrations in milk that are similar to, or *higher* than those in plasma

breastfeed her baby, who should, however, be protected with iso-niazid-resistant BCG and also treated with isoniazid (10 mg/kg/day orally in three doses) for the first few months of life.

The key to successful breastfeeding is a relaxed mother. To achieve such relaxation in a hospital ward requires care, consistent, research-based advice and patience from all those who attend her.

Breast milk drug excretion

Surprisingly little is known about the excretion of many drugs in breast milk. It seems likely that virtually all substances given to the mother will be excreted in some form, in greater or lesser concentration, in her breast milk. How much depends on the size of the drug molecule, its solubility in water and fat, its acidity and its degree of ionization at physiological pH. Excretory mechanisms are summarized in Table 7.4. As a general rule, the amounts of drugs excreted are usually small, do not affect the baby clinically, and are not a contra-indication to continuing breastfeeding. The only important exceptions to this rule are mothers who have been given radioactive iodine for thyrotoxicosis and possibly other drugs affecting thyroid function, and those on cytotoxic drugs. The midwife and doctor should be particularly aware of possible complications when the drugs listed in Table 7.5 are being taken over a long period of time by the breast-feeding mother. Table 7.6 gives more information about the potential toxicity of a number of drugs now in common use or where information is available. Many lactating mothers receive drugs without particular justification. Paracetamol and nitrazepam should not be routinely prescribed to all postpartum obstetric patients.

Table 7.5 Drugs believed to have serious adverse effects in breast-fed babies when taken by the mother.

Drug	May cause
Sulphonamides	Neonatal jaundice
	Haemolysis in infants with glucose-6-phosphate dehydrogenase deficiency
Chloramphenicol	Possibility of grey baby syndrome and bone marrow toxicity
Phenindione	Increased prothrombin time
Indomethacin	Single report of convulsions in an infant
Thiouracil	Goitre
	Agranulocytosis
Radioactive iodine	Goitre
	Late risk of thyroid cancer
Cyclophosphamide and other anti-neoplastic drugs	Bone marrow depression
Ergot alkaloids	Ergotism
High doses benzodiazepines	Hypotonia
Lithium	Hypothermia
	Cyanosis
Amiodarone	Present in milk in significant amounts. Theoretical risk from release of iodine
High dose steroids	Affect adrenal function
High dose oestrogen	May suppress lactation
High dose diuretics	May suppress lactation
High dose barbiturates	Sedation

Expressing

Establishing and maintaining lactation can prove extremely difficult for mothers of very preterm babies, particularly as it is strongly influenced by stress and fatigue. All mothers wishing to breastfeed should be taught hand expression by their midwife, as well as being instructed in the importance of breast hygiene and the use of breast pumps. Facilities for borrowing or hiring pumps must be readily available, and mothers should be encouraged to start expressing as soon as possible. It is important to explain the physiology of lactation to enable them to understand the factors which influence it, such as poor diet, smoking, fatigue and stress. The effectiveness of stimulation provided by electric and manual breast pumps gradually reduces

Table 7.6 Potential toxicity to the baby of various commonly prescribed drugs taken by breastfeeding mother.

Antibacterial drugs

Sulphonamides	Milk/plasma (M/P) ratios vary from 0.08 to 0.97 depending on ionization at plasma pH. Theoretical risk of neonatal jaundice by competition with bilirubin for protein binding sites. Haemolytic anaemia has been reported in a G-6-PD-deficient baby breastfed while the mother was taking sulphamethoxypyridazine
Penicillins	Amounts too small to have antimicrobial effect, but rarely may provoke antigenic response. Safe
Ampicillin	May cause diarrhoea and candidiasis
Isoniazid	High M/P ratio (too little information to be categoric about safety)
Tetracycline	High M/P ratio (too little information to be categoric about safety)
Streptomycin	Mother with normal renal function may take up to 1 g daily without causing ototoxicity in infant. Maternal renal failure increases milk concentrations up to 25-fold. Safe
Metronidazole	High concentrations in milk and plasma. No harmful effect when mother receives 200 mg three times a day for seven days, but avoid high dosages (metallic taste may put baby off breastfeeding)
Nalidixic Acid	One report of haemolysis in infant with normal enzymes whose mother was uraemic
Nitrofurantoin	Small amounts found in breast milk
Erythromycin	Occurs in small amounts in milk if taken orally by mother. Amounts increase 10-fold when it is given intravenously. Safe
Cephalexin/Cephadrine	Trace amounts may occur in milk. Safe
Ciprofloxacin	Animal data demonstrate potential accumulation in milk. Not recommended

Hormones

Insulin Adrenaline ⎫ ACTH ⎭	Destroyed in infant's gut

Table 7.6 (cont.) Potential toxicity to the baby of various commonly prescribed drugs taken by breastfeeding mother.

Thyroxine } Corticosteroids }	If given in moderate amounts, are found in the milk in significant quantities
Oral Contraceptives	Theoretical risk that male babies may develop gynaecomastia; females may show proliferation of vaginal epithelium. Infant is unlikely to be affected provided drug is withheld until third or fourth week post partum. Combined pills are usually avoided because of potential risk of suppressing lactation
Anticoagulants Heparin	Destroyed in gut. Safe
Warfarin	Not detected in milk; baby's prothrombin time remains normal. Anticoagulant of choice in breastfeeding mothers
Phenindione	Increased prothrombin time reported; also large postoperative haematoma. Not recommended
Anticonvulsants Sodium Valproate	Amount too small to be harmful
Phenobarbitone	Probably no adverse effects when taken in anticonvulsant doses
Phenytoin	No ill-effects. Insignificant amounts excreted. One child developed methaemoglobinaemia while mother was taking large doses of phenytoin and phenobarbitone
Carbamazepine	Recently has been licensed for use in breastfeeding mothers. Single report of skin reaction in a breastfed baby
Psychotherapeutic drugs Diazepam	Diazepam and its active metabolite found in milk and in infant's serum and urine. Infants' EEGs show changes characteristic of sedative medication. Sedation and lethargy. Not recommended
Chlordiazepoxide	Minimal amounts in milk. Not considered to be harmful
Chloral hydrate	Enter in sufficient amounts to cause minimal sedation after larger feeds
Imipramine	Small amounts found in milk. Probably safe

Table 7.6 (Cont.) Potential toxicity to the baby of various commonly prescribed drugs taken by breastfeeding mother.

Chlorpromazine	Evidence conflicting. Probably best to limit maternal dose to less than 100 mg/day
Lithium	Concentration in milk about one-half to one-third that in plasma. Complete absorption from gastrointestinal tract. Hypotonia and cyanosis observed in the baby of a mother taking lithium during pregnancy. Breastfeeding is contraindicated if treatment is essential. Patients on low doses with good control of plasma concentration may safely breast-feed provided infant is closely monitored
Haloperidol	No reports of ill-effects
Narcotics	
Heroin Methadone	Enter milk, and infant probably already tolerant *in utero*. Nevertheless withdrawal symptoms common even in breastfed. Breastfeeding during maintenance on Methadone is permissible provided the infant is closely monitored
Morphine	Traces only. Safe, if indicated
Analgesics	
Codeine	Amount too small to be detected
Salicylates	Present in breast milk. CSM advises avoid in children under 12 years due to risk of Reye's syndrome. Not recommended
Paracetamol	Amount too small to be harmful
Iodides and thiouracil	
Propylthiouracil	The infants of mothers who have to take this drug should have thyroid function closely monitored
Iodides	Actively transported and goitrogenic. Sensitize infant's thyroid to co-goitrogens such as chlorpromazine, lithium and methylxanthines
Radioactive iodine	28% of dose may enter milk and be completely absorbed by baby. Stop breast-feeding for 10 days after use. Also increases risk of later thyroid cancer. BNF advice is stop BH after therapeutic dose. Withhold BH for 48 hours after diagnostic dose

Table 7.6 (Cont.) Potential toxicity to the baby of various commonly prescribed drugs taken by breastfeeding mother.

Technetium	Stop breastfeeding for up to 24/48 hours
Alkylating agents	
Cyclophosphamide	Do not breastfeed depending on radiopharmaceutical used
Methotrexate	Weak organic acid with low M/P ratio but possible long-term effects on baby unknown
Miscellaneous	
Digoxin	Amount too small to be harmful
Propranolol Atenolol	Found in significant quantity in milk. Infants should be assessed regularly for signs of B-blockade
25-Hydroxycholecalciferol	Large doses may cause hypercalcaemia in baby. Monitor calcium levels
Antihistamines	Low levels. Unlikely to be significant (this may not be true for some of the newer agents, e.g. Astemizole)
Tolbutamide	Found in milk. Could cause hypoglycaemia but it seems safe
Fluoride	Accepted daily dose for optimal tooth development under two years is 0.25 mg. This is provided in breast milk if local water supply provides 1 part per million. London water is not fluoridated. Mottling of the teeth may occur if extra fluoride is taken or if local water concentration exceeds this level
Laxatives	Do not cause purgation except, possibly, for anthraquinone derivatives, e.g. cascara, senna, rhubarb, danthrone and aloes. In fact anthraquinone has not been shown to have any definite effect on the infant's bowel
Alcohol Nicotine	Probably not harmful in moderate quantities
Caffeine	Not enough occurs in milk to affect infant (heavy coffee drinkers would dispute this)
Gold	Trace amounts in infant's serum
Thiazides	Small amounts not harmful

over a period of time, with a resulting decline in the volume of expressed breast milk (EBM).

There are several ways in which lactation can be boosted:

1 Allowing the baby to suck at the breast, even if it is non-nutritive or inefficient sucking.

2 Expressing or feeding from the breast more frequently, ideally at least six to eight times in 24 hours (Hopkinson et al., 1988).

3 Expressing next to the baby to encourage the let-down reflex.

4 Expressing from both breasts simultaneously, or swapping from one breast to the other at five-minute intervals over a total of about 20 minutes, both of which boost prolactin levels.

5 Kangaroo care – cuddling the baby with skin-to-skin contact.

6 Aromatherapy – fennel or geranium oil mixed with a carrier oil, massaged into the breasts. It must be washed off prior to feeding or expressing.

7 Prescribing oral metoclopramide (10–15 mg tds) or domperidone. Although not yet formally approved for this purpose, they are widely used in many neonatal units. Controlled trials into the usage of these drugs have shown an increased milk yield of up to 30 ml at each expression (Ehrenkranz & Ackerman, 1986).

These measures are usually effective in sustaining lactation until the baby can be fully breastfed.

Fresh EBM may be fed to the baby immediately, in which case it retains all its immunological properties. In many developing countries mothers express at each feed time, and give the fresh milk to their baby using a cup. These practices have greatly reduced the incidence of infection and subsequent mortality in preterm infants.

EBM may also be frozen for future use. It is recommended that the maximum time it is frozen is six months, although due to space and infection risks most neonatal units do so for only three months. If mothers are only expressing small volumes, the use of a sterilized ice-cube tray to freeze milk cubes may be useful.

Unfortunately, EBM may not contain sufficient calories or protein for adequate nutrition in a small baby. The nutritional content can be boosted by adding powders such as 'Duocal' – which consists of 43% fat and 57% carbohydrate, providing 19.74 kJ/g (4.7 kcal/g). 'Caloreen' is a carbohydrate which is also used in doses of up to 5 g/kg. The quantity of such additives should be gradually increased as tolerated, as they can cause diarrhoea if given in excessive amounts. This obviously counteracts the purpose of the supplement.

The use of these increases the weight gain velocity and this should be remembered when the baby starts fully breastfeeding, and supplements are no longer given. It is important to have realistic expectations of weight gain at this time, and explain this to the parents. Milk fortifiers are now widely used in Europe, but only one has been subjected to trials in the UK to date, with good results (Warner *et al.*, 1993). They are marketed by baby milk companies. Milk that is collected from the breast while the baby sucks the opposite breast, 'drip milk', has a very low fat content and about two-thirds the energy content of EBM.

Milk banks

It is sad that the advent of HIV infection has reduced the number of milk banks in the UK considerably over the past decade (Williams *et al.*, 1985). Strict screening for milk donors is required, just as for blood donors (Balmer & Wharton, 1992). The Department of Health and Social Security published a document in 1988 advising on how to protect babies from accidental transmission of HIV in donor breast milk. Pasteurization at 56°C for 30 minutes has been shown to inactivate the virus (Eglin & Wilkinson, 1987), and does not destroy as much IgA as older, fiercer methods, such as boiling. Drip milk can be used despite its low energy content, as pooling of the milk donated evens out such variations.

There is much evidence that breast milk is better tolerated by sick, preterm infants than formula, and that it can prevent necrotizing enterocolitis (Lucas & Cole, 1990). Long-term benefits are also apparent (Lucas *et al.*, 1989, 1992). Its use should therefore be actively encouraged, and NICU feeding policies should reflect this. With adequate screening, pasteurization and nutritional boosting human donor milk also has many benefits; milk banks have a place in providing optimum nutrition for these babies.

Feeding Techniques

Breastfeeding

Even with a mature, healthy newborn baby it can take several weeks before breastfeeding is truly established and the mother feels confident feeding her baby. Inevitably this process is much more protracted and difficult with a preterm or sick infant, where both physical and psychological influences may have adverse effects on lactation.

The benefits of breastfeeding for preterm and SFGA babies in particular are well documented. Research has shown the incidence of Necrotizing enterocolitis (NEC) to be much reduced in infants fed purely on EBM (Lucas *et al.*, 1992) and enteral feeding can therefore be introduced sooner. The benefits to the mother in terms of early physical contact and having an exclusive role in her baby's care are invaluable.

The establishment of breastfeeding is an important role for neonatal staff, and one that is sadly undervalued in many units. Education in the physiology and practical aspects of breastfeeding should be a part of all neonatal nursing staff's training, as adequate support early on has been shown to be a vital factor in establishing feeding successfully. The mother must be taught the technique of fixing her baby to the breast properly, and shown different positions for feeding to ensure maximum comfort for both herself and the baby. The principles behind breastfeeding and the production of milk should be explained to the mother, to enable her to understand the process and what influences it.

Bottle feeding

If the mother has decided to bottle feed, it is usually possible to establish this in a term baby without much difficulty. The occasional baby needs a change of teat; preterm babies born at less than 34 weeks gestational age usually need special techniques of tube feeding before progressing to bottle feeding. The choice of milk needs a little thought; in general, it seems reasonable to choose a milk that is chemically similar to breast milk. Table 7.3 shows the composition of breast milk. The figures refer to pooled mature breast milk and there is, in fact, a lot more variation than is suggested by average figures. The concentration of chemicals looks very similar in some artificial baby milks and breast milk but there are still important differences, particularly in immunoglobulins and, of course, in the live cells which breast milk contains. It is important that the amount of sodium should be very little higher than in breast milk since hypernatraemia used to be a common complication of gastroenteritis in the early months of life before milks were modified to contain less sodium. However, very small newborn babies may develop hyponatraemia and often need sodium supplements (3 mmol/kg/day or more).

Soya milk has a high aluminium concentration, and is not indicated for feeding the preterm baby.

Intragastric feeding

Naso/orogastric feeding

Indications for intragastric feeding include any baby who has considerable difficulty in sucking or is unable to suck. This commonly means the preterm baby, generally less than about 34 weeks gestation, an ill baby of any size or maturity and babies with difficulty in breathing such as those with heart failure. Such infants may be gradually introduced to breast or bottle feeding at the appropriate time with the frequency of intragastric feeds gradually reduced. The aim is to achieve a weight gain of about 200 g/week.

Technique.   A tube is inserted through the baby's nostril or mouth and passed down the oesophagus into the stomach. Different size tubes are now available for babies of different weights: FG4 for babies of less than 1.2 kg, FG5 for 1.2–1.7 kg and FG6 for greater than 1.7 kg. FG8 gastric tubes are used for orogastric feeding only. The nose–umbilicus length is a good guide to how far to insert the tube. It is wise to choose the smaller nostril so as to leave the larger one for the baby to breathe through. There may particularly be a case for passing the tube through the mouth if the baby has respiratory problems. When it is thought to be in the stomach, a syringe is attached and an attempt made to aspirate stomach contents. The liquid from the stomach is acid and will turn blue litmus paper red. If there is any doubt about the position of the tube, air can be gently blown down with a syringe while listening with a stethoscope over the upper abdomen. Once the correct position of the tube has been confirmed, it can be fixed in position by strapping on the baby's cheek.

Amounts of feed for the preterm baby (usually full-strength expressed breast milk):

60 ml/kg/24 hours on Day 1
90 ml/kg/24 hours on Day 2
120 ml/kg/24 hours on Day 3
150 ml/kg/24 hours on Day 4

These amounts should be increased as shown and the intake may need to exceed about 200 ml/kg/day before the very tiny baby will grow adequately.

Very preterm babies may need oral sodium supplements after the first week. Babies of less than 1 kg or in whom the plasma sodium is less than 125 mmol/l need about 6 mmol/kg/day of extra sodium. The plasma sodium should be measured at least every day.

Feeds can be given as often as hourly to reduce the risk of aspiration. For similar reasons, the baby may be nursed prone.

Expressed breast milk should be used when available. There seems to be no ideal milk for very preterm babies because they need the anti-infection qualities of fresh breast milk but with a higher energy and protein content for growth (see above).

Dangers.   There is some evidence that a baby who is tube fed for a long time may be slow to learn sucking. For this reason, it is useful to allow even a very small baby a little time for sucking at the mother's breast well before this is likely to be the normal means of feeding.

Trauma from the tube is uncommon if the tube is passed gently. If resistance is met, the tube should be withdrawn slightly and a further attempt made at re-insertion.

Airway obstruction may occur in the smallest babies, as the diameter of the tube may approach that of the nasal passages. As the young baby is an obligatory nose breather, care must be taken to ensure that a small enough tube is used, and that the opposite, larger, nostril is never allowed to block. An orogastric tube may be preferable.

Aspiration of feeds should largely be prevented if babies are fed upright, prone or on their sides. In addition, particular care should be taken when passing the tube that it has actually reached the stomach. The risks of aspiration into the lungs of feed from a tube which is coiled up in the oropharynx are considerable. Nasogastric feeding is not suitable for babies with respiratory problems; it should certainly not be used for 24 hours after endotracheal extubation or when giving continuous positive airways pressure (CPAP) (see Chapter 8).

Continuous intragastric feeding

This method has proved extremely useful for the small preterm baby. It may well be more physiological than the large bolus feeds described above as such babies would normally take very small amounts of feed at very frequent intervals. The overall amounts given are similar to those given by intermittent feeding. Because the baby is handled less, there is less likelihood of infection. A constant infusion pump is used to regulate the rate that the milk is given. It is vital that babies fed in this way are nursed prone, otherwise the risk of aspiration of feed into the lungs is very high. Once again, care must be taken that the nasogastric tube is in the stomach and not coiled up in the oropharynx. If these precautions are taken, this is an extremely simple and safe technique to use in small babies. It is wise to aspirate every three hours to ensure that milk is not collecting in the stomach. Agitate the bottle or syringe fairly often to keep the fat mixed with the rest of the milk and keep the pump below the level of the baby or most of the fat (and therefore calories) will be left in the syringe. Alternatively place the barrel exit uppermost.

Naso/orojejunal (NJ/OJ) feeding

Indications.   Naso/orojejunal feeding is used to maintain full nutrition in small babies who are ill and not receiving sufficient energy. This includes those being ventilated or receiving CPAP by nasal prongs, where there would be a serious risk of aspiration with gastric feeds. Sometimes, also in very small babies, it may offer an alternative to intravenous feeding. Therefore it should be considered in babies weighing less than 1.25 kg, those with respiratory distress syndrome, congenital heart disease, septicaemia, some surgical conditions, seizure disorders and sedated babies.

The method of passing a nasojejunal tube is as follows:

1 A 125 cm FG silicone coated Vygon tube is selected.
2 The baby's nose-to-pubis (gastric mark) and chin-to-heel (jejunal mark) lengths are measured and the tube is marked with pen at these distances from the tip.
3 The infant is turned onto the right side and the attendant's hand is placed in the left hypochondrium to compress the stomach gently.
4 The nasojejunal tube is passed through the smaller nostril and into the stomach until resistance is felt at the nose-to-pubis length.
5 The tube is aspirated to see whether acid gastric juice or bile is obtained. If bile is obtained the tube is advanced to the chin-to-heel mark over five minutes, aspirating occasionally. Once the tube has reached the stomach it can be flushed with 1 ml of sterile water to keep the tube patent and, by stimulating peristalsis, to allow the tube to advance further.

6 If bile is not obtained, the infant is kept on the right side. Every 15 minutes a further attempt is made to advance the tube.

7 When bile is obtained and the tube is advanced to the second mark, a supine radiograph is taken of the baby's abdomen. Successful passage of the tube is indicated by: (a) the tube crossing the mid-line and traversing the duodenal loop into the proximal jejunum; (b) aspiration of bile; and (c) aspiration of a nasogastric tube before feeding shows no residual volume present on successive occasions.

8 A little air should then be blown in to clear the end of the tube.

9 Pass a nasogastric tube through the same nostril (so as not to produce respiratory obstruction). This tube should be tied to the nasojejunal tube.

10 A radiograph of the abdomen should be taken after two hours.

It is important that a silicone-coated or silastic tube is used. Polyvinylchloride tubes, which were used for this purpose, became rigid within a few days of being passed and led to a risk of bowel perforation. Silastic or silicone tubes should probably be changed about every 10–14 days.

Most naso/orojejunal tubes pass within eight hours. The best feed for the baby is expressed breast milk which may conveniently be given by infusion pump. The baby's total fluid requirements should not be given immediately. The feed should be increased by 1–2 ml per hour until the baby's calculated requirement is reached within 12–24 hours.

Precautions. A number of precautions should be taken with the baby being fed naso/orojejunally:

1 The nasogastric tube should be aspirated between two- and four-hourly. If there is no aspirate, blow 0.5 ml of air to clear the tube, and re-aspirate. Aspirates may be replaced down the tube, but this should be done slowly. If the aspirate is not replaced remember to include it as fluid deficit. If milk is aspirated through the nasogastric tube check to see if the aspirate is acid in case the naso/orojejunal tube has slipped into the stomach.

2 The girth should be measured eight-hourly. Mild distension is fairly common. If it becomes progressive or marked, a jejunal feeding may have to be discontinued for 8–12 hours. An abdominal radiograph will be necessary to detect any evidence of necrotizing enterocolitis (see p. 354).

3 Record the size and frequency of any vomit and whether the fluid vomited has been replaced. If vomiting is excessive in frequency or quantity the position of the tube should be checked.

4 The frequency and characteristics of the stools passed should be recorded. Test them daily for blood.

5 Blood for electrolytes and calcium should be checked twice weekly, or if the volume of aspirate is particularly large.

Naso/orojejunal feeding is a useful way of giving feeds to small, sick babies over long periods of time. In most units it is less risky than intravenous alimentation and, if the precautions described above are taken, it is a relatively safe procedure. However, the following complications have been reported: abdominal distension, altered gut flora, gastric reflux, frequent loose stools, disturbance of peristalsis, bowel perforation, peritonitis, necrotizing enterocolitis and intussusception.

Total parenteral nutrition (TPN)

Indications. It is not always possible to feed a baby enterally, particularly after abdominal surgery, or those who are very small (less than 800 g). Attempts should always be made to give babies expressed breast milk, as even small quantities have advantages in preventing necrotizing enterocolitis and in encouraging growth and development of the gut.

One should balance the possibility of serious complications from intravenous feeding against the need for improved nutrition. It is, however, important to avoid severe weight loss and maintain growth by using intravenous feeding, if enteral nutrition is not sufficient. The common indications for intravenous feeding are:

1 Extreme prematurity, with failure to establish feeding by means of a gastric or jejunal tube.

2 Respiratory disorders lasting four or more days, including repeated apnoeic attacks.

3 Necrotizing enterocolitis.

4 Prolonged diarrhoea or malabsorption.

5 After serious neonatal surgery, particularly intestinal operations.

6 Seriously ill babies.

In order to provide intravenous feeding it is essential to have strict aseptic techniques and skilled nursing care. Frequent biochemical monitoring is required and any acidaemia or electrolyte disturbances must be corrected. Fat emulsions should not be used if there is hyperlipidaemia, hypoglycaemia or impaired bone marrow function.

As always, remember to explain to the parents what is being done and why. It is useful to have an information leaflet for parents.

Preparation of intravenous feeding.   It is essential that the solution should be aseptically prepared. There are two major possibilities: (a) prepared solutions from a pharmaceutical company; and (b) solutions prepared in the hospital pharmacy. The second method is the cheaper and is preferable, because individual solutions can be made for babies when necessary. A Class I aseptic suite is required and the feeds are prepared in laminar flow cabinets or isolators. Strict aseptic techniques are employed by trained pharmacy staff in the preparation of these solutions.

Great care must be taken in prescribing the solution accurately and this should be checked by the pharmacy. Schedules of prescription are extremely valuable and the use of modern personal computers has allowed prescribing on the neonatal unit. The formula is checked automatically by the software program. It is then possible to send the prescription on-line from one hospital to another through a network or by a telephone line to speed up the process of prescribing the solutions and to allow time for preparation.

Choice of constituents.   The contents of the fluid given to the baby must supply adequate energy, water, essential fatty acids, nitrogen, vitamins, electrolytes and trace elements:

1 *Water.* The preterm baby has a proportionately higher water content than older infants or children. Careful attention must be given to the fluid requirements of the baby by assessing the electrolytes and the baby's weight. A standard schedule for a preterm baby used to be 60 ml/kg/24 h on the first day, 90 ml/kg on the second day, 120 ml/kg on the third day and 150 ml/kg on the fourth day and subsequently. However, this longstanding schedule is no longer used. This is partly because some of the very smallest infants – those under 25 weeks gestation – have a very high water loss through the skin and require much higher quantities; this water loss may also be increased by phototherapy. Other infants may have impaired renal function and require much less fluid to allow only for basic water loss only of about 20–40/ml/kg/day. The very smallest infants in the first two days need to be reassessed every six to eight hours to make sure the water intake is sufficient.

2 *Glucose.* This is the commonest substance used for energy intake in the preterm, but by itself will not be sufficient to deal with the baby's needs. It is commonly prescribed as 10 mg/kg/min. The solutions available vary from 5% to 50%. The amount prescribed needs to reflect the blood glucose estimations which should be done frequently in any baby needing intravenous feeding. When the blood glucose is above 10 mmol/l, the glucose concentration of the intravenous fluid should be reduced; of course, any hypoglycaemia needs to be corrected. Glucose is an acidic solution and can cause sclerosis in a vein; thus, any solution above 15% must ideally be given into a central vein rather than a peripheral vein.

3 *Amino acids (protein).* In the past, the amino acid solutions were the same as those used for older children and adults. However, special solutions are now available for the newborn baby to mimic the pattern of amino acids seen in cord blood or breast milk (Heird *et al.*, 1987; Puntis *et al.*, 1989). These solutions contain more taurine and cystine than adult solutions and less phenylalanine and methionine. Examples of the contents of a standard solution are shown in Table 7.7. Amino acids are commonly prescribed according to nitrogen content. Normal requirements are 400–480 mg/kg/day, this is equivalent to 2.5–3.0 g of protein/kg/day (Zlotkin *et al.*, 1981). As with most intravenous fluids, one starts with relatively small amount of amino acids and increases rapidly over three days. Neonatal units vary in the amount of monitoring that they do for amino acids. With the modern solutions there is little danger of reaching toxic levels of the most dangerous amino acids, such as phenylalanine. However, some units do weekly amino acid chromatograms on blood to detect any possible toxicity, whilst others use a weekly Guthrie test which would detect high levels of phenylalanine.

Table 7.7 Suggested TPN solutions (all per kg/24 h).

	Glucose (g)	Fat (g)	Amino acid (g protein)	Non-protein energy (kcal)
Day 1	15	0	0.7	56
Day 2	15	0.5	1.4	61
Day 3	15	1	1.4	66
Day 4	15	1.5	2.2	71
Day 5	15	2	2.8	76
Day 6	15	2.5	2.8	81
Day 7	15	3	2.8	86

4 *Fat.* This is given as an emulsion, usually prepared from soya bean. The emulsions are isotonic and therefore do not have some of the problems associated with glucose administration. It is usual not to start lipids on the first day of TPN. It used to be common practice to leave the administration of lipids for several days, but this had the risk of giving insufficient energy to infants. Lipids have 42 kJ/g (10 kcal/g) compared to 14.7 kJ/g (3.5 kcal/g) for glucose; they therefore provide more energy than other substances. It has now become common to start lipids on the second day of intravenous feeding. At one time lipids were given intermittently, but now they are infused continuously over 24 hours (Kao *et al.*, 1981). The maximum fat dose is 0.15 g/kg/h which is equivalent to 0.7 ml/kg/h of Intralipid 20%. The aim is to provide up to 3.5 g of fat/kg/24 h. We start at 1.0 g/kg/ 24 h, and build up over four days. The fat emulsion is given in a separate syringe and the infusion line is connected to the other infusion fluids very near the hub of the intravenous cannula. Interesting developments are being made with a view to providing all intravenous nutrition in one fluid. Such *all-in-one* fluids may prove to be extremely valuable and are being studied. Like other solutions in intravenous feeding, the frequency of monitoring has not yet been completely established; most units monitor triglyceride levels on a weekly basis. The target is not to exceed a triglyceride concentration of 150 mg/l. Other methods have been used, such as looking for turbidity of fat in plasma. The problem is that a baby receiving intravenous lipids has rather turbid plasma because of the fat emulsion and the old practice of stopping the infusion to see whether the lipidaemia disappeared deprived the baby of energy over several hours. We suspect that weekly triglyceride levels will become the standard method of monitoring. Intravenous fat needs to be reduced in some circumstances. There is evidence that, during sepsis, lipids cannot be metabolized adequately and therefore the rate of administration should be reduced. There is similar evidence that, during hyperglycaemia, fat is not tolerated and again its administration should be reduced. The fat infusion should not be stopped completely or the baby will be deprived of essential fatty acids – linolenic and linoleic acids (Table 7.8).

5 *Vitamins.* It is essential to give complete supplementation of vitamins for babies, particularly if they are to be on intravenous feeding for any length of time. We use Solivito-N and Vitlipid-N Infant (both of these are made by Pharmacia) (Table 7.9). Solivito is a yellow mixture of water-soluble vitamins (thiamine, riboflavine, pyridoxine, cyanocobalamin, nicotinamide, folic acid, biotin, pan-

Table 7.8 Constituents of Intralipid (20%).

Fractionated soybean oil		100 g
Fractionated egg phospholipids		6 g
Glycerol		11 g
Water for injection	to	500 ml

tothenic acid and ascorbic acid) and is added to the glucose solution. Vitlipid is a white, sterile emulsion containing the fat-soluble vitamins A, D_2 (calciferol), E and K_1 (phytomenadione); this is added to the fat emulsion.

6 *Electrolyte solutions.* Electrolytes must include sodium, potassium, magnesium, calcium and phosphorus (Table 7.10). Very preterm babies are usually hypocalcaemic in the first 48 hours of life and many of them are hypoproteinaemic and thus many of them have a limited calcium-carrying capacity. The sodium content of the fluid needs to be adjusted according to the plasma sodium concentration which is monitored at least daily, but three to four times a day in the first two days of life or when the baby is ill. The normal range of sodium is regarded as 135–145 mmol/l. It is usual to take action to provide more sodium when it falls below 130 mmol/l, and to provide

Table 7.9 Constituents of Solivito-N and Vitlipid-N Infant.

	Solivito-N added at 1.0 ml/kg	Vitlipid-N Infant added at 1.0 ml/kg
Thiamine (B_1)	0.31 mg	
Riboflavine (B_2)	0.49 mg	
Nicotinamide	4.00 mg	
Pyridoxine (B_6)	0.49 mg	
Pantothenic acid	1.50 mg	
Biotin	6 mcg	
Folic acid	40 mcg	
Cyanocobalamin (B_{12})	0.50 mcg	
Ascorbic acid (C)	10 mg	
Retinol (A)		230 iu
Ergocalciferol (D_2)		40 iu
Phytomenadione (K_1)		20 mcg
α-tocopherol (E)		0.7 iu

Table 7.10 Suggested electrolytes (added from day 1).

Electrolyte	Basal level	Nomal range
Calcium	1	0–4 mmol/kg/24 h
Sodium	4	0–15 mmol/kg 24 h
Potassium	2	0–6 mmol/kg/24 h
Phosphate	1	0–3 mmol/kg/24 h
Magnesium	0.3	0–1 mmol/kg/24 h
Zinc	0.6	0–1.0µmol/kg/24 h*

*Suggested zinc level increased to 1.0 µmol/kg/24 h on day 42 of TPN.

sufficient fluid and less sodium if the value rises above 145 mmol/l. It is essential to avoid hypernatraemia – over 150 mmol/l – as this could cause serious derangement of the brain.

Phosphorus and calcium have to be given very carefully as they can precipitate in the infusion fluid; on the other hand, their administration is essential for bone growth and development. The calcium to phosphate ratio in intravenous fluid ideally should be 1.3:1 in mmols (the ratio in grams is 1.7:1). It is usual to take action when the plasma calcium falls to 1.5 mmol/l and phosphorus when it falls below 1.2 mmol/l. Glycerophosphate solutions are being developed which will overcome the problems of precipitation with calcium.

7 *Trace elements.* Some of these are provided in other ways; for instance, most ill newborn babies need repeated small blood transfusions which will provide sufficient iron for their needs. Trace elements are now most conveniently given as a solution, such as Ped-El (Table 7.11); this will cover the daily losses of electrolyte and trace elements. This solution was developed for adults and contains excessive amounts of manganese and too little zinc for infants. A further solution is being developed and Ped-El will be replaced by Pedi-Trace. Selenium is not contained in Ped-El and some units provide this in a separate solution, but selenium will be contained in the Pedi-Trace. We start trace element administration as soon as intravenous feeding is begun.

Parenteral nutrition

Methods of administration.   Parenteral nutrition may be given:

1 Into a peripheral vein using a short cannula. Intravenous feeding can be continued in this way for several weeks, though the cannula

Table 7.11 Constituents of Ped-El (per ml).

Calcium	0.15 mmol
Sodium	0.075 mmol
Phosphorus	0.075 mmol
Magnesium	0.025 mmol
Iron	0.5 μmol
Zinc	0.15 μmol
Manganese	0.25 μmol
Copper	0.075 μmol
Fluoride	0.75 μmol
Iodide	0.01 μmol
Chloride	0.35 mmol
Potassium	0.05 μmol

will need resiting fairly frequently. It is usual to say that the infusion should be resited every 48 hours, but in practice it is usual to wait until the drip tissues (the fluid leaks subcutaneously). The greatest care should be taken to stop the infusion promptly if the cannula becomes displaced from a vein as a hypertonic solution can cause severe tissue necrosis. The infusion should be resited fairly soon after it tissues to prevent hypoglycaemia.

2 Into a central vein. This method of infusion has the advantage that the cannula does not need frequent resiting so there is less handling. The major disadvantage is serious infection, sometimes with a fungus such as *Candida albicans*, or bacteria resistant to the common antibiotics. The commonest organism now, by far, is *Staphylococcus epidermidis* (also known as coagulase-negative staphylococcus). It has been shown that infection with these organisms can be reduced by meticulous attention to aseptic technique when inserting or handling catheters, and when changing the intravenous infusion. It is important that umbilical vessels should not be used because of the risk of portal vein or aortic thrombosis, necrotizing enterocolitis, and septicaemia.

The following technique can be used for placing a catheter in a large vein or right atrium:

1 The baby should be assessed and adequate analgesia given.
2 Scrub up and wear mask, gown and gloves.
3 Open pack and assemble equipment: cut-down pack, 19 FG butterfly needle, 25 FG butterfly needle, syringe and needle, heparinized

saline, chlorhexidine in spirit, pointed scalpel blade, adhesive tape, splint and dressing, silastic catheter and sterile tape measure.

4 Measure the silastic catheter with sterile tape measure and note length.

5 Connect silastic catheter to 25 FG needle and run through heparinised saline (0.5 iu/ml). Thread the plastic needle cover back over the needle to protect it from cutting through the catheter.

6 Suitable veins in order of preference are antecubital, saphenous, scalp, external jugular.

7 Having chosen a vein in advance and prepared the skin, an assistant must apply a suitable tourniquet to fill the vein and hold the baby still.

8 Clean the skin carefully with chlorhexidine in spirit and allow to dry. Measure the distance from the chosen vein to the right atrium.

9 Cut the tubing off the butterfly needle. Pass the needle under the skin to enter the vein, taking care not to transfix the vein.

10 Blood will flow freely back out of the needle. Stem the flow by pressing with a finger on the skin over the tip of the needle. Thread the silastic catheter through the needle and into the vein; blood should flow back into the catheter if the end is open.

11 Thread the catheter into the vein until sufficient has been passed to reach the right atrium (the length remaining can be measured with the sterile tape measure).

12 Fix the catheter to the skin with tape leaving the entry point open. Apply a sterile dressing and splint as required.

13 Do not use the line for feeding until the position has been confirmed radiographically. This is done by injecting 0.7 ml of Conray 280 through the 25 FG butterfly needle and silastic tube. Take a radiograph of the limb and chest just as the injection finishes.

14 If necessary withdraw the catheter until the position is correct. It is not usually possible at this stage to push the catheter in further, so it is important to be generous in the initial measurements; however, do not be too generous or you may knot the catheter in the right atrium.

Precautions and monitoring. A baby who is being fed intravenously must be carefully observed clinically for signs of complications (see below). The baby should be weighed daily to assess fluid balance, and have head circumference and length measured weekly to assess growth. Fluid intake and output must also be recorded scrupulously.

Intravenous drugs should not be infused into the central line. Penicillin, fusidic acid, adrenaline, papaverine and many other drugs are of low pH and may be unstable in infusions.

Urine is tested eight-hourly for sugar, and more frequently in tiny infants, as blood sugar may rise very rapidly. Blood sugar should be estimated (using test-strips) at least daily and if there is glycosuria. Electrolytes, calcium and acid–base status are estimated daily. Phosphorus, magnesium, amino acids, albumin, total protein, bilirubin and transaminases are measured weekly. Chromatography of urinary amino acids may also be helpful for the detection of hyperaminoacidaemia, including tyrosinaemia which may respond to high doses of vitamin C. A Guthrie test may be a useful way of detecting hyperphenylanalaemia, which may occur during the use of TPN.

A full blood count, including packed cell volume, should be performed twice a week.

The complete intravenous infusion set tubing is changed every 24 hours using an aseptic technique.

Intralipid fat infusion can be stopped every day at 5 a.m., so that one may be certain that the fat is being cleared from the blood. A blood sample is taken at 8 a.m. and spun in a centrifuge; the plasma is examined for a milky appearance (see p. 156).

Bacteriological monitoring demands appropriate cultures from the intravenous site, blood and catheter if it appears infected. Blood culture should be done if there is any clinical deterioration, and urine sent for *Candida* culture. All babies on antibiotics are given oral nystatin in addition.

Complications.

1 *Septicaemia* is usually caused by *Staphylococcus epidermis*, *Candida albicans*, staphylococci, *Pseudomonas aeruginosa*, *E. coli* or diphtheroids. It may follow contamination during insertion of the intravenous line but is more likely to occur if catheters are left in place for prolonged periods.

2 *Hypoglycaemia* can follow abrupt termination of intravenous feeding, possibly due to high levels of endogenous insulin. Therefore, reduce the intravenous input gradually whilst simultaneously increasing oral feeds. Do frequent blood glucose estimations during the transition.

3 *Hyperglycaemia* can cause osmolar diuresis and dehydration.

4 *Heart failure* may occur, since acid solutions contain relatively high sodium concentrations, as do several antibiotics such as ampicillin and cloxacillin.

5 *Hypophosphataemia* may occur even if phosphate is being given in

theoretically adequate amounts. This problem is associated with osteopaenia and rickets.

6 *Trace metal deficiencies* such as zinc.

7 *Mechanical complications* from catheter malpositioning or dislocation may include thromboembolism, thrombophlebitis, intracardiac curling or knotting of the catheter, arteriovenous fistula, pneumothorax, haemothorax or hydrothorax.

References and Further Reading

Ball, P., Booth, I.W. & Puntis, J.W.L. (1990) *Paediatric Parenteral Nutrition.* KabiVitrum Ltd.

Balmer, S.E. & Wharton, B.A. (1992) Human milk banking at Sorrento Maternity Hospital, Birmingham. *Arch. Dis. Child.,* 67, 556–559.

Cesar, G.V., Tomasi, E., Olinto, M.T.A. *et al.* (1993) Use of pacifiers and breastfeeding duration. *Lancet,* 341, 404–406.

Cochran, E.B., Phelps, S.J. & Helms, R.A. (1988) Parenteral nutrition in pediatric patients. *Clin. Pharm.,* 7, 351–366.

Cunningham *et al.* (1992) *Breastfeeding, Growth and Illness.* New York: UNICEF.

Department of Health and Social Security (1988) *HIV Infection, Breastfeeding and Human Milk Banking.* London: HMSO.

Eglin, R.P. & Wilkinson, A.R. (1987) HIV infection and pasteurisation of breast milk. *Lancet, i,* 1093.

Ehrenkranz, R.A. & Ackerman, B.A. (1986) Metoclopromide effect on faltering milk production by mothers of premature infants. *Pediatrics,* 78(4), 614–620.

Haggkvist, A.P. (1990) *What Factors Influence the Breast Feeding Prevalence of Mothers to Premature Babies?* Proceedings of the International Conference of Maternity Nurse Researchers. Goteborg, Sweden.

Heird, W.C., Dell, R.B., Helms, R.A. *et al.* (1987) Amino acid mixture designed to maintain normal plasma amino acid patterns in infants and children requiring parenteral nutrition. *Pediatrics,* 80(3), 401–408.

Hopkinson, J.M., Schanler, R.J. & Garza, C. (1988) Milk production by mothers of premature infants. *Pediatrics,* 81, 815–819.

Howie, P.W., Stewart Forsyth, J., Ogston, S.A. *et al.* (1990) Protective effect of breastfeeding against infection. *BMJ,* 300, 11–15.

Kao, L., Cheng, M.H. & Warburton, D. (1981) Triglycerides, free fatty acids/albumin molar ratio, and cholesterol levels in serum of neonates receiving long-term lipid infusions: controlled trial of continuous and intermittent regimens. *J. Pediatr.,* 104, 429–435.

Lucas, A. & Cole, T.J. (1990) Breast milk and neonatal necrotising enterocolitis. *Lancet,* 336, 1519–1523.

Lucas, A., Morley, R., Cole, T.J. *et al.* (1989) Early diet in preterm babies and developmental status in infancy. *Arch. Dis. Child*, *64*, 1570–1578.

Lucas, A., Brooke, O.G., Morley, R. *et al.* (1990) Early diet of preterm infants and development of allergic and atopic disease: randomised prospective study. *BMJ*, *300*, 837–840.

Mathur, G.P., Mathur, S. & Khanduja, G.S. (1990) Non-nutritive suckling and use of pacifiers. *Indian Pediatr.*, *27*, 1187–1189.

Mitchell *et al.* (1991) *N.Z. Med. J.*, *104*, 71–76.

OPCS (1990) *Infant Feeding Practices*. London: HMSO.

Puntis, J.W.L. *et al.* (1989) Egg and breast milk based nitrogen sources compared. *Arch. Dis. Child.*, *64*, 1472–1477.

Royal College of Midwives (1991) *Successful Breastfeeding*. London: Churchill Livingstone.

Thiry, L., Sprecher-Goldberg, S., Jonckneer, T. *et al.* (1985) Isolation of AIDS virus from cell free breast milk of three healthy virus carriers. *Lancet*, *ii*, 891–892.

Van de Perre, P., Simonon, A., Msellati, P. *et al.* (1991) Postnatal transmission of human immunodeficiency virus type 1 from mother to infant. *New Engl. J. Med.*, *325*, 593–598.

Warner, J.T., Lintou, H.R. & Cartlidge, P.H.T. (1993) Human milk fortification in preterm infants. Abstract (available from Milupa, Milupa House, Uxbridge Road, Hillingdon, Uxbridge, Middlesex UB10 0NE).

WHO/UNICEF (1989) *Protecting, Promoting and Supporting Breastfeeding – A Global Initiative*. WHO; London: HMSO.

Williams, A.F., Fisher, C., Greasley, V. *et al.* (1985) Human Milk Banking. *J. Trop. Pediatr.*, *31*, 185–190.

Yu, V.Y.H. & MacMahon, R.A. (eds) (1992) *Intravenous Feeding of the Neonate*. London: Edward Arnold.

Zlotkin, S.H., Bryan, M.H. & Anderson, G.H. (1981) Triglycerides, free fatty acids/albumin molar ratio, and cholesterol levels in serum of neonates receiving long-term lipid infusions: controlled trial of continuous and intermittent regimens. *J. Pediatr.*, *104*, 429–435.

8

Respiratory Problems

Breathing difficulties are the most common problems of newborn babies. For example, respiratory distress syndrome (RDS), due to lack of surfactant in the lungs, is common in babies born early, but it can be confused with a large number of other problems in the first few days of life. It is often very difficult to make a clear diagnosis even after examining the baby and having seen the chest radiograph. It is also difficult to exclude infection and this means that many babies have to be treated with antibiotics initially until the results of cultures are known.

A clue to diagnosis is the time of onset of the respiratory problem. *RDS* and *transient tachypnoea of the newborn* begin during the first four hours of life. *Pneumonia* can occur at any time during the newborn period. *Pneumothorax* often causes a sudden deterioration in a baby who has had a respiratory problem. *Bronchopulmonary dysplasia* or *chronic lung disease*, appears insidiously after the first week or two and is often a complication in a baby who has required ventilation at high pressures for respiratory problems such as RDS or recurrent apnoeic attacks. *Apnoeic attacks* can occur as part of any respiratory problem, but are particularly common in babies born at less than 32 weeks gestation and who may be otherwise completely well, or in those with a periventricular haemorrhage. *Meconium aspiration* is an important cause of respiratory distress in small-for-gestational-age (SFGA) babies or where there has been intrapartum asphyxia. One of the most difficult problems may be the differential diagnosis of cyanosis, which may be due to any of a number of respiratory problems or to some forms of congenital heart disease (see Table 11.2, p. 271).

Hyaline Membrane Disease (HMD)

Hyaline membrane disease is common in preterm babies, but it is a diagnosis made at post-mortem. The clinical syndrome is called RDS. It is rare after 37 weeks gestation. It is still the largest single cause of death in babies born alive without major congenital defects.

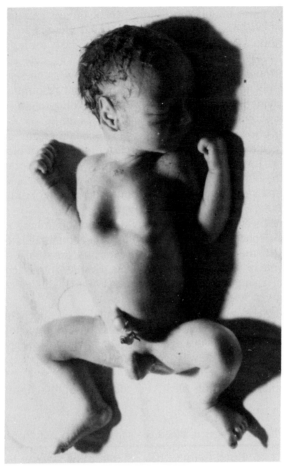

Fig. 8.1 A baby with respiratory distress syndrome (RDS). Note marked
sternal recession.

Clinical features

Affected babies may not show any respiratory problems at birth but,
asphyxia during birth or a delayed onset of breathing makes the
condition more severe. Gradually, over the next few hours, the
baby becomes increasingly tachypnoeic with increased respiratory
effort and expiratory grunting. Conventionally, the diagnosis is

restricted to those infants who show two of three signs (tachypnoea greater than 60/min, expiratory grunting and chest wall recession) within four hours of birth, and when the illness lasts for more than 24 hours (Fig. 8.1).

The small and very sick babies may not show all these signs and may be deeply cyanosed with gasping or absent respirations. Since many babies are put straight on to a ventilator following resuscitation they do not show the classical earliest signs.

Over the following few hours, the baby needs a greater concentration of oxygen to prevent cyanosis. An arterial sample of blood shows hypoxaemia (low Pa_{O_2}). On listening to the chest there are diminished breath sounds, and there are also usually oedema and oliguria. The problems are greatest at 48–72 hours of age after which gradual recovery starts.

The cyanosis is caused by shunting of blood in the lung itself, past collapsed air spaces, with the result that reduced amounts of oxygen are carried in the blood. A shunt also occurs through a re-opened foramen ovale or patent ductus arteriosus. Besides hypoxaemia, other biochemical changes include acidaemia (low pH), high P_{CO_2} (Table 8.1), hypoglycaemia and hypocalcaemia.

A typical chest radiograph shows a ground-glass appearance of the lungs with an ill-defined heart border and an air bronchogram (air visible in the larger airways against the shadowing of collapsed small airways). In the most severe cases the lung fields appear virtually opaque (Figs. 8.2 and 8.6).

The diagnosis is often clear, but differential diagnoses include

Table 8.1 Plasma changes in blood gas and acid–base disturbances.

	Partial pressure of CO_2 (Pa_{CO_2})	Blood pH	Plasma bicarbonate (HCO_3)
Respiratory acidosis (impaired CO_2 excretion)	↑	↓	Normal or ↑
Respiratory alkalosis (excessive CO_2 excretion)	↓	↑	↓
Metabolic acidosis (acid retention or alkali loss)	Normal or ↓	↓	↓
Metabolic alkalosis (alkali retention or acid loss)	Normal	↑	↑

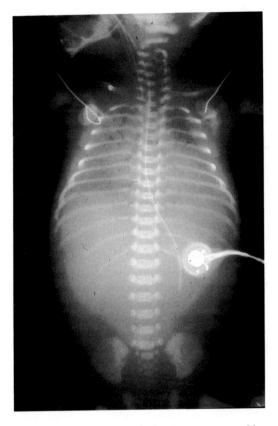

Fig. 8.2 Chest X-ray showing 'ground-glass' appearance of lungs in hyaline membrane disease.

meconium aspiration, pneumonia, pneumothorax, pulmonary haemorrhage, cyanotic congenital heart disease, oesophageal atresia and diaphragmatic hernia. The immotile cilia (Kartagener) syndrome may cause prolonged tachypnoea in the newborn. Dextrocardia is the clue to this diagnosis in a proportion of cases.

A post-mortem examination shows that the infant's lungs have collapsed and contain no air. The 'hyaline membrane' consists of fibrin with entrapped red cells, protein and necrotic alveolar epithelium.

Surfactant

The anatomy of the normal lung provides a large surface area for gaseous exchange so that breathing air provides effective oxygenation of blood. The lungs of the fetus are filled with fluid; at birth, the first breath fills the lungs with air and the production of lung liquid ceases.

Surface tension in the fluid-filled lungs would be very high if surfactant were not present to allow the lungs to expand with air. It is secreted by the lung from about 22 weeks gestation, and increases in quantity thereafter with surges at about 33–35 weeks and also at birth. Thus preterm infants are at risk because they have less surfactant present in their lungs.

Susceptibility depends on lung maturation. Babies who are especially at risk include those born before 37 weeks gestation, boys, second twins and babies of diabetic mothers. After birth, the high surface tension causes alveoli to collapse at the end of expiration; this is the basis of RDS. Recovery is associated with increased surfactant production.

Surfactant is a collection of fatty substances, which include large amounts of surface-active lecithins. Trials have shown that surfactant introduced into the trachea for treatment of RDS definitely improves survival (Hallman *et al.*, 1985; Gitlin *et al.*, 1987). The treatment is thought to shorten the length of the illness, improve oxygenation, and reduce the risks of bronchopulmonary dysplasia, pneumothoraces and subsequent periventricular haemorrhages. Some trials using bovine surfactant have suggested that patent ductus arteriosus (PDA) is more common (Raju *et al.*, 1987). Also, there are problems with hypoxaemia when a relatively large volume of fluid containing the surfactant is introduced into the trachea.

Three types of natural surfactant have been assessed in trials. Human surfactant can be obtained from amniotic fluid, but is expensive to produce. Two types of animal surfactant have been widely used, obtained either from cattle (bovine) (Shapiro *et al.*, 1986; Raju *et al.*, 1987), or pigs (porcine) (Robertson, 1983). Since some people may not like the use of animal products, it is important to always discuss their origin with parents. Artificial surfactant has also been used in trials (Ten Centre Study Group, 1987; Morley *et al.*, 1988), and is now licensed for use. Surfactant is still expensive but it is hoped that it will become much cheaper in the future, particularly artificial surfactant.

It has been common to use surfactant in hypoxaemic babies. This is assessed by comparing the oxygen tension in the alveoli and in arterial blood (a:A). The a:A ratio is usually less than 0.22 before surfactant is given. The formula for calculation of a/A ratio is

$$\text{a/A ratio} = \frac{P\text{ao}_2}{713 \times \dfrac{\text{Fi0}_2}{100} - P\text{co}_2}$$

Note: 1 kPa = 7.5 mmHg. Figure 8.3 shows a graph for calculating the a:A ratio:

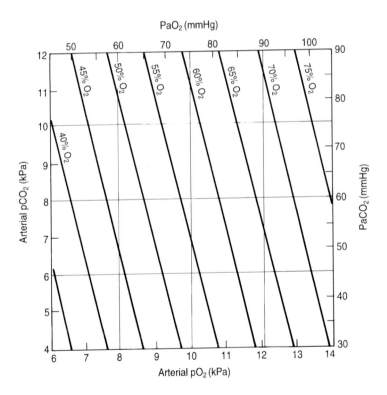

Fig. 8.3 Graph for calculating the a:A ratio

1 Plot P_{CO_2} and arterial (or trancutaneous) P_{O_2} on the graph.
2 Note the inspired oxygen concentration. If the plotted value lies to the left of the diagonal inspired oxygen line, the a/A ratio is less than 0.22.
3 If unsure, check by using the formula above.

Some events affect the rate of surfactant production in the fetus. Sudden intrapartum asphyxia resulting from antepartum haemorrhage or maternal hypotension impairs the production of surfactant. Some chronic problems seem to increase lung surfactant: for example, ruptured membranes for more than 24 hours, placental infarction and pre-eclampsia or hypertension with intrauterine growth retardaton. This may be because stress to the fetus causes glucocorticoids to be released from the adrenal glands, and these steroids stimulate surfactant release. This now has clinical application; several trials indicate that treatment of a mother in premature labour with betamethasone (a steroid) decreases the incidence of RDS and its mortality (Collaborative Groups, 1981).

In utero, lung fluid containing surfactant flows up the trachea, out of the mouth and into the amniotic fluid. It is possible to measure the concentration of surfactant in amniotic fluid. Amniocentesis thus provides a clinical measure of fetal lung maturity before birth. This is expressed as the ratio of surface-active agents to sphingomyelin (a substance in lung secretions that remains relatively constant in concentration in the third trimester of pregnancy). This is known as the lecithin: sphingomyelin (L:S) ratio. A ratio greater than 2 indicates a low risk of RDS; under 2% of babies develop RDS with a ratio above 2. Over 75% develop RDS when the ratio is below 1:5; therefore a ratio of less than 1.5 indicates a high risk (Table 8.2). The obstetrician may therefore with more accuracy weigh the risk of a baby developing RDS after early delivery against the dangers of non-delivery. This is particularly useful in such situations as intrauterine growth retardation and rhesus disease.

Very often spontaneous premature delivery cannot be prevented. Sometimes a cervical suture, intravenous salbutamol, or ritodrine, which inhibit uterine contractions, may delay birth to allow steroids to be given or the baby to become more mature.

Management

After birth, prompt resuscitation with early endotracheal intubation reduces anoxia, acidaemia and therefore the incidence and severity of

Table 8.2 The L/S ratio and the risk of RDS.

L/S ratio	Incidence of RDS (%)	Mortality from RDS (%)
> 2.5	0.9 (0.7 diabetes)	nil
> 2.0	2.2	0.1
1.5–2.0	40	4
< 1.5	75	14

RDS (Robson & Hey, 1982; Drew, 1982). Hypoxia immediately after birth must be avoided since it will reduce surfactant production. Every baby of 30 weeks gestation or less, and any baby of less than 35 weeks gestation who has respiratory difficulty, should be intubated.

Surfactant has also been proposed as a prophylaxis for RDS (Halliday *et al.*, 1984), and could be given into the trachea immediately after birth. When used in this way the incidence of RDS and its severity are reduced. At the moment it cannot be recommended for all preterm babies owing to the cost.

Supportive measures

General supportive measures should include the following:

1 *Adequate warmth.* In practice abdominal skin temperature should be maintained between 36.5°C and 37.0°C.
2 *Feeding.* Feeds given by mouth may well be aspirated into the lungs with lethal consequences. It is therefore usual initially to avoid gastric feeds. Adequate calories and fluid should be given through a peripheral vein or a nasojejunal tube. A prolonged illness must be managed with total intravenous nutrition or jejunal feeding (see Chapter 7).
3 *Minimal disturbance or handling.* Feeding and crying have been shown to cause a fall in arterial Po_2, as does any handling. Manoeuvres such as over-vigorous suction, frequent cleaning, nappy changing or repositioning should be avoided. Temperature, heart and respiratory rates, inspired oxygen concentration, arterial Po_2 and blood pressure should be monitored continuously without disturbance. Routine procedures should be re-assessed frequently to ensure they are not being done unnecessarily, causing disturbance to the baby (Danford *et al.*, 1983).
4 *Infection.* Scrupulous attention to procedures to prevent infection,

such as handwashing, must be followed by all medical and nursing staff, and taught to parents. Tracheal toilet needs to be performed with gloved hands. It is not possible to be sure that a baby with severe respiratory problems does not have pneumonia, and therefore antibiotics are almost always given. Some organisms, for example group B β-haemolytic streptococcus, can cause a severe illness in the neonatal period, with a high mortality. A cephalosporin, such as cefotaxime, with ampicillin to cover listeria infection, are probably the commonest antibiotics used in the newborn today. An alternative combination is ampicillin (or penicillin) and an aminoglycoside, such as gentamicin or netilmicin (see also Chapter 16).

5 *Parental visiting*. It is important for nurses and doctors to explain to parents what the extensive and frightening equipment is, what it does and why it is being used.

Oxygen therapy

The temperature, humidity, flow rate and concentration of inspired oxygen must be adequately controlled and monitored. Oxygen concentrations above 30% cannot be effectively maintained in an incubator without the use of a headbox because the oxygen concentration drops when the doors are opened. It is convenient to use piped air and oxygen. The flow rate should be between 3 and 7 l/min, sufficient to prevent CO_2 accumulation in the headbox. Headbox oxygen should be used in conjunction with a humidifier.

The inspired oxygen concentration is adjusted to maintain the Pa_{O_2} in the normal range. Satisfactory levels of a baby's arterial blood gases are: pH 7.3–7.4; oxygen (Pa_{O_2}) 7–10 kPa (50–75 mmHg); carbon dioxide (Pa_{CO_2}) 4.5–6 kPa (35–45 mmHg). They are best checked by continuous monitoring, using umbilical arterial catheters with oxygen electrodes at their tips, or transcutaneously. When the infant is shocked, intra-arterial monitoring is more satisfactory than transcutaneous monitoring. Less ideally, intermittent samples can be taken four-hourly (but more frequently when the infant's condition is changing rapidly or adjustments are made to therapy) from indwelling umbilical catheters or a radial artery. A small cannula can be placed in the radial artery by percutaneous insertion to monitor oxygen levels. Capillary blood gas analysis is not satisfactory particularly for P_{O_2} estimation. If a good flow is obtained it can give a reasonable estimation of pH and P_{CO_2}.

An umbilical arterial catheter is inserted with full aseptic precautions so that the lip lies approximately at the level of the fourth lumbar vertebra. It should be tied in position and taped to the abdominal wall away from the perineum to minimize risks of contamination. The position must be checked by radiography. There is a characteristic downward loop on the X-ray as the catheter passes down into the pelvis via the umbilical artery into the common iliac artery. A catheter in the umbilical vein passes directly upwards.

As many as 10% may have a complication from an arterial catheter. Nurses should look particularly for disconnected tubing, through which the baby may bleed to death. A blue foot is an initial and commonly noticed sign of obstructed blood flow with insertion of umbilical artery catheters. The foot must be observed closely, and if there is no improvement within 15 minutes, the catheter will need to be removed or gangrene may ensue. White leg is associated with arterial spasm at the time of insertion or with a catheter which has passed down into the femoral artery so obstructing blood flow to the leg. Other complications include infection and thrombosis. To reduce these risks catheters are best removed as soon as possible.

Transcutaneous monitoring is now in widespread use for oxygen but has not proved so valuable for CO_2. Readings must be checked regularly by measurement from arterial samples. *Transcutaneous oxygen monitoring (TCPO$_2$)* is accurate because local heating is applied which causes vasodilatation and thus, particularly during the recovery phase of RDS, a close approximation to true arterial Po_2 is obtained. Monitors which measure continuously the saturation of oxygen in blood (Sao_2) are now widely available. It is usual to aim at a saturation between 92 and 95% to avoid hypoxaemia or hyperaemia. Saturations above 95% may be associated with Pao_2 levels which are very high indeed (Southall *et al.*, 1987). It is important to recognise that Pao_2 and Sao_2 give different information, and should both be obtained if possible.

The danger of uncontrolled oxygen therapy with prolonged high arterial Po_2 levels is that retinopathy of prematurity (ROP) (see Plate III) will develop. In affected babies there is initial vasoconstriction of retinal arterioles which, after some hours of exposure, becomes irreversible. On returning to normal oxygen tensions, the vessels proliferate intensely with new capillary formation which may result in retinal detachment and blindness (Committee for the classification of ROP, 1984).

It is important to realise that it is not high inspired oxygen concentrations in themselves that are dangerous; it is inappropriately high concentrations leading to high Pao_2 levels which cause the damage. Thus oxygen therapy must be closely controlled to prevent this serious complication on the one hand and death or brain damage from hypoxaemia on the other. ROP has become more common once again with the survival of very small babies. It is possible that there may be factors other than oxygen in its aetiology (Prendeville & Schulenberg, 1988).

All preterm babies born at less than 32 weeks gestation should have their eyes examined regularly by an ophthalmologist, until they reach 39 weeks gestation. When ROP is discovered, it is possible to improve the prognosis by cryotherapy (Cryotherapy for ROP Cooperative Group, 1988).

Continuous inflating pressure

Many babies with RDS will require further respiratory support to prevent hypoxaemia, apnoeic attacks or rising P_{CO_2} levels. The expiratory grunt of a baby with RDS is an attempt to prevent alveolar collapse, by breathing out against a partially closed glottis (vocal cords). This keeps the alveoli expanded for as long as possible during expiration. The asthmatic or chronic bronchitic patient who purses lips and puffs out cheeks during expiration is doing the same thing.

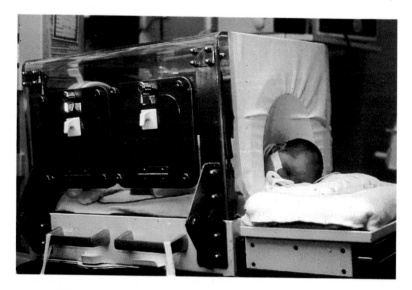

Fig. 8.4 Continuous negative extra thoracic pressure box.

This effect may be obtained artificially by applying a continuous inflating pressure against which the baby breathes spontaneously. Many techniques have been used for applying a continuous inflating pressure, either with continuous positive airways pressure (CPAP) by headbox with neck seal, intranasal catheters, face mask or by applying continuous negative extrathoracic pressure (CNEP) with subatmospheric pressure around the chest by means of a negative pressure body box (Fig. 8.4).

All studies confirm a significant increase in Po_2 with CPAP or

Table 8.3 Methods of applying continuous inflating pressure.

Method	Advantages	Disadvantages
Continuous positive airway pressure (CPAP)		
Face mask	Easy to apply	Leaks may occur if mask does not fit well. Stomach may be distended. Looks frightening to parents. Now rarely used
Nasal catheters	Easy to apply, free access to baby's mouth	Ulceration of nasal passages if catheters used for a long time. Air may escape from the mouth. Stomach may be distended
Endotracheal tube	Artificial ventilation can be used quickly if needed	Complications of endotracheal tubes, trauma and lung infection
Head box		Tight seal around neck may traumatise skin and obstruct venous return from the head, leading to cerebral haemorrhage and hydrocephalus. Now rarely used
		Poor access to baby's head. High noise level in box. Stomach may be distended
Continuous negative extrathoracic pressure (CNEP)		
Body box	Easy access to baby's head	Tight seal around neck may traumatise skin and obstruct venous return from head. Air leak may cool the baby. Poor access to baby's body. Babies in the box for prolonged periods may suffer from lack of stimulation, and lie continuously in one position.
		Box looks frightening to parents

CNEP in spontaneously breathing infants. CNEP may also improve ventilation since it allows lower inspiratory pressures to be used. CPAP is still commonly employed in weaning babies off the ventilator. Some argue that CPAP should be used early in RDS to limit surfactant reduction, therefore reducing the length and severity of the illness. It may be possible to reduce the risk of bronchopulmonary dysplasia in this way, and in most units mechanical ventilation is used from the start.

Complications may occur (Table 8.3). Pneumothorax is more common than in babies breathing spontaneously, but less common than in those mechanically ventilated. Some indications for CPAP include:

1 Recurrent apnoeic attacks.
2 Pao_2 less than 6 kPa (45 mmHg) when the baby is breathing 40% oxygen.
3 To assist in weaning babies from the ventilator.

Pneumothorax and CO_2 retention are commoner above 5 cm of water and much commoner above 10 cm, and such pressures are no longer used.

Apart from its use with an endotracheal tube, it is important when using CPAP to have an open naso/orogastric tube in place. This prevents gastric rupture if gas should be blown into the stomach and reduces the likelihood of aspiration of stomach contents in to the lungs.

Mechanical ventilation

Babies with severe RDS often need mechanical ventilation to prevent hypoxaemia. Indications are:

1 Prolonged apnoea with bradycardia unresponsive to stimulation.
2 Frequent or recurrent apnoeic attacks unresponsive to theophylline or CPAP.
3 Pao_2 less than 8 kPa (60 mmHg) in 80% oxygen with or without CPAP, indicating severe respiratory failure.
4 $Paco_2$ greater than 9 kPa (70 mmHg).

The ventilator must be carefully adjusted so that the baby's blood gases are normal at the least possible pressure. Ventilators suitable for newborn babies allow independent adjustment of respiratory rate, inspiratory and expiratory times, inspiratory–expiratory ratio (I:E), peak inspiratory pressure (PIP) and positive end expiratory pressure (PEEP). CPAP should be available at the turn of a switch.

Several strategies are needed to deal with hypoxaemia and hypercapnia. Hypoxaemia is initially treated by increasing the oxygen concentration (FiO_2; a value of 1 is equivalent to 100% oxygen). If this is insufficient to correct the hypoxaemia, it is necessary to increase the mean airway pressure (MAP), which can be done in a number of ways. The simplest is to increase the PIP. Other methods, increasing the inspiratory time to allow inspiration to have more of the respiratory cycle, or increasing PEEP, are much less used.

It was common at one time to use an inspiratory time of one second, or even longer, with an I:E ratio of 1:1 or more. It is now usual to keep the inspiratory time to less than 0.5 seconds, and times of 0.3 seconds and 0.4 seconds are common.

Hypercapnia can be treated by increasing the rate, but may also require an increase in the PIP. Overventilation with a low Pco_2 may be treated by decreasing the rate, or decreasing the PIP. The least PIP necessary to produce good chest movement and breath sounds should be used. High pressures damage the lungs and pressures above 30 cm of water are seldom necessary.

It is becoming commoner to use a higher frequency of ventilation with rates over 60/min (Greenough & Milner, 1987; Greenough et al., 1987). In this situation an I:E ratio of 1:1.5 or 1:2 is required. Higher pressures can be used since they are only applied for a small proportion of the ventilatory cycle.

Such ventilation is thought to reduce the incidence of pneumothorax and bronchopulmonary dysplasia (BPD). It is thought that BPD (see below) is largely due to ventilation at high pressures, for a large proportion of the ventilatory cycle. The most satisfactory machines are the constant flow, pressure-limited, time-cycled ventilators developed especially for the newborn. Reasonable initial ventilator settings are summarised in Table 8.4. A recent develop-

Table 8.4 Suggested initial ventilator settings.

Rate	60 per min
Inspiratory time	0.4 s
Peak pressure	15–20 cmH$_2$O
PEEP	3 cmH$_2$O

The initial oxygen concentration should be that which the baby is already receiving and the peak inspiratory pressure the minimum which gives adequate chest expansion and air entry, as assessed clinically. Larger babies may be ventilated at a slower rate.

ment is the introduction of equipment which allows trigger ventilation (Mehta *et al.*, 1986). These ventilators respond to a pressure change in the airway, produced by the baby, and this causes the ventilator to produce an inspiration in time with the baby's own breathing movements. It is possible to set a background rate, to ensure that the baby is ventilated even during long apnoeic pauses. One method of this is called synchronous intermittent mandatory ventilation (SIMV) (South & Morley, 1986). The problem with trigger ventilation is that small babies, particularly those under 28 weeks gestation, do not produce strong enough respiratory efforts to trigger the ventilator.

It is important to assess ventilation clinically (chest wall movement, auscultation, colour) and blood gases must be checked, at least four-hourly or within 15 minutes of any adjustments in ventilator settings (if electrodes for continuous monitoring are not in place). Necessary clinical observations are summarised in Table 8.5. It is important to monitor the baby's blood pressure. This is best done via an intra-arterial transducer, but it can be measured using a cuff and ultrasound sensor. A small transfusion of blood or plasma (10 ml/kg) can be given if the blood pressure is low (mean pressure less than 30 mmHg).

Adequate humidification helps to prevent the accumulation of sticky secretions. Tracheal toilet should be performed as often as necessary using an aseptic technique. On each occasion the baby may become hypoxic therefore suction should be performed as quickly as possible. All babies on ventilators should be given regular physiotherapy, with frequent changes of position to assist drainage of secretions from the lungs, together with stimuli to dislodge secretions so that they can be coughed up or sucked up the endotracheal tube. A

Table 8.5 Clinical observations that should be made of a baby on a ventilator.

1 Temperature	**9** General activity
2 Heart rate	**10** Blood gases
3 Blood pressure	**11** Tracheal aspirate
4 Respiratory rate	**12** Urine passed
5 Colour	**13** Bowel actions
6 Chest movement	**14** Concentrations of inspired oxygen
7 Breath sounds, whether equal both sides of the chest	**15** Ventilator settings
	16 Physiotherapy
8 Peripheral circulation	**17** Drugs

useful method is using a Bennet face mask which gives a cupping action, which physiotherapists find is effective and comfortable for the baby.

Most neonatal units use endotracheal tubes. This is partly because they are used during emergency resuscitation and it is easier to secure in place than replace it. Some units, however, prefer nasal tubes for prolonged ventilation, as they can be secured more effectively. Nasal tubes have been reported as causing pressure necrosis of the margin of the nose, and therefore need careful management. Oral tubes may cause palatal grooves, which are preventable if dental plates are fitted early on. Orotracheal tubes should not have a shoulder or change in

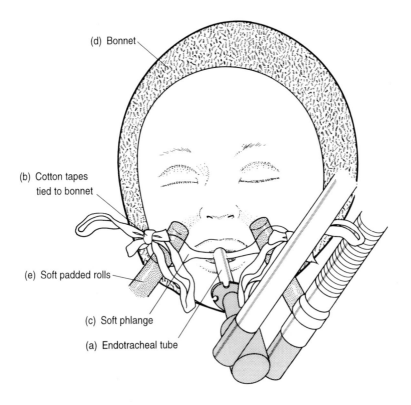

Fig. 8.5 Fixing of an endotracheal tube (ETT).

diameter, as they have been thought to cause tracheal stenosis, although there is some controversy over this. It is important that the tube should be fixed firmly. The simplest method is to use a tube with wings fixed to the side, which can be secured firmly to a bonnet over the head.

Complications of ventilation are common, and include pneumothorax, which must always be suspected if there is a sudden deterioration, particularly if high pressures have been used; pneumonia; lobar or pulmonary collapse from mucous obstruction; bronchopulmonary dysplasia (see below); mechanical failure and dislodged tube.

A summary of the action to be taken if a baby deteriorates while being ventilated is shown in Table 8.6.

The baby should be weaned off the ventilator as soon as possible. A good time to start is when oxygen requirements start falling or if there are signs of spontaneous breathing. The simplest way is to reduce the ventilatory pressure gradually and then the respiratory rate settings, or by intermittent mandatory ventilation (IMV), in which the ventilatory rate is slowly decreased. When a rate of 15–20 breaths per minute is reached, it is usually appropriate to try extubation. It is sometimes very difficult to ventilate a big baby. Initially, one can try abolishing the baby's respiratory efforts by increasing the rate to 90–100 per minute. An alternative is sedation with a drug like chloral, or intravenous narcotics. If these are not successful, it is necessary to paralyse the baby with a drug such as pancuronium (dose 0.02 mg/kg intravenously and repeat as necessary) (Pollitzer et al., 1981). This appears to reduce the incidence of pneumothorax. Hypoxaemia can occur when the drug is given, so monitor the Po_2 closely. If the baby is paralysed care should be taken to change the position of the baby regularly to relieve pressure areas and also to perform passive limb exercises. The effects of paralysis must be explained carefully to the parents. Quite often they feel the baby appears more peaceful and comfortable once paralysed. It is, of course, essential to sedate the baby during periods of paralysis, and eye drops, such as hypromellose, will be needed to prevent corneal damage.

There are many new developments in ventilation of the newborn. CNEP reduces the PIP needed for ventilation, trigger ventilation is proving very useful, and very high frequency oscillation with rates over 1000 per minute shows promise. Extracorpeal membrane oxygenation (ECMO) is used widely in North America for hypoxic, full-term babies, who have suffered meconium aspiration. The technique involves cannulating a major artery and vein, and circulating the

Table 8.6 Action to be taken if the baby deteriorates while being ventilated.

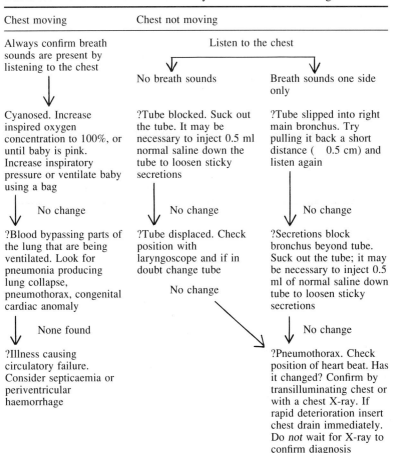

Chest moving	Chest not moving

Always confirm breath sounds are present by listening to the chest

Listen to the chest

No breath sounds

Breath sounds one side only

Cyanosed. Increase inspired oxygen concentration to 100%, or until baby is pink. Increase inspiratory pressure or ventilate baby using a bag

?Tube blocked. Suck out the tube. It may be necessary to inject 0.5 ml normal saline down the tube to loosen sticky secretions

?Tube slipped into right main bronchus. Try pulling it back a short distance (0.5 cm) and listen again

No change

?Blood bypassing parts of the lung that are being ventilated. Look for pneumonia producing lung collapse, pneumothorax, congenital cardiac anomaly

?Tube displaced. Check position with laryngoscope and if in doubt change tube

No change

?Secretions block bronchus beyond tube. Suck out the tube; it may be necessary to inject 0.5 ml of normal saline down tube to loosen sticky secretions

None found

?Illness causing circulatory failure. Consider septicaemia or periventricular haemorrhage

?Pneumothorax. Check position of heart beat. Has it changed? Confirm by transilluminating chest or with a chest X-ray. If rapid deterioration insert chest drain immediately. Do *not* wait for X-ray to confirm diagnosis

blood through an oxygenator. A UK multicentre national trial is underway at present (Pearson, 1992).

Alkali therapy

The correction with alkali (e.g. 8.4% sodium bicarbonate) of the metabolic acidaemia associated with RDS was popular when there was no really effective treatment. Hypoxia causes lactic acidaemia and the best treatment is to improve tissue oxygenation to allow the baby to correct the blood pH. Respiratory acidosis can be corrected by ventilation; sodium bicarbonate may increase the P_{CO_2}. It is possible that the over-enthusiastic use of alkali therapy in the past was responsible for many deaths from periventricular haemorrhage (PVH).

Careful resuscitation of all preterm babies at birth and the prevention of hypoxaemia and acidaemia almost certainly reduce the incidence of PVH and a reasonable indication for using alkali would be persistent acidaemia after attention to ventilation with a pH below 7.2 and base excess more than -7 mmol/l. Give sodium bicarbonate, 2–3 mmol/kg, slowly over about 30 minutes. THAM is sometimes used to correct acidaemia. It reduces the P_{CO_2} unlike sodium bicarbonate and does not contain sodium, which is another advantage.

Pneumothorax

Pneumothorax can occur at any time during the newborn period but it usually appears as a complication of some other respiratory problem. For instance, it is common in babies who have been resuscitated at birth, especially if high pressures have been used to expand the lungs, and it often occurs as a result of ventilation or CPAP in a baby with RDS or after meconium aspiration. A significant reduction in the incidence of pneumothoraces has been reported from trials into the effects of surfactant, particularly human surfactant (Merritt *et al.*, 1986). The usual presentation is sudden collapse and cyanosis. The classical physical signs found in adults are not always present in babies. If the pneumothorax is under tension and is on only one side of the chest, there may be mediastinal shift so that the heart sounds are displaced. Unfortunately, the diagnosis can often be difficult because these signs are not present. A major help in diagnosis is transillumination using a cold light source. Using this technique the chest will transilluminate brightly if there is a lot of air around the lung. It is only really satisfactory in very small babies (under 1300 g), although it can be useful in larger babies. In babies over about 2500 g the technique may not show any transillumination even though a large pneumothorax is present. If a pneumothorax can be found on transillumination, it is reasonable to drain the chest immediately if the baby is obviously very ill. Otherwise it is helpful to obtain a chest radiograph which usually makes the diagnosis quite

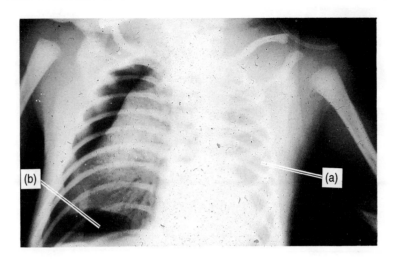

Fig. 8.6 Chest X-ray showing opaque appearance of severe hyaline membrane disease (a) and right pneumothorax (b).

clear (Fig. 8.6), although small pneumothoraces are sometimes difficult to diagnose because skin folds or items of clothing may give confusing shadows on a radiograph. In an emergency, when the baby has suddenly collapsed, it may be necessary to put a needle into the chest in order to see if a pneumothorax is present and to provide some instant relief. It is important to have an underwater seal and this is most easily done using a butterfly type of needle with the end of the plastic tubing under sterile distilled water. If a stream of bubbles appears, a chest drain can be inserted without radiographic confirmation because the baby may die without immediate treatment. Indiscriminate needling of the chest should not be done since it is very easy to damage the lung of a newborn baby and to *cause* a pneumothorax.

It is important to prevent pneumothoraces by avoiding pressures above 30 cm of water during resuscitation, or to use a ventilation bag properly constructed for neonates. One should choose the lowest pressure that will provide adequate mechanical ventilation of the lungs. It is common to see interstitial emphysema before the pneumothorax actually occurs. The radiographic picture is then very remarkable, with areas of translucency and collapse scattered through the lung so that it looks almost like a snowstorm. The air often escapes from the small alveoli into the substance of the lungs

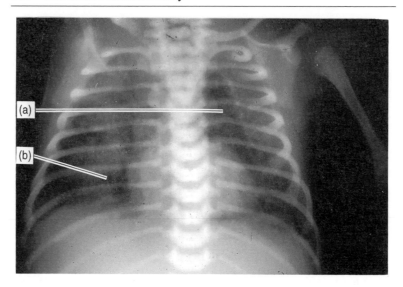

Fig. 8.7 Chest X-ray showing pneumomediastium (a) and pulmonary interstitial emphysema (b)

surrounding the bronchi; it then tracks up to the hilum of the lung and into the mediastinum. A lateral radiograph is essential whenever a pneumothorax is suspected because a pocket of air behind the sternum indicates that a pneumomediastinum (see Fig. 8.7) is present. Sometimes radiographs show an even more dramatic picture with air in the pericardium or in the peritoneum (Fig. 8.8). When a very large amount of air has escaped into the mediastinum one may be able to feel the crackle of subcutaneous air around the neck or over the chest wall.

Careful thought should be given to the treatment of a pneumothorax. If the baby is in good condition, draining the air is not necessary. In a full-term baby, who is not at risk of retinopathy of prematurity, the use of high concentrations of oxygen will probably allow the pneumothorax to absorb more quickly. The baby's arterial oxygen tension should be monitored and the pneumothorax is drained only if satisfactory Po_2 levels cannot be maintained. If the pneumothorax needs draining, it is important that a fairly large tube should be used. We suggest a proper chest drain; these are available in pre-packed disposable units, with a metal stilette down the middle of the catheter. There are various sites where the drain can be

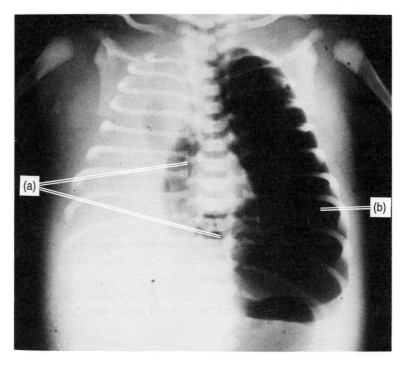

Fig. 8.8 Pneumopericardium (a) with a large left pneumothorax (b)

inserted. It is commonest to use the front of the chest in the second or third interspace in the middle clavicular line. However, this has problems particularly in a girl; the hole produced by the chest drain will leave a scar which will be visible later and if the drain is inserted anywhere near the breast there is a danger that a part of the breast may not develop normally. It therefore seems reasonable to use the anterior axillary line in the fourth or fifth intercostal spaces. Adequate local anaesthetic must be used prior to this procedure. A small incision should be made through the skin, one intercostal space below the proposed site of insertion. The drain and stilette can then be passed through the skin and manoeuvred over the point of insertion through the intercostal space. It is wise to put artery forceps on the catheter as a guard, so that when the drain is pressed into the chest it does not suddenly go too far. When the chest has been entered, the stilette is withdrawn and the plastic catheter advanced upwards and anteriorly.

The proximal end of the chest drain must be attached to some form of seal to prevent air entering the pleural space during inspiration. The most convenient seal is a Heimlich flutter valve which is available as a pre-packed disposable unit. An alternative is to use the simple under-water seal, but it is important to keep this below the level of the baby, otherwise water may enter the chest. We usually find that it is necessary to put a pump on the other end of the seal with a pressure of about 3–5 mmHg in order to drain the air satisfactorily. Plate IV shows a baby who has a right pneumothorax and is being artificially ventilated. A right intercostal drain has been inserted.

It is often difficult to decide when to remove the chest drain:

1 The chest radiograph should show that the pneumothorax has absorbed completely.
2 The drain should be clamped with artery forceps and the radiograph taken about six hours later.
3 If the pneumothorax has reformed, further drainage will be necessary but if there is no air in the chest it is reasonable to remove the drain.

If two pneumothoraces are present, an attempt should be made to remove only one drain at a time. The second drain could be examined about 24 hours after the first.

Pneumopericardium is often lethal. If it is diagnosed, an attempt should be made to drain the air using a needle passed under the xiphisternum into the pericardium.

Meconium Aspiration

This subject is also discussed in Chapters 3 and 6. It can be a major problem and is particularly likely to occur in babies born at term and SFGA babies who have suffered from intrapartum asphyxia. When a baby does not have enough oxygen before birth meconium is passed into the amniotic fluid and the baby makes gasping movements. Meconium is present in the liquor in about 10% of deliveries at term, but a much smaller proportion of babies develop meconium aspiration. If meconium is present in the liquor, the mouth should be sucked out at delivery. It is best to clear the mouth completely as soon as the head is born so that it is done before the first breath when the chest is still in the birth canal. If the baby is covered with thick meconium, the larynx must be inspected so that any meconium on the vocal cords can be removed. If there is any suspicion that meconium has been aspirated into the trachea, the essential prophylactic measure is to suck out the trachea under direct vision. The routine use of tracheal lavage should be avoided (Hodge, 1991; Shorten *et al.*, 1991). If it is used, 0.1–0.2 ml/kg normal saline 0.9% should be instilled just prior to suctioning (Hodge, 1991).

If aspiration is suspected, it is important to observe the baby carefully for 12–24 hours as insidious deterioration may take place. The baby with meconium aspiration usually shows an increase in respiratory rate and cyanosis. The chest radiograph is very variable but often shows large fluffy opacities in many parts of the lung field (see Fig. 6.9). The standard method of treatment is to give sufficient oxygen to keep the baby's arterial Po_2 between 7 and 10 kPa (50–75 mmHg). It is common to use antibiotics as pneumonia may follow. Pneumothorax is also a common complication.

In severe meconium aspiration, ventilation is often required but there is still doubt about the best way of ventilating the baby. It is common to use a rather higher rate than is usual for hyaline membrane disease. One of the major problems is a marked right-to-left shunt of blood as a result of persistent fetal circulation. This has been treated by over-ventilation to reduce the Pco_2 below normal, but this reduces cerebral blood flow and is not usually recommended. The use of a vasodilating drug such as tolazoline (dose 1–2 mg/kg bolus, then 1 mg/kg/h by intravenous infusion) may be particularly useful if the Po_2 remains low. It can produce a dramatic improvement in oxygenation, but it may cause hypotension. Prostacycline is another drug which can be used, but it has not been fully evaluated, and is very expensive.

The baby may remain ill for several days. The course of the illness is often complicated by pneumothorax, but if the baby survives the first few days, the tachypnoea will gradually reduce. The babies do not have any prolonged respiratory problems.

Pneumonia

Pneumonia is also discussed in Chapter 16. It may occur any time during the newborn period but is commonest shortly after birth, as a result of infection of the amniotic cavity. It should be suspected in any baby whose mother has had ruptured membranes for longer than 12 hours, is pyrexial or has had a long, difficult labour. Examination of gastric aspirate at birth gives a clue to the diagnosis since pus cells may be seen in large numbers in a baby who has pneumonia, but, since pus cells are often seen without infection, it may cause confusion, and many units no longer rely on this. A vaginal swab from the mother and a swab from the external ear of the baby may identify the causative organism. Babies with RDS or meconium aspiration may develop pneumonia, particularly if they are intubated or ventilated. The greatest danger is in babies with group B β-haemolytic streptococcal pneumonia and septicaemia. These infected babies are often rather larger than those who have hyaline membrane disease and they may be extremely ill and shocked. The chest radiograph may show patchy opacities but very often the picture is indistinguishable from hyaline membrane disease. If there is any suspicion that the baby might have pneumonia, it is important to start antibiotics very early. Ampicillin and cefotaxime, or ampicillin and gentamicin, are standard combinations of drugs.

Transient Tachypnoea of Newborn (TTN)

This is an ill-defined but common syndrome. It is often diagnosed in babies who would not be expected to have RDS, for example, a term baby who is breathing rapidly; the essential criterion for the diagnosis is a respiratory rate of more than 60/min. There may be recession, slight grunting or even cyanosis. The illness disappears by 24 hours and therefore does not fulfil the criteria for hyaline membrane disease. Some babies may have tachypnoea alone for longer than 24 hours but do not have the other criteria of grunting, recession, characteristic chest radiograph and cyanosis which would suggest a diagnosis of RDS. It may be that such babies have only mild surfactant deficiency and that this is the pathological mechanism underlying transient tachypnoea.

Another possible cause is failure to absorb lung fluid satisfactorily after birth, for example, after a caesarian section delivery. Characteristic chest radiographs have been described; they show increased markings and opacification of the transverse fissure, suggesting oedema between the lobes of the lung on the right. Other characteristics are streaks which spread out from the hilum; it is suggested that these represent enlarged lymphatic vessels which are draining lung fluid. If the lungs were wetter than normal they would probably be stiffer and this could account for the fast breathing.

These babies need very little treatment apart from good standard incubator care and small and appropriate quantities of added oxygen to relieve cyanosis. If there are any opacities in the lung fields on the chest radiograph, it is wise to give antibiotics until the results of the cultures are known. Pneumonitis from chlamydial or cytomegalovirus infection has been described in newborn babies. These infections may be commoner than we suspect so antibody tests should be done in any baby with an unusual respiratory illness.

Neonatal Myasthenia Gravis

This is a rare transient disorder which occurs in about 10–15% of babies born to mothers with myasthenia. Antibodies to striated muscle acetylcholine receptors cross the placenta and may cause muscle weakness, feeding difficulties and respiratory problems, usually in the first 24 hours of life. Intravenous edrophonium (1 mg) will confirm the diagnosis by producing a marked improvement in respiratory effort and spontaneous limb movements, and less pooling of pharyngeal secretions. However, respiratory arrest may occasionally occur. Treatment with the anti-cholinesterase drug, neostigmine, is then necessary. This may be needed for only a few days or as long as several months.

The prognosis in terms of neuromuscular function is excellent. However, associated congenital deformities such as joint contractures may occur and require treatment in their own right with physiotherapy.

Bronchopulmonary Dysplasia (BPD)

This condition has been seen more frequently in recent years as more small babies have been ventilated for long periods or have needed prolonged oxygen therapy.

The typical case is a baby under 1500 g who required prolonged ventilation for RDS and apnoeic attacks. Oxygen dependency then continues, and cyanosis occurs if no added oxygen is given. There is usually intercostal recession, a high respiratory rate and a very abnormal chest radiograph showing streaking of the lung fields alternating with translucent areas probably representing cystic or over-inflated parts of the lung (see Fig. 8.9). There is a high mortality and at post-mortem examination the histology of the lung shows focal areas of emphysematous alveoli, bronchiolar smooth muscle hypertrophy and perimucosal fibrosis.

There has been a lot of controversy about the cause of the

Table 8.7 Some important causes of apnoeic attacks in the newborn.

Respiratory
Exhaustion (severe RDS, bronchopulmonary dysplasia)
Pneumonia – viral or bacterial; tracheo-oesophageal fistula
Pneumothorax – meconium aspiration; resuscitation; spontaneous; ventilation
Aspiration – blood; meconium; feed; vomitus
Vagal or pharyngeal stimulation (deep suction, passage of tubes)

Central
Apnoea of preterm infant (immature respiratory centre)
Seizures
Excess sedation with drugs (mother or baby)
Cerebral haemorrhage
Cerebral birth trauma
Kernicterus
Meningitis or other severe infections

Metabolic
Hypoglycaemia
Hypocalcaemia
Hypothermia
Acidosis, metabolic or respiratory
Hyponatraemia
Giving intravenous or intra-arterial calcium or potassium too rapidly

Obstructive
Choanal or oesophageal atresia
Tongue (in Pierre Robin syndrome)
Mechanical (face accidentally covered during procedures)

breathing. In this way periods of prolonged apnoea with possible cerebral hypoxia are avoided and babies can be more easily resuscitated.

Treatment

Prevention

Apnoeic attacks are better prevented than treated:

1 Minimal handling.
2 An appropriate environmental temperature.
3 Nurse prone when possible.
4 Nurse with apnoea alarm set to a 20-second delay and use a heart rate monitor alarm set at 100 beats/min.

After the first attack consider nursing prone, removing nasal tubes, nursing on a sheepskin and adjusting environmental temperature. Intravenous alimentation may be necessary.

Do not give oxygen routinely: during an apnoeic attack the baby is not breathing so that it would have no effect. After the attack, breathing oxygen-enriched gases may be dangerous as the baby's Pao_2 may rise to very high levels.

Physical stimulation can be given by stroking or patting the baby and changing the position. Suction of the posterior pharynx may provoke apnoea and clearing the airways should therefore involve suction only of the mouth. The baby can then be rapidly intubated if necessary.

If there is continued apnoea with bradycardia and physical stimulation fails, intubation and hand ventilation are needed (for technique see Chapter 3). If regular spontaneous respirations with a normal heart rate return the baby can safely be extubated.

Recurrent apnoeic attacks

There is good evidence that the use of the respiratory stimulant theophylline may prevent or greatly reduce the incidence of apnoeic attacks in preterm babies. It is important to check blood levels regularly, so as to reduce the risks of toxicity – the most common of which are cardiac arrhythmias. A dose is omitted if the heart rate is persistently above 180 bpm. The drug is converted into caffeine in the neonate, and many therefore use caffeine instead (Table 8.8). So far there have not been any reports of long-term side effects.

Continuous positive airways pressure (see earlier in this chapter for the possible techniques) can be used. There is good evidence that this method, however applied, prevents apnoeic attacks. The technique has its own dangers, however, and these are described above. There is evidence that theophylline is more effective and is certainly easier to administer than CPAP.

Mechanical ventilation is indicated if adequate respiration is not maintained between attacks with or without the use of CPAP (for details, see Table 8.8).

Investigations

Any baby who needs treatment for apnoea should be investigated.

1 *Exclude infection* by blood culture, urine analysis, culture swabs from any obviously infected area and white blood cell count. A

Table 8.8 Management of recurrent apnoeic attacks.

Theophylline	Give the loading dose of 6.2 mg/kg either intravenously over 20 minutes or orally as choline theophylline. Then give maintenance dose of 4.4 mg/kg/day intravenously or Choledyl 1.5 mg/kg six-hourly. Plasma theophylline level should be checked the following day
Caffeine	Loading dose of 10 mg/kg. Maintenance dose of 2.5–5 mg/kg every 24 hours. May need to be given every 12 hours in babies over 28 days old
CPAP	Administer via tube or endotracheal tube depending on infant's condition and size. Start at 2–4 cmH$_2$O and increase to a maximum of 4–6 cm. Pass nasogastric tube to aspirate stomach
Ventilation	If apnoea is causing persistent acidosis (pH < 7.2) and hypoxaemia (Pao_2 < 6 kPa) ventilate by endotracheal tube or facemask. Keep peak pressure low (< 15 cmH$_2$O) or use with Intermittent mandatory ventilation (IMV). Monitor response by blood gas analysis

lumbar puncture may often be indicated, but this may precipitate a further severe apnoeic attack. Be prepared for this.
2 *Exclude hypoglycaemia* with glucose monitoring strips and a blood glucose estimation if the glucose monitoring strip result is low.
3 An *electroencephalogram* may reveal evidence that convulsions are presenting as apnoeic attacks.
4 *Ultrasound scanning* may demonstrate periventricular haemorrhage or other cerebral abnormalities.

Appropriate specific treatment (such as antibiotics, dextrose or anticonvulsants) may need to be given. If infection is suspected, do not await the culture results before starting treatment. Treatment should be started as soon as specimens have been obtained.

Diaphragmatic Hernia

This subject is discussed in Chapter 3 (p. 66).

References and Further Reading

Collaborative Groups in Antenatal Steroid Therapy (1981) Effect of antenatal dexamethasone administration on the prevention of respiratory distress syndrome. *Am. J. Obstet. Gynecol.*, *141*, 276–287.

Committee for the classification of ROP (1984) The international classification of ROP. *Pediatrics*, *74*, 127.

Cryotherapy for ROP Cooperative Group (1988) Multicenter trial of cryotherapy for ROP: preliminary results. *Pediatrics*, *81*, 697.

Danford, D.A., Miske, S., Headley, J. *et al.* (1983) Effects of routine care procedures on transcutaneous oxygen in neonates: a quantitative approach. *Arch. Dis. Child.*, *58*, 20.

Drew, J.H. (1982) Immediate intubation at birth for very-low-birthweight infants. *Am. J. Dis. Child.*, *136*, 207–210.

Gitlin, J.D., Soll, R.F., Parad, R.B. *et al.* (1987) Randomized controlled trial of exogenous surfactant for the treatment of Hyaline Membrane Disease. *Pediatrics*, *79*, 31–37.

Greenough, A. & Milner, A.D. (1987) High frequency ventilation in the neonatal period. *Eur. J. Pediatr.*, *146*, 446–449.

Greenough, A., Greenall, F., Pool, J. *et al.* (1987) Comparison of different rates of artificial ventilation in preterm infants with respiratory distress syndrome. *Acta. Paediatr. Scand.*, *76*, 706–712.

Halliday, H.L., McClure, G., Reid, M. *et al.* (1984) Controlled trial of artificial surfactant to prevent respiratory distress syndrome. *Lancet*, *i*, 476–478.

Hallman, M., Merritt, T.A., Jarvenpaa, A.L. *et al.* (1985) Exogenous human surfactant for treatment of severe respiratory distress syndrome: a randomized prospective clinical trial. *J. Pediatr.*, *106*, 963–969.

Hodge, D. (1991) Endotracheal suctioning and the infant: a nursing care protocol to decrease complications. *Neonatal Network*, *9*(5), 7–15.

Mehta, A., Wright, B.M., Callan, K. *et al.* (1986) Patient-triggered ventilation in the newborn. *Lancet*, *i*, 17–19.

Merritt, T.A., Hallman, M., Bloom, B.T. *et al.* (1986) Prophylactic treatment of very premature infants with human surfactant. *N. Engl. J. Med.*, *315*, 785–790.

Morley, C., Greenough, A., Miller, N.G. *et al.* (1988) Randomized trial of artificial surfactant (ALEC) given at birth to babies from 23 to 24 weeks gestation. *Early Human Development*, *17*, 41–54.

Ng, P.C. (1993) The effectiveness and side effects of dexamethasone in preterm infants with bronchopulmonary dysplasia. *Arch. Dis. Child.*, *68*, 330–336.

Ng, P.C., Thomson, M. & Dear, P.R.F. (1989) Dexamethasone and infection in preterm babies: a controlled study. *Arch. Dis. Child.*, *65*, 54–58.

Pearson, G. (1992) UK experience in neonatal extracorporeal membrane oxygenation. *Arch. Dis. Child.*, *67*(7), Foetal/neonatal supplement: 822–825.

Pollitzer, M.J., Reynolds, E.O.R. & Shaw, D.G. (1981) Pancuronium during mechanical ventilation speeds recovery of lungs of infants with hyaline membrane disease. *Lancet*, *i*, 346–348.

Prendiville, A. & Schulenberg, W.E. (1988) Clinical factors associated with retinopathy of prematurity. *Arch. Dis. Child.*, *63*, 522–527.

Raju, T.N.K., Vidyasagar, D., Bhat, R. *et al.* (1987) Double blind controlled trial of single-dose treatment with bovine surfactant in severe Hyaline Membrane Disease. *Lancet, i,* 651–656.

Robertson, B. (1983) Lung surfactant for replacement therapy. *Clin. Physiol., 3,* 97–110.

Robson, E. & Hey, E. (1982) Resuscitation of preterm babies at birth reduces the risk of death from Hyaline Membrane Disease. *Arch. Dis. Child., 57,* 184–186.

Shapiro, D.L., Notter, R.H., Morin, F.C. *et al.* (1986) Double blind, randomizes trial of calf lung surfactant extract administered at birth to very premature infants for prevention of respiratory distress syndrome. *Pediatrics, 76,* 593–599.

Shorten, D.C., Byrne, P.J. & Jones, R.L. (1991) Infant responses to saline installation and endotracheal suctioning. *J. Obstetrics, Gynaecology and Neonatal Nursing,* 20(6), 464–469.

South, M. & Morley, C.J. (1986) Synchronous mechanical ventilation of the neonate. *Arch. Dis. Child., 61,* 1190–1195.

Southall, D.P., Bignall, S., Stebbens, V.A. *et al.* (1987) Pulse oximeter and transcutaneous arterial oxygen measurements in neonatal and paediatric intensive care. *Arch. Dis. Child., 62,* 882–888.

Ten Centre Study Group (1987) Ten centre trial of artificial surfactant (artificial lung expanding compound) in very premature babies. *BMJ, 294,* 991–996.

9

Congenital Disorders: General Principles

Congenital malformations are common (Fig. 9.1) and are a major cause of death in the perinatal period. Some children who survive are left with very little handicap because the abnormality can be corrected, but many children have lasting problems. In the past congenital abnormalities have been a particular problem as a cause of perinatal death in the British Isles because of the high incidence of neural-tube defects. Antenatal screening and selective termination have reduced the numbers in recent years. The overall incidence of congenital malformations is about 2%. There appear to be major differences in the incidence of congenital malformations around the world and in different parts of the British Isles (Young & Clarke, 1987). In general, neural-tube defects, including anencephaly and myelomeningocele, are commoner in western Europe; in the British Isles they are commoner in the north and west. There appear to be more neural-tube defects in cities where there is a large population of Irish descent and this has been shown in some of the large cities of North America. Cleft palate and cleft lip appear to be commoner in East Asia. The incidence of malformations also shows a difference depending on the mother's country of birth (Balarajan *et al.*, 1989).

Many surveys are difficult to interpret because one cannot establish the true incidence of congenital abnormalities at birth. Some abnormalities are immediately obvious, like anencephaly or cleft lip, whereas others are obvious only later, such as a ventricular septal defect which may not be accompanied by a murmur in the newborn period but only several weeks later. The prevalence of congenital abnormalities varies according to the age at which a survey is taken because, for example, dislocation of the hips is relatively common at birth but becomes less common as the child grows older, particularly if treatment is used. Some congenital malformations correct themselves, for example, a ventricular septal defect which may close spontaneously.

The incidence of some important congenital malformations and inborn errors is shown in Tables 9.1 to 9.3. These figures,

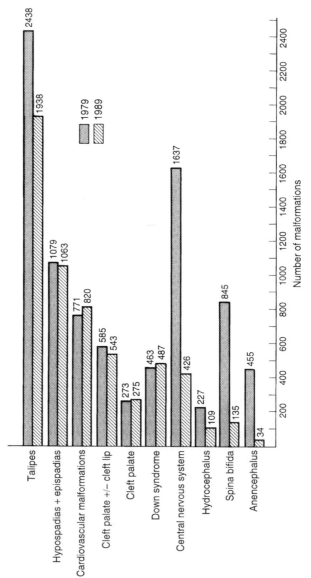

Fig. 9.1 Changes in number of births with selected conditions 1979–1989 (OPGS)

Table 9.1 Approximate incidence of some important congenital
abnormalities and inborn errors with multifactorial inheritance.

Abnormality	Incidence (in total births)	Risk to siblings
Myelomeningocele		
South-east England	1/600	1/30 (3.4%) for either myelomeningocele or anencephaly, i.e. 1 in 40 for each
South Wales/Ireland	1/250	1/18 for either myelomeningocele or anencephaly, i.e. 1 in 35 for each
Anencephaly		
South-east England	1/800	1/30 (3.4%) for either myelomeningocele or anencephaly, i.e. 1 in 40 for each
South Wales/Ireland	1/300	1/18 for either myelomeningocele or anencephaly, i.e. 1 in 35 for each
Cleft lip and palate		
Whites	1/750	1/25 (4%)
Chinese	More common than in Caucasian	
Blacks	1/2500	
Cleft palate only	1/2000	1/33 (3%)
Congenital heart disease		
Overall	1/150	
VSD	1/400	1/23 (4.4%)
ASD	1/1000	1/30 (3.3%)
PDA	1/2000	1/70 (1.4%)
Tetralogy of Fallot	1/3300	1/100 (1%)
Congenital dislocation of the hip		
Newborn (dislocatable or dislocated)	1/200	
Established (untreated)	1/1000	If ♀, risk for next ♀ 1/20 (5%), risk for next ♂ 1/60 (1.6%). If ♂, higher risks. Overall about 1/25 (4%)
Talipes equinovarus	1/1000	1/35 (2.9%)
Hirschsprung's disease	1/5000	If brother affected: 1/25 (4%) If sister affected: 1/8 (12.5%)
Hypospadias		
Whites	1/120	1/14 (7%)
Blacks	1/500	

Table 9.2 Approximate incidence of some important congenital abnormalities and inborn errors with inheritance by single mutant gene.

Abnormality	Incidence	Incidence of heterozygotes
Autosomal recessive (recurrence risk 1 in 4)		
Cystic fibrosis		
Whites	1/1500 to 1/7200	1/20 (5%)
Black Americans	1/17 000	
Africans	Rare	
Orientals	Rare	
Congenital adrenal hyperplasia (21 hydroxylase deficiency)		
Western Europe	1/5000 (50% are salt-losers, cf. USA 30%; Alaska 100%)	1/37 (2.7%)
Autosomal dominant (recurrence risk 1 in 2 if a parent is affected)		
Achondroplasia	1/10 000	
X-linked recessive (if mother is a carrier 1/2 daughters are carriers and 1/2 sons have the disease)		
Glucose-6-phosphate dehydrogenase deficiency		
African type		1/4 (25% of black American ♀)
Black Americans	1/8	
Whites	Rare	
Factor VIII deficiency (haemophilia A)	1/4000 ♂	

particularly the risk of a sibling being affected, are useful when counselling for future pregnancies. In most cases, however, it would be wise to seek the advice of a clinical geneticist, especially where there is some complication such as consanguinity, several cases of an abnormality within a family or several abnormalities in one baby.

Aetiology

A few congenital abnormalities have a well-known aetiology:

Rubella, particularly in the first trimester of pregnancy, usually produces abnormalities. The babies have microcephaly, retinal pigmentation, patent ductus arteriosus or other heart anomalies, mental handicap, deafness and are small-for-gestational-age (SFGA) at birth.

It is interesting that the incidence of congenital abnormalities is less if the virus invades the fetus later in pregnancy.

A large dose of *radiation* in mid-trimester is well known to produce severe damage to the brain. Microcephaly was seen in the fetuses in the survivors of radiation from atomic bombs in Japan in 1945.

Some *drugs* produce congenital abnormalities but the list is relatively short. The most famous and disastrous example is thalidomide, which produced congenital limb deformities in the babies of women who took this sleeping tablet around 1960 (see Fig. 2.9). Other drugs which are known to cause congenital abnormalities are listed in Chapter 2. Thalidomide produced obvious and unusual abnormalities but it can be very difficult to know whether a drug causes abnormalities because the number produced could be very small and the abnormality is otherwise common. Thus very careful studies are needed before a drug can be used widely in pregnancy.

Poorly controlled *diabetes mellitus* is associated with a higher

Table 9.3 Incidence of some common chromosomal abnormalities.

	Incidence in total liveborn births	Risk if sibling affected (apparently normal parents)
Down syndrome (trisomy 21)		
Overall	1/700	1/65 depends on chromosome type and maternal age
Regular (non-disjunction) depends on mother's age:		
< 25 years	1/2000	1/100
25–34 years	1/1300	1/100
35–44 years	1/250	1/90
45 years+	1/40	greater if maternal age > 40 years
14;21 translocation	About 4% of all babies with Down syndrome	1/5 if maternal translocation 1/100 if paternal translocation
Trisomy-18 (*Edwards syndrome*)	1/3000 increases with advancing maternal age	1/100 for chromosome abnormality
Trisomy-13 (*Patau syndrome*)	1/5000 increases with advancing maternal age	1/100 for chromosome abnormality
Turner syndrome	1/10 000	Not increased

incidence of congenital abnormality; several surveys have suggested 6% rather than 2% for the general population. It is now clear that careful control of diabetes early in pregnancy reduces the incidence of congenital malformations (Fuhrman *et al.*, 1983). Prepregnancy clinics for diabetic women have been established in many areas (see Chapter 15).

Some abnormalities appear to be commoner in one *social class* rather than another. The most well-known example is anencephaly, which is commoner in social class V than in social class I.

A single *mutant gene* can produce a congenital abnormality, such as achondroplasia, polydactyly or some types of hydrocephalus. However, it is probable that many congenital abnormalities, for example, neural tube defects, are produced by a number of genes acting together – polygenic inheritance.

There are many conditions with a rather more doubtful aetiology. Women anaesthetists are said to have babies with a higher incidence of congenital anomalies and this may be related to the anaesthetic gases which they accidentally inhale during induction of anaesthesia. Many hypotheses have been made about items of diet such as blighted potatoes, corned beef or even tea as an aetiological factor of neural-tube defects, but these have been disproved. It is possible that some environmental factors such as an item of diet could act together with genetic factors. Vitamin supplements, specifically folic acid (The Medical Research Council, 1991) before conception have been shown to reduce the incidence of neural tube defects and some other major non-genetic congenital abnormalities (Czeizel, 1993).

Classification

There are many ways of classifying congenital malformations; the most usual is according to the part of the body where the anomaly occurs. A useful scheme for those looking after newborn babies is to divide the lesions into those that need immediate treatment, usually meaning an urgent referral to a neonatal surgical unit, those requiring early treatment within the first week of life, and those where treatment can be left for some time or which may need no treatment at all. Many of the problems listed below are discussed in more detail elsewhere in the text.

Problems requiring immediate treatment

1 *Tracheo-oesophageal fistula with or without oesophageal atresia.* It is essential to avoid feeding the baby, who must be transferred rapidly to a surgical centre for closure of the fistula and repair of the oesophagus. A Replogle tube attached to continuous suction apparatus should be passed into the oesophageal pouch, to drain it during transfer. The operation is often done within the first 24 hours.

2 *Congenital diaphragmatic hernia* produces a characteristic syndrome of cyanosis and dextrocardia immediately after birth. It requires urgent surgical attention; unfortunately, the results may be poor because of pulmonary hypoplasia underneath the herniated gut in the thorax.

3 *Pierre Robin anomaly.* Affected babies can easily die from asphyxia because the tongue falls back into the pharynx. The baby needs careful nursing in the prone position and may require an airway *in situ.*

4 *Choanal atresia.* When this is complete and bilateral, the baby cannot breathe satisfactorily and an oral airway should be passed until an opening can be made in the nose.

5 *Gastroschisis and exomphalos* need urgent referral.

6 *Spina bifida.* A decision should have been made within 24 hours of birth, whether or not a surgeon is to be consulted about closing the lesion. A baby with meningocele should be referred immediately; in a baby with myelomeningocele, there should be careful discussion with the parents about possible treatment.

7 *Talipes equinovarus.* If the deformity is not reducible, there should be an urgent referral to an orthopaedic surgeon, as early strapping is thought to improve the prognosis.

Lesions requiring early treatment (within the first week)

1 *Imperforate anus.* Some would include this in the urgent group, but in fact one often waits for one to two days to allow air to reach the lower end of the rectum so that a radiograph can be taken to estimate the length of the atresia. Some babies have only a covered anus with a flap of skin over the anus.

2 *Abnormal external genitalia.* Only rarely is there a reason for operating on these babies but investigations should be started within the first few days and careful discussions held with the parents.

3 *Cleft lip and palate.* In many units the lip is closed during the first week and a dental prosthesis is fitted into the cleft.

4 *Teeth*. A congenital tooth can often cause an ulcer on the tongue and may need to be removed.

5 *Congenital adrenal hyperplasia* in a girl can usually be suspected at birth from ambiguous genitalia, but may present more difficulties in a boy.

6 *Intestinal obstruction*. The higher the obstruction, the more likely that bilious vomiting will occur, unless the atresia is in the first part of the duodenum; the lower the obstruction the more likely that distension will occur. Any baby with definite intestinal obstruction should be referred for treatment at once. In some cases it is now possible to make the diagnosis even before birth by the use of ultrasound.

Lesions requiring treatment later or not at all

There are many congenital abnormalities that require very little attention. Some of those that will need attention but only after the first week, include:

1 *Cleft lip*, which is often closed within the first six months. Some surgeons will repair it even within the first few weeks.

2 *Hydrocephalus*. Where this is present at birth, the prognosis is often poor and no operation is done, but progressive hydrocephalus that develops in the first few weeks needs a shunt.

3 *Hypospadias*.

4 *Urethral valves* causing urinary obstruction in boys. If detected by ultrasound these may be treated by prenatal surgery.

5 *Birth marks*.

Most babies with a congenital malformation can be nursed at their mother's bedside. Parents of a baby born with a congenital abnormality should have every opportunity to get to know and learn how to look after their baby. The family is then in a better position to decide whether they will be able to cope with the baby at home. We separate mother and baby only if there is an abnormality that requires surgical or intensive care, in particular a condition where the baby's airway may suddenly become obstructed.

Surgery

Surgery on the newborn baby is technically extremely demanding, and the paediatric care must also be highly skilled. The baby is vulnerable to heat loss and, because of the baby's small blood volume, measurement of blood loss and total fluid and electrolyte replacement must be scrupulous. The baby is also vulnerable to infections.

Many babies will require transfer to a regional neonatal surgical unit for operation. The greatest risks to such a baby are aspiration pneumonia and hypothermia. It is usually advisable to take time at the referring hospital to stabilize the baby by correcting hypoxaemia, acidosis or hypothermia. No baby requiring surgery should be transferred without a nasogastric tube *in situ* and ideally body temperature should be normal. The latter may be difficult to achieve if there is massive heat loss from a large gastroschisis, and urgent transfer may then be preferable.

Frequent or continuous oral and pharyngeal suction may be necessary. Vitamin K should be given (see below). Ensure that a specimen of maternal blood and a parental consent form accompany the baby. There must be a full referral letter with details of the obstetric history, delivery, birthweight and gestational age, nature and sequence of symptoms, family and social background, drugs given and investigations performed with their results.

The general principles of management prior to surgery involve two main areas: (a) Explain to the parents what is involved. Tell them why the operation is necessary, what the risks are and what the prognosis is. (b) Anticipate and prevent predictable complications. In particular:

1 Ensure that the baby's airway is clear and that there is adequate oxygenation.
2 Have crossmatched blood available by the time the baby goes to theatre. The newborn baby's blood volume is only 80 ml/kg (100 ml/kg in the preterm baby). It is easy, therefore, to underestimate the need for replacement.
3 Reduce the risk of bleeding from hypoprothrombinaemia by giving vitamin K (Phytomenadione): 0.5 mg should be given to all babies before operation.
4 Pay careful attention to reducing heat loss and keeping the room warm (see Chapter 6).
5 Replace fluid and electrolyte losses correctly. The baby's maintenance requirements are 60–80 ml/kg on Day 1, 80–100 ml/kg on Day 2 and 100–120 ml/kg on Day 3. About two-thirds of these totals should be given during the first 24 hours after operation. The baby will need approximately 3 mmol/kg/day of sodium and 2 mmol/kg/day of potassium. Energy requirements (500 kJ/kg daily or more;

about 120 kcal) are best given as 10% dextrose. Abnormal fluid losses (e.g. aspirate) will need to be added to these basic requirements when the total fluid volume required is calculated. If the bowels are not working (e.g. following a gastrointestinal resection), the fluid must be given intravenously. Once there is normal gastrointestinal function, fluid may be introduced orally starting with 30 ml/kg on Day 1 and increasing by 30 ml/kg per day until a total of 150 ml/kg/day is reached on Day 5. 150ml of milk contains about 480 kJ (about 115 kcal). The intravenous fluid should be reduced by an equivalent amount as the oral feed is increased.

6 Keep a careful watch for metabolic abnormalities such as hypoglycaemia, hypocalcaemia, or acidosis. The specific treatment for each is discussed elsewhere.

7 Prevent infection first by aseptic theatre technique and postoperative care and secondly with early investigation by swabbing, blood culture and suprapubic aspiration of urine, and the use of appropriate antibiotics if there is any deterioration in the baby's condition.

Many doctors and nurses find the management of families of infants with congenital abnormalities difficult. Some ways of helping the staff to support and care for these families are described in Chapter 19

References and Further Reading

Balarajan, R., Raleigh, V.S. & Botting, B. (1989) Mortality from congenital malformations in England and Wales: variation by mother's country of birth. *Arch. Dis. Child.*, *64*, 1457–1462.

Czeizel, A. (1993) Prevention of congenital abnormalities by periconceptual multivitamin supplementation. *BMJ*, *306*, 1645–1648.

Emery, A.E. & Rimoin, D.L. (eds) (1990) *Principles and Practice of Medical Genetics*, vol. 1, 2nd ed. Churchill Livingstone.

Fuhrman, N.K., Reiher, H., Semmler, K. *et al.* (1983) Prevention of congenital malformation in infants of insulin-dependent diabetic mothers. *Diabetes Care*, *6*, 219–223.

Harper, P.S. (1988) *Practical Genetic Counselling*, 3rd ed. Edinburgh: Wright.

Jones, K.L. (1988) *Smith's Recognizable Patterns of Human Malformation.* 4th ed. Philadelphia: W.B. Saunders.

McKusick, V.A. (1992) *Mendelian Inheritance in Man*, 10th ed. Baltimore: The Johns Hopkins University Press.

Oates, J.N. (1991) *Diabetes in Pregnancy*. London: Ballière Tindall.

OPCS (1989) *Notification of Congenital Malformations.* MB3 Series. London: HMSO.

OPCS (1989) *Cause of Death.* DH3 Series. London: HMSO.

The Medical Research Council Vitamin Study Group (1991) Prevention of neural tube defects: Results of the Medical Research Council Vitamin Study. *Lancet, 238,* 131–137.

Young, I.D. & Clarke, M. (1987) Foetal malformations and perinatal mortality: A ten year review with comparison of ethnic differences. *BMJ, 295*(6590), 89–91.

─10 ─────────────────

Congenital Disorders: Specific Conditions

Some individual congenital abnormalities are now discussed (for congenital heart disease see Chapter 11). Many of them require surgical intervention.

Alimentary System

Cleft lip and palate

Cleft lip, whether unilateral (Fig. 10.1) or bilateral (Fig. 10.2), is among the most immediately obvious and distressing abnormalities to the parents. It may occur on its own or associated with cleft palate. Cleft palate may itself occur alone and its detection at the first postnatal check is extremely important. The embryological development of the nose and mouth region is complex and specific causes for such defects are seldom present. Genetic factors clearly play a part; these defects are commoner in some families, and there is an increased risk of producing subsequent affected babies (see Table 9.1). There are also ethnic variations in incidence (Manchester *et al.*, 1991). Associated malformations are not uncommon, sometimes as part of a chromosomal disorder such as Patau syndrome (see below).

Cleft lip, with or without cleft palate, occurs about once in every 1200 births. Cleft palate alone occurs about once in 2500 births. The chance of having another baby with cleft lip is about 1 in 25 if both parents are normal, but 1 in 10 if one parent has a cleft lip. The chance of an affected parent having an affected child is about 1 in 50. With isolated cleft palate the recurrence risk is about 1 in 30 with normal parents, but as high as 1 in 6 if both parent and older child are affected (see Chapter 9). There is no evidence that barbiturates taken in the first trimester of pregnancy are associated with cleft palate.

Unilateral or bilateral cleft lip virtually never produces any feeding problems. It is very reassuring to the parents to be shown photographs of previous babies, before and after surgical correction, so that they

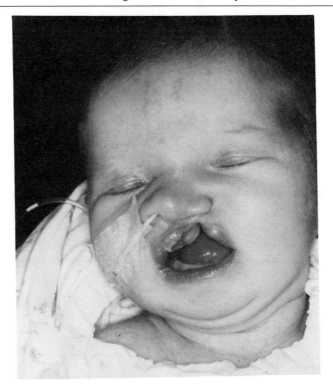

Fig. 10.1 Unilateral cleft lip

may see the excellent results that modern plastic surgery can produce. The timing of surgery is a matter for the individual surgeon. Bilateral defects are usually closed one side at a time.

The management of cleft palate is more difficult. Many mothers, given the proper encouragement and support, are able to breastfeed, but some babies with large defects may be unable to suck as they cannot create the negative pressure necessary because of the palatal defect. There is in addition an increased risk of aspiration of feeds. The baby must then be taught to swallow feeds delivered to the back of the tongue. This may be done using a Habermann bottle, by cup or spoon feeding, or by using a lamb's teat wth a large hole.

Subsequent management requires a multidisciplinary approach. A plastic surgeon repairs the defect; this is often done at about the age of one year. An orthodontist makes sure that the alveolar arch

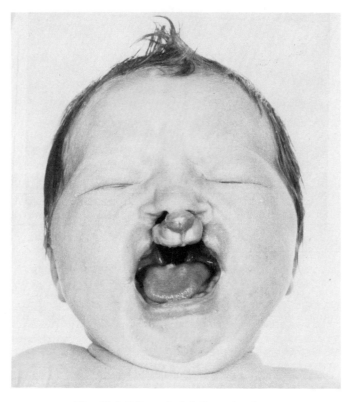

Fig. 10.2 Bilateral cleft lip and palate

develops normally with correct alignment of teeth; some recommend
fitting dental plates soon after birth to stimulate forward growth of the
upper jaw, and cover the defect to allow more efficient suction during
feeds.

A speech therapist corrects defective speech which results from the
inability to prevent air from escaping into the nose during phonation.
An ENT surgeon will be required because of the likelihood of
recurrent and frequent attacks of otitis media; these may be associated with high-frequency deafness. Adenoids should only very
rarely be removed, as they help ensure an airtight fit between the
posterior pharynx and palate. The paediatrician is responsible for
explaining to the parents what is involved and coordinating the

efforts of the other specialist members of the team. The parents will need considerable support over many years.

Congenital teeth

Normally the first dentition begin to erupt at about the age of six months. From time to time, a baby has one or more lower incisors present at birth (Fig. 10.3). They may need to be removed to prevent aspiration into the lungs or tongue ulceration.

Pierre Robin anomaly

This condition is discussed below under Respiratory system (p. 221).

Neonatal intestinal obstruction

There may be a block anywhere in the baby's bowel, from oesophagus to anus. Early diagnosis is important. The problem is best considered according to the region affected.

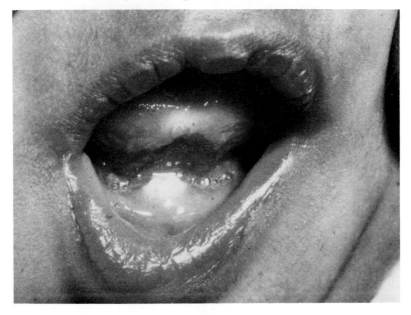

Fig. 10.3 Congenital teeth

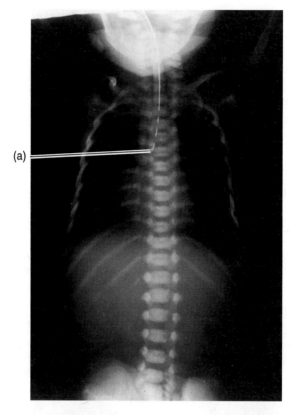

Fig. 10.4 X-ray showing oesophageal atresia without fistula. Note no air in the abdomen. Replogle tube in blind end of oesophagus (a)

Oesophageal atresia

There is usually a blind-ending oesophagus with a fistula between the upper trachea and lower oesophagus (Fig. 10.4). A number of variations may occur (Fig. 10.5).

It is important that the diagnosis is made before the first feed. If not, the feed will cause acute choking, coughing and cyanosis. If the diagnosis is still not made, dehydration, electrolyte disturbances and starvation will follow. Once lung complications have occurred, the baby's prognosis is much poorer and surgery is less successful.

Three clues should lead to the diagnosis before the first feed:

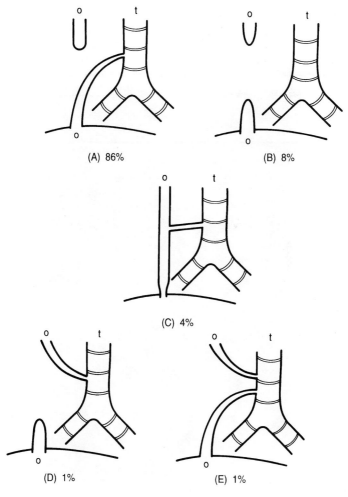

Fig. 10.5 Types and relative incidence of oesophageal atresia and tracheo-oesophageal fistula. o, oesophagus; t, trachea

1 Maternal polyhydramnios, which is present in two-thirds of cases, sometimes predisposing to preterm delivery.
2 Noisy breathing after birth with bubbly or frothy mucus regurgitating from the mouth.
3 Frequent cyanotic attacks during the early minutes and hours of life.

If the diagnosis is suspected, it can be confirmed by passing a catheter down the oesophagus. It is important not to push too hard and also to use a catheter which is not so thin that it coils up, giving the erroneous impression that the tube has passed further than it has.

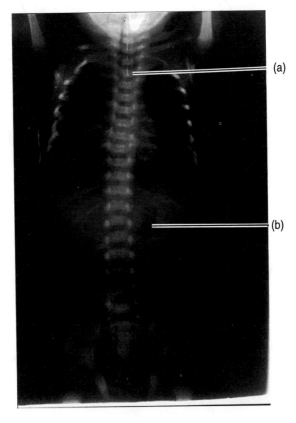

(a)

(b)

Fig. 10.6 X-ray showing oesophageal atresia with fistula. Repogle tube in oesophageal pouch (a). Note air in the abdomen (b).

In practice a size 12 FG catheter is best. In oesophageal atresia it will not pass more than 5–10 cm from the mouth. A radiograph will confirm that the tip is in the upper oesophagus (see Fig. 10.6). Confirmation may also be obtained by aspiration; the contents of the pouch contain no acid. Alternatively, a little air can be blown down the tube, and no sounds will be heard in the abdomen. The use of radio-opaque material should be avoided because of the risk of aspiration of oily material into the lungs with subsequent pneumonia.

If one congenital abnormality has been demonstrated, others are more likely to be present (Chittmittrapap et al., 1989). In the case of oesophageal atresia associated abnormalities include those of the heart, lower bowel and skeleton.

Before surgery a double lumen (Replogle) tube should be passed into the upper oesophageal segment and continuous suction applied to prevent aspiration of saliva into the lungs. This is particularly important during transfer of the baby to a surgical unit. Antibiotic cover should be given. Full-term babies in whom the diagnosis is made early often have an operation within 24 hours. Usually the fistula is closed through a right thoracotomy and in the majority of cases an end-to-end anastomosis of the two oesophageal segments can be made. Postoperative feeding is initially by gastrostomy. Preterm babies, or those diagnosed late and showing lung complications, may need to be fed intravenously or by gastrostomy before surgery is feasible. Sometimes the gap is too wide to be anastomosed at the first operation, and gastrostomy feeds need to be continued until significant growth occurs. In some cases grafts are necessary to join the two ends of the oesophagus. A transanastomotic tube may be passed through the newly repaired oesophagus at the time of surgery. The mortality among full-term babies diagnosed before the first feed is less than 2%; however, the overall survival rate is only 85%. This emphasizes the importance of early diagnosis before the first feed is given and also the worse prognosis in preterm babies.

Small and large bowel obstruction

These lesions may be considered in two groups – high and low obstructions – as the timing of onset of signs may differ in the two groups (see below). The obstruction may be within the lumen of the bowel (e.g. meconium ileus from cystic fibrosis) (Fig. 10.7), an abnormality of the bowel wall (e.g. duodenal atresia) or an extrinsic lesion constricting the bowel (e.g. peritoneal bands).

Early diagnosis is possible on the basis of findings on examination

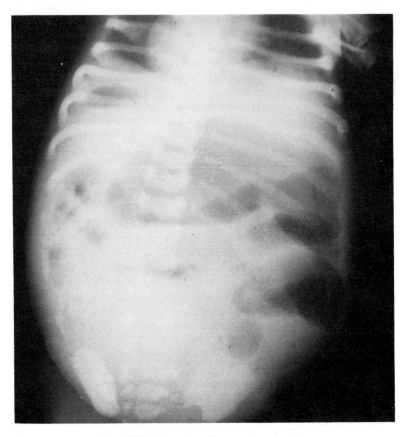

Fig. 10.7 Meconium ileus and peritonitis

at birth or subsequently, and certain pointers in the maternal or family history. A maternal history of polyhydramnios suggests the possibility of intestinal obstruction; upper bowel distension *in utero* can even be seen by ultrasound. Ganglion-blocking agents or other drugs such as methyldopa given to the mother to treat hypertension cross the placenta and may cause paralytic ileus in the baby. A family history of gastrointestinal abnormalities or cystic fibrosis may be relevant.

Early symptoms and signs are:

1 *Vomiting.* Depending on the level of lesion, the vomitus may or may not contain bile. Bile is present if the obstruction is below the bile ducts.

2 *Delayed or absent passage of meconium* (particularly in low lesions).

3 *Abdominal distension* (most noticeable with low lesions).

4 *Respiratory distress* following aspiration into the lungs (particularly with high lesions).

5 *Dehydration* with acid–base or electrolyte disturbances.

6 *Septicaemia*, particularly following bowel perforation.

As the obstruction has often been present for some time by the time of birth, bowel perforation may well have taken place *in utero*. The most useful investigation is a plain erect abdominal radiograph. This may show either fluid levels due to obstruction or air under the diaphragm if perforation has taken place. The presence of grey, inspissated meconium containing air bubbles indicates the presence of meconium ileus (Fig. 10.7). Intraperitoneal calcification indicates previous perforation and meconium peritonitis.

In *duodenal atresia* the plain abdominal radiograph is characteristic, with a double bubble of gas visible in stomach and dilated duodenum but no air below this level (Fig. 10.8).

Imperforate anus (Fig. 10.9) must always be specifically excluded by testing the patency of the anus as part of the routine examination of every newborn baby. Thus delayed diagnosis should not occur. Should this happen, the baby will present with bile-stained vomiting and abdominal distension. Meconium is not passed. Occasionally the presence of a rectovaginal or rectourethral fistula causes meconium to be passed from vagina or urethra. Sometimes the anus is covered by a triangle of skin which allows meconium to be passed.

In all these conditions the key to a successful outcome is to make the diagnosis early. Babies who develop electrolyte abnormalities or an aspiration pneumonia are much less likely to survive. In the case of imperforate anus, it is useful to know the length of terminal bowel that is absent. To demonstrate this, time must be allowed for air to reach the lower bowel (usually 24–48 hours). The infant is then suspended head downwards for several minutes and a lead marker is placed on the perineum. A plain radiograph shows gas in the blind rectal pouch and the distance between the gas and the anal skin can be estimated. The scale of the operation will, of course, depend on the length of the gap demonstrated.

In *Hirschsprung's disease* the defect is a congenital absence of

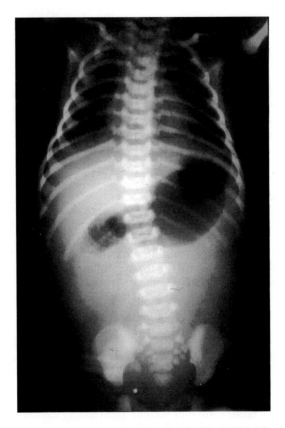

Fig. 10.8 Abdominal X-ray showing classic 'double bubble' in duodenal atresia. Note absence of gas in abdomen

ganglion cells of the myenteric parasympathetic nerve plexus of Auerbach from a segment of colon. This extends from the internal anal sphincter for a variable distance up through the rectum and often lower colon. This aganglionic segment is narrow, but there is great hypertrophy and distension of the normal colon above it. On rectal examination a tight sphincter is often found, but this is not an infallible sign. Passage of the finger often produces a rush of faeces and gas. The diagnosis is confirmed by rectal biopsy and balloon studies which show that the anal sphincter will not relax normally. With modern surgery these infants usually do extremely well, but a

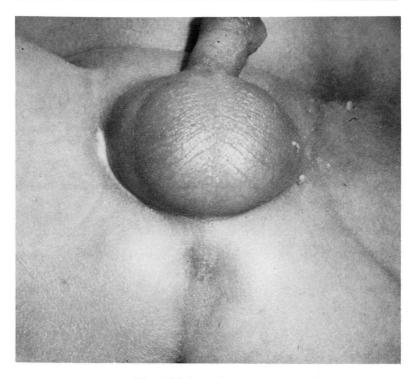

Fig. 10.9 Imperforate anus

colostomy is required to allow the abdominal distension to subside before a definitive procedure is undertaken. The most serious post-operative complications are necrotizing enterocolitis and incontinence of faeces. The characteristic presentation is delay in the first passage of meconium; a rectal examination should be done in any baby who has not passed meconium by 24 hours of age.

Diaphragmatic hernia

This condition is discussed in Chapter 3.

Exomphalos

This is a rare abnormality involving herniation of bowel and other viscera into the base of the umbilicus (Fig. 10.10) (Lafferty *et al.*,

1989). It is covered by fused layers of amnion and peritoneum, not skin. Rupture and evisceration can occur after birth with secondary infection. Associated abnormalities are present in three-quarters of the affected babies. Look out for Beckwith's syndrome: exomphalos, large tongue and internal organs, plus severe hypoglycaemia (1 in 7 affected) (see Chapter 15). Complete repair is possible when there is a small defect in an otherwise healthy baby. Larger lesions may be covered by skin to provide protection and definitive repair deferred until the peritoneal cavity is larger (by about one year of age). Alternatively a tent of inert material may be sewn over the lesion. There is a considerable mortality in those babies most severely affected. (For early management see Chapter 3.)

It is common to see babies of African descent with umbilical hernias, sometimes containing gut or omentum. The sac is completely covered by skin. No treatment is required because the hernias disappear spontaneously by about three to five years of age.

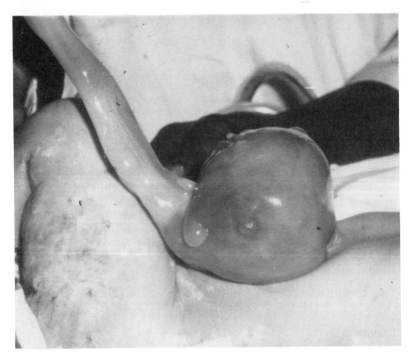

Fig. 10.10 Exomphalos

Gastroschisis

Gastroschisis is antenatal evisceration of abdominal contents through a defect to one side of a normally inserted umbilical cord (Torfs *et al.*, 1990). There is no covering membrane sac and the defect is usually small. Associated anomalies are much less frequent than with exomphalos, but resultant malrotation and intestinal atresia are common. Gastroschisis is particularly common among preterm babies, but in the best hands about three out of four babies survive surgical repair (Stoodley *et al.*, 1993). The acute management of the condition in the labour ward is described in Chapter 3.

Respiratory System

Choanal atresia

This condition is discussed in Chapter 3.

Congenital laryngeal stridor

Some babies have a low-pitched stridor on inspiration. The common variety from a soft collapsing larynx is not usually noticed until after the first week of life. Many babies have a short-lived stridor after endotracheal intubation, and if ventilated for a prolonged period, stridor may persist for many months, recurring during episodes of respiratory illness. Since there are some important, though rare, causes of stridor, such as laryngeal webs, polyps or haemangioma, direct laryngoscopy should be performed for any persistent stridor.

Pierre Robin anomaly

This consists of (Fig. 10.11):

1 Small lower jaw (micrognathia).
2 Midline cleft palate without cleft lip.
3 Glossoptosis (an abnormal attachment of the genioglossi muscles allows the normally sized tongue to fall back and block the airway, especially during feeding).

It is likely that the primary abnormality is hypoplasia of the mandibular area before the ninth week of intrauterine life. This

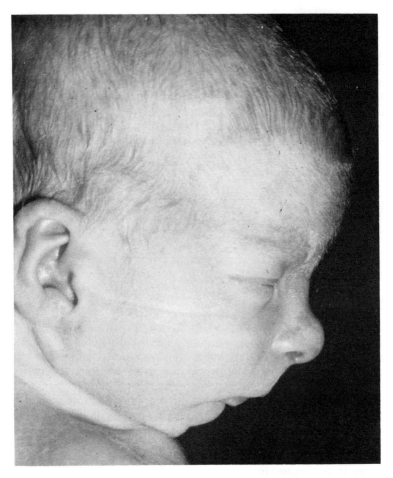

Fig. 10.11 Pierre Robin anomaly

allows the tongue to be pushed backwards and prevents the normal closure of the posterior palate.

Cyanotic and choking episodes with the risk of bronchopneumonia are prevented by nursing these babies in a prone position. Anterior fixation of the tongue surgically may sometimes be necessary. Alternatively, in some centres a dental prosthesis is used to fill in the cleft and prevent the tongue falling into the nasopharynx. The Pierre Robin anomaly is most commonly seen in otherwise normal babies. If they survive the neonatal period without episodes of hypoxia and aspiration pneumonia, the prognosis is extremely good. The retrognathia improves with time. Occasionally the anomaly is but one feature in a syndrome of multiple defects, for example, trisomy 18 (see below).

Congenital lobar emphysema

This results from a congenital abnormality of bronchial cartilage causing bronchomalacia and therefore air-trapping in the affected lobe (usually left upper lobe). The obstructive emphysema presents with rapid breathing, cough, stridor, and shortness of breath during feeds. Sometimes the significance of these symptoms is not realized for many weeks or even months as they may be attributed to recurrent chest infections if a careful history is not taken. On chest radiography there is distension of the affected lobe, with herniation across the midline and compression of remaining lung tissue. Treatment is by resection of the affected lobe.

Potter's syndrome

This name is used for babies whose mothers had oligohydramnios, usually because the baby had passed very little urine *in utero*, for example due to renal agenesis. There is amnion nodosum, small nodules of desquamated skin on the fetal surface of the placenta. The baby has a squashed face (Fig. 10.12) with a flattened nose and

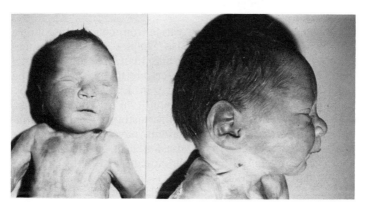

Fig. 10.12 Potter's syndrome (renal agenesis)

grooves below the eyes. Other compression effects are seen, such as talipes equinovarus and dislocation of the hips. The baby often dies immediately after birth because the lungs do not grow normally in such fetuses (pulmonary hypoplasia) and resuscitation is therefore impossible.

Central Nervous System

Neural tube defects

The nervous tissue in the embryo forms as a neural plate and then a tube which develops from the head downwards and is complete by the fourth week of intrauterine life. The spinal cord is derived from the surface of the embryo (neuroectoderm). The meninges and vertebral column come from tissue below the surface (mesenchyme) (Moore, 1988).

A bifid lumbosacral vertebra occurs in 10% of the normal population. There is no underlying abnormality of meninges or spinal cord and the condition is known as spina bifida occulta. Its presence may be marked by an overlying patch of hair, lipoma, naevus, dermal sinus or other abnormality, usually minor.

In contrast, spina bifida cystica occurs when there is protrusion and dysplasia of the meninges only (meningocele) (6%) or of meninges and spinal cord (myelomeningocele) (94%). These are much more serious conditions and are colloquially referred to as spina bifida (Fig. 10.13). A myelomeningocele is usually accompanied by neurological signs.

The incidence of the condition varies from country to country and regionally within countries (see also Chapter 9). For example, it is much commoner in Ireland and Wales than in south-east England. Both genetic and environmental factors are thought to play a part in its aetiology. The overall incidence in England and Wales has dropped over the past decade to about 1 in 5000 total births. The risk increases when there is a family history of babies born with neural tube defects. When the parents have already had a child with a neural defect they have about a 1 in 20 chance of having another such baby and of these approximately half will have anencephaly and half spina bifida. The risk is higher in some areas. When the parents have had two affected children the risk is 1 in 8.

The defect is always in the midline. It may be anywhere from the head (encephalocele) to the sacrum (Fig. 10.14). Defects are com-

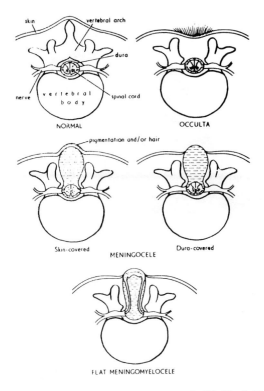

Fig. 10.13 Various forms of spina bifida. From S. Wallis & D. Harvey (1979) *Nursing Times* by permission of the authors and editor

monest in the lumbosacral region. This is probably because it is this area which, embryologically, is the last to form the neural tube by fusion of the neural plate. A sac of variable size is then seen on the baby's back (Fig. 10.15). It is covered by a thin neuroepithelium (arachnoid membrane) rather than skin, with neural tissue on the surface. Many myelomeningoceles do not have a sac at all, so the spinal cord is exposed and only about 15% of spina bifida are closed by a membrane.

The natural history of such lesions is that the sac becomes infected within a few days or months of birth with meningitis and eventual death. Thus until about 30 years ago such lesions were almost always fatal. Only about 5% survived the first year, the lesion becoming

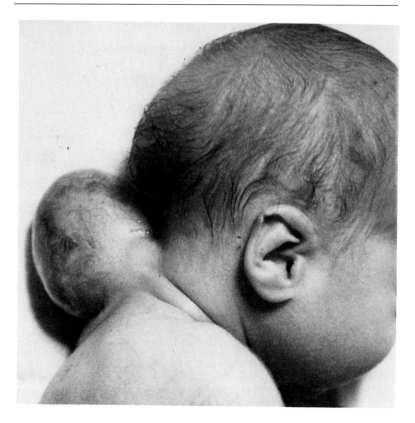

Fig. 10.14 Cervical meningocele

covered by skin within the first few months. During the 1960s it was found that early closure of the defect surgically (within 24 hours of birth) would prevent the onset of meningitis and death.

Many of these surgically treated infants have considerable further problems:

1 There is often extensive flaccid paralysis, depending on the level of the lesion, with associated sensory loss. Such children are therefore often confined to wheelchairs.
2 There is commonly dribbling incontinence of urine without normal control due to loss of parasympathetic outflow to the bladder. The anal sphincters are similarly affected with resulting incontinence of faeces. There is a high incidence of ureteric reflex and ascending

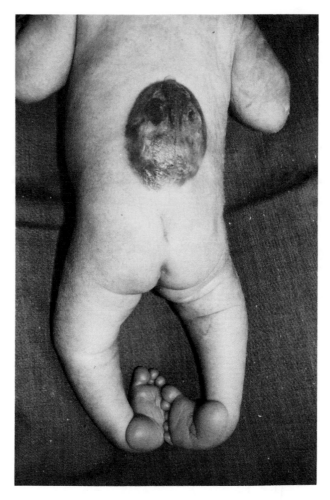

Fig. 10.15 Myelomeningocele with bilateral severe talipes

urinary tract infection resulting in renal damage and eventual renal failure. To prevent this, many urological operations are necessary.
3 Hydrocephalus is commonly associated; it is present in about 75% of babies with myelomeningocele. It is due to the so-called Arnold–Chiari malformation which is a protrusion of the cerebellum through the foramen magnum at the base of the skull (Fig. 10.16). This causes

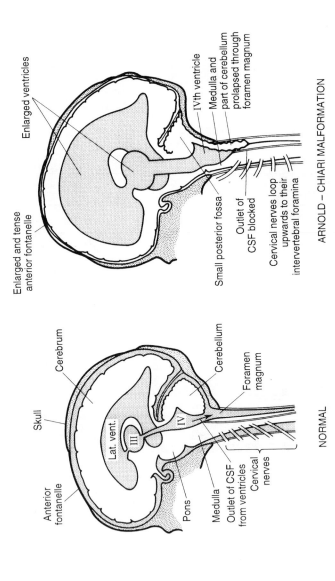

Enlarged ventricles

Enlarged and tense anterior fontanelle

IVth ventricle

Medulla and part of cerebellum prolapsed through foramen magnum

Small posterior fossa

Outlet of CSF blocked

Cervical nerves loop upwards to their intervertebral foramina

ARNOLD – CHIARI MALFORMATION

Cerebrum

Skull

Cerebellum

Foramen magnum

Lat. vent.

III

IV

Anterior fontanelle

Pons

Medulla

Outlet of CSF from ventricles

Cervical nerves

NORMAL

Fig. 10.16 Normal circulation of the cerebrospinal fluid and the development of hydrocephalus following obstruction of the circulation by the Arnold–Chiari malformation. From S. Wallis & D. Harvey (1979) *Nursing Times* by permission of the author and editor

obstruction to the downward flow of cerebrospinal fluid (CSF) so that its pressure rises within the head. To allow CSF to circulate freely, shunt operations were devised but they have a significant morbidity. Severe mental handicap is also often present.

4 Orthopaedic deformities, for example kyphoscoliosis, congenital dislocation of the hips and talipes equinovarus (Fig. 10.15), are common in this condition and may require many operations for their correction.

It is felt by many that the quality of life of these children is extremely poor. For this reason the policy of automatic operation was reviewed.

A decision should be made at birth about the baby's prognosis. Criteria, following the work of Lorber in Sheffield (1971), have been developed to enable a more rational decision to be made. Meningocele has a very good prognosis. The presence of any of the following adverse factors increases the chance of early death or poor quality of life and would tend to make the paediatrician advise against surgery for a myelomeningocele:

1 Flaccid paralysis of the lower limbs, often with urinary incontinence with dribbling and a patulous anus.
2 Hydrocephalus (defined as 2 cm above the 90th centile for the baby's gestational age).
3 Other congenital abnormalities.
4 Kyphosis.
5 Large lesions (more than 5 cm in diameter).
6 High lesions (thoracolumbar or higher).
7 Meningitis.

It now seems that a very early decision regarding the need for surgery may not be as crucial as used to be thought. When a decision is made that immediate surgery is not indicated, it is usual to avoid other active treatment such as antibiotics. Such babies should be kept warm, fed and free from pain but they will probably die within days or weeks. It is kindest to feed the baby on demand and sedation may be appropriate. Strong analgesia is often required. Some babies do not die; this must be explained to the parents before any decision is made. A number of parents make the decision to take the baby home. A baby may need an operation later, either to correct hydrocephalus or to make nursing easier by closing the back.

Parents must be fully informed about the prognosis for their baby. It seems wrong, however, to expect them to make a decision for or against surgery. This is made by the paediatrician in consultation with the parents. A decision should be proposed which they are free to accept or reject, but in their emotional state of grief and anxiety the onus of treating or not treating should not be placed on their shoulders. In this way we hope to reduce the strength of parental guilt feelings when the baby does die.

Those children who undergo surgery will require prolonged follow-up by the paediatrician, neurosurgeon, urologist, orthopaedic surgeon and psychiatrist acting as a team. The parents will also require a great deal of support.

These agonizing decisions now have to be made less commonly. The birth of a baby with spina bifida is now preventable provided the parents are willing to accept termination of pregnancy. The amniotic fluid surrounding babies with open spina bifida or anencephaly contains raised concentrations of alpha-fetoprotein (AFP). AFP can also be measured in maternal blood, so screening of the whole maternal population is now possible, and this is done between 16 and 18 weeks gestation. This unfortunately means two visits to clinic or hospital early in pregnancy; the earlier (at about 12–14 weeks) is for booking and taking blood for basic serology. An ultrasound scan is often performed at this visit to assess the gestation. If abnormally high levels of AFP are found, the patient is examined by ultrasound again to exclude wrong gestation, multiple pregnancy, fetal death or anencephaly. It is often possible to scan the back for spina bifida. An amniocentesis is performed for estimation of AFP when two samples suggest a high plasma AFP concentration. Clearly not every pregnant mother should have an amniocentesis, since the procedure carries at least a 1% risk of subsequent abortion and a small increased risk of respiratory distress and congenital abnormalities (congenital disloca-tion of the hips or talipes equinovarus), but where there is a family history of the condition it should be carried out. If amniotic fluid is obtained for another reason, for example to do a chromosome analysis, the AFP concentrations should always be measured.

Anticholinesterase levels are now also measured on amniotic fluid. Raised levels are found in open spina bifida. If AFP or anticholines-terase levels in the amniotic fluid are high, termination of pregnancy may be offered as the fetus is very likely to have a neural-tube defect. A few other conditions may give rise to high levels of AFP in blood and amniotic fluid. As these are all extremely serious, there is little risk of terminating normal babies or babies with only minor abnorm-alities. Real-time ultrasound is useful in assessing movements of the legs and in allowing a lesion to be seen *in utero* (Campbell & Pearce, 1983).

Recent controlled trials have shown that some cases of neural tube defect can be prevented by multivitamin supplementation of the mother before conception (Czeizel, 1993).

Cardiovascular System

Congenital heart disease is discussed in Chapter 11.

Single umbilical artery

After delivery, the vessels should be counted on the cut end of the cord. There are normally two small thick-walled arteries pouting above the cut surface and one large thin-walled vein. Sometimes (in about 0.5% of all deliveries) a single artery is present. About one-third of these babies have congenital malformations, especially of the gut (e.g. oesophageal atresia or imperforate anus), heart or kidneys. Such babies should therefore be examined carefully for detectable lesions and observed closely during the newborn period for signs such as heart murmurs or those of urinary tract infections. It is now usual to perform a renal ultrasound scan on all babies with a single umbilical artery.

Skeletal System

Congenital dislocation of the hip

A check for dislocated hips is one of the most important parts of the routine examination of the newborn. Repeated checks are necessary, but even so it is likely that not every case can be diagnosed during the newborn period. Those not detected may not present until toddler age when the child will walk with a limp, or may be diagnosed during later checks in infancy by finding limited abduction of the thigh. Treatment of those diagnosed late is much less satisfactory and involves orthopaedic operations. Diagnosis during the newborn period and treatment by splinting is often successful in saving the baby from surgery and a possibly permanent disability.

Congenital dislocation is commoner in girls, following breech presentations or oligohydramnios, and, for reasons that are

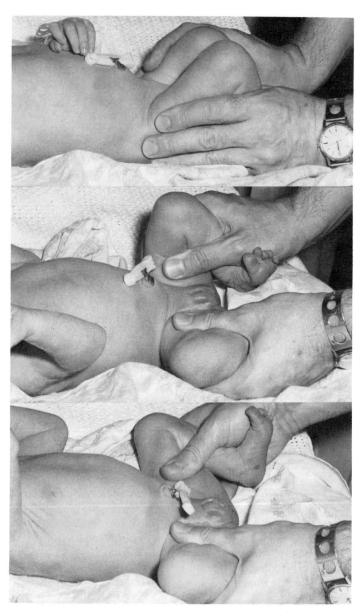

Fig. 10.17 Examination of the hips to exclude congenital dislocation

unknown, in the left hip. It seems that such things as the amount of amniotic fluid and intrauterine posture are relevant to the aetiology.

The diagnosis is made as follows (Fig. 10.17): the baby is laid supine with the feet facing the examiner on a flat surface. The legs are grasped with the thumbs along the inner side of the thigh and the middle fingers over the greater trochanters. The bent knees are held comfortably in the palm of the examiner's hands. Each hip is tested individually. The hip is gradually abducted while the middle finger presses upwards on the greater trochanter. If a hip is dislocated it will be felt to 'clunk'; this must not be confused with the much more commonly detected tendinous click which does not represent true dislocation. Further signs of true dislocation are that the dislocatable hip will not abduct fully and that the skin creases over the thighs are asymmetrical. These signs are often absent in the newborn.

Radiographs are usually unhelpful until five months of age when the femoral heads have calcified. Ultrasound scanning of the femoral head (Fig. 10.18) will detect abnormalities of the acetabulum and whether the femoral head is displaced or dislocated. Many now feel that this could be done routinely in the newborn, but this would require considerable resources. A selective policy of scanning high

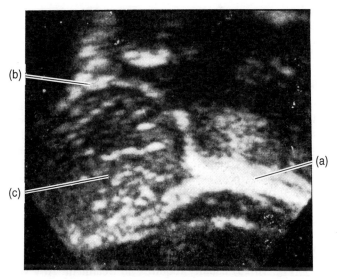

Fig. 10.18 Normal ultrasound scan of head of femur (a) showing femoral head in socket (b) in acetabulum (c).

risk groups is usually applied – breech presentation, positive family history, or where there is any clinical abnormality on examination. When a dislocatable or dislocated hip is confirmed, the baby's legs should be kept in abduction by the use of a brace or harness. An orthopaedic opinion will be needed as early as possible.

Talipes

This type of club foot (see Fig. 4.8) is not uncommonly seen in newborn babies. Usually the foot is plantar flexed (equinus) and inverted (varus). Less commonly the foot is dorsiflexed (calcaneous) and everted (valgus). Both deformities probably derive from mechanical pressure *in utero* and if the foot can be over-corrected into the opposite position easily the defect is said to be 'positional' and will get better without treatment. If correction is not possible by manipulation a permanent deformity may result if treatment is not started as soon as possible. In this case an orthopaedic opinion should be sought urgently. Initial treatment is usually by manipulation which can be taught to the parents by the physiotherapist. Careful follow-up will detect those babies who require operations to produce a satisfactory result.

Talipes is a common finding in severe myelomeningocele and a quick check of the back should always be made in case a cystic lesion there has been overlooked.

Extra digits

Extra digits are quite common in babies whose parents come from the West Indies and they have an autosomal dominant inheritance. The fingers vary in size from tiny bumps to miniature fingers with a nail (Fig. 10.19). They are almost always attached to the ulnar side of the hand. If there is a tiny pedicle, the finger can be tied off with silk. The finger then becomes gangrenous and drops off. When there is a thick base, a formal removal by a surgeon is necessary. Analogous deformities may occur in the feet.

Syndactyly

Syndactyly (Fig. 10.20) usually requires no treatment. Any webbing of the fingers will need attention by a plastic surgeon. In some cases, all, or almost all, of the digits are joined together. This may be

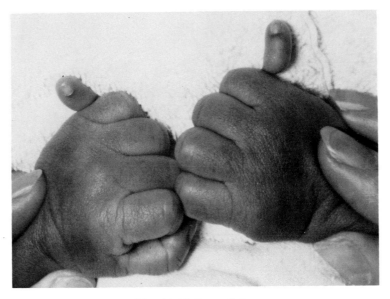

Fig. 10.19 Extra digits

associated with other congenital abnormalities, for example in Apert's syndrome, which includes cleft palate and craniofacial synostosis.

Skin

Birth marks

These are blemishes on the baby's skin and are present at birth or from a few days afterwards. They are a common source of concern to the infant's parents (Thomas *et al.*, 1992).

Local blood vessel malformations. There are three types of abnormality involving localized malformation of blood vessels in the skin.

1 *Naevus simplex* ('stork bite') is so common that it could be considered normal. It consists of a pink capillary haemangioma on the upper eyelids, in a V shape on the forehead, on the nose and upper lip or often at the back of the head just above the hair-line. The marks almost always disappear within the first year but, even if not, are

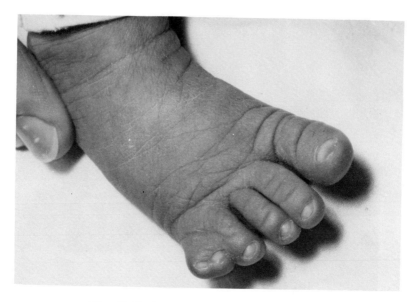

Fig. 10.20 An extra digit with syndactyly

nearly always practically invisible. Those on the nape of the neck do not fade but are covered by hair.

2 *Port-wine stains* are very different from simple lesions in their poor prognosis. Although they are capillary haemangiomata, they are much denser and better defined, as well as being larger and blue or purple in appearance. Unfortunately they are permanent. Treatment in later life has been revolutionized by laser treatment, although not all lesions respond equally well. A plastic surgeon will give advice. Port-wine stains of one side of the head and face (usually confined to one branch of the fifth cranial nerve) are particularly serious as they are often associated with a similar underlying abnormality of the meningeal coverings of the brain. These intracranial haemangiomata may give rise to fits on the opposite side of the body. This combination of port-wine stain and fits is known as the Sturge–Weber syndrome.

3 *Strawberry naevi* are also capillary haemangiomata but, because they are more cavernous in nature, are usually raised above the level of the surrounding skin, looking like small strawberries (Plate V). They are not obvious at birth, but appear only during the early days or weeks of life. They start as tiny flattened lesions which escape notice.

They can occur on any part of the body and there are often many lesions. They continue to grow during the early months of life, but gradually they begin to epithelialize from the middle, becoming bluer and then whiter, and gradually flatter and fading away altogether. As they nearly always disappear on their own without treatment before the age of about five years, they are best left untreated. Surgical excision always leaves a scar and may be hazardous as quite large blood vessels are sometimes involved. The only indication for surgery is for those which press on vital organs such as the eye. Some are easily abraded and are commonly rubbed, causing bleeding and secondary infection. In other cases bleeding from lesions is uncommon and usually insignificant. Occasionally, it may be necessary to reduce the growth of the rapidly expanding lesion with steroids. Very rarely, in the case of enormous naevi, coagulation occurs in the naevus and thrombocytopenia may result.

Pigmented naevi (common brown moles) are less often a source of concern to the parents; they will often have many such small lesions themselves. They usually grow with the infant and are permanent. Some hairy moles can be very big and unsightly. They are difficult to treat by surgery when they are large, but abrasion produces impressive results. When they occur over the scalp there are sometimes lesions on the meninges.

'Mongolian' blue spot (see Plate I). These spots are found on babies of African or Asian descent. They appear as poorly defined blueish areas of pigmentation which are described as being confined to the sacral area. In practice they are often multiple and may extend well up the back or even on to the shoulders and limbs. It is important to recognize such lesions for what they are, as at first glance they look rather like areas of bruising. It has not been unknown for parents to come under suspicion of having caused non-accidental injuries to their infants when such lesions have been misdiagnosed at routine follow-up examinations. The lesions usually become less obvious as the babies grow.

Remember that many parents tend to brood about what, to the doctor, may seem to be trivial blemishes. These worries must be appreciated and full reassurance given. For advice on talking to the parents of the more severely handicapped or abnormal child, see Chapter 19.

Milia

These are small white sebaceous spots present on the nose, forehead or cheeks of practically every newborn baby. They are harmless and gradually disappear.

Toxic erythema (urticaria of the newborn)

This rash is common in babies after the first 48 hours of life. It usually disappears by seven to ten days. At first, the lesions are white papules with a red flare, as if the baby has been stung by a nettle, but they then develop a central yellow vesicle like a pustule. They seem to be rare in the preterm baby. They are most frequent on the trunk, followed by the face. Occasionally severe examples may be confused with infected pustules, but the lesions characteristically change their position within a few hours and scrapings from the central spot show eosinophils rather than organisms or pus cells. No treatment, other than explanation, is necessary.

Genitourinary System

Hypospadias

In babies with hypospadias, the external urethral meatus opens on the ventral aspect of the penis (glans or shaft) or on the perineum (see Fig. 4.6). In the worst cases, the scrotum is bifid and the sex of the genitalia may look ambiguous. When necessary surgical repair is carried out in several stages during the second or third years of life. Such babies should not be circumcised as the surgeon requires the redundant foreskin to fashion a urethral passage.

At birth, some babies look as if they have been inexpertly circumcised. On closer inspection they are found to have a mild degree of glandular hypospadias. The penis may be bent (chordee) (Fig. 10.21), but do not make the diagnosis before an erection has been seen, as the penis may straighten properly. Some babies in this group do not require surgery. Others, and some of those in the more severe groups, may require an operation soon after birth for correction of chordee and meatotomy for meatal stenosis.

Before surgery is contemplated for the perineo-scrotal type of severe hypospadias, the baby's karyotype should be checked. In

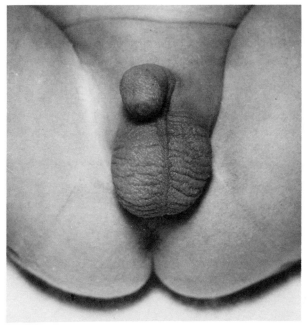

Fig. 10.21 Chordee

this way, the occasional girl virilized *in utero* due to congenital adrenal hyperplasia will not be misdiagnosed (see below).

Congenital adrenal hyperplasia (CAH)

This is due to an enzyme defect which interferes with the synthesis of cortisol in the adrenal glands. This leads to overproduction of adrenocorticotrophic hormone (ACTH) by the pituitary gland because cortisol does not inhibit the hypothalamus or pituitary from producing it in excessive amounts. Abnormal steroids are formed by the uncontrolled stimulation of the gland by ACTH (Fig. 10.22). The commonest variety is 21-hydroxylase deficiency which occurs in about 1 in 5000 live births. The lack of the enzyme leads to hormones (androgens) being produced which masculinize the female fetus and infant (ambiguous genitalia) (Fig. 10.23). There is no obvious change in boys in the newborn period. Some of these infants cannot make the hormone aldosterone and therefore cannot retain

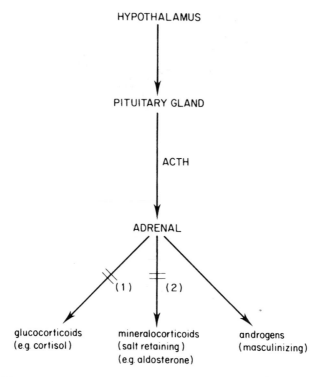

Fig. 10.22 Congenital adrenal hyperplasia. (1) A block in cortisol biosynthesis, often associated with (2) a block in aldosterone biosynthesis. Raised ACTH levels thus result in raised adrenal androgen levels (see text)

salt. They become dehydrated, hyponatraemic and hyperkalaemic within the first few weeks of life – the so-called salt-losing crisis. Two clues to the diagnosis are therefore ambiguous genitalia in a female infant or a salt-losing crisis during the early weeks of life. A family history of CAH or of any unexplained neonatal death should also be sought. Most babies who present with dehydration will be losing fluid into the gut due, for example, to gastroenteritis. Sodium loss in the urine may be due to a renal problem or to CAH. A useful distinction is that there is hyperkalaemia and low aldosterone levels in CAH – they will be high in renal disease. An ultrasound scan of the renal tract will provide valuable information whilst the results of electrolyte and hormone levels are awaited. Treatment of the salt-losing crisis is a matter of urgency; this is best done by simple salt

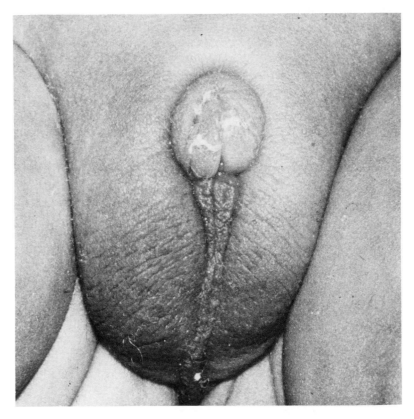

Fig. 10.23 Ambiguous genitalia in a female infant with congenital adrenal hyperplasia

replacement. Once this has been achieved, full investigation and diagnosis can be made. Long-term replacement steroid therapy is then necessary. In 21-hydroxylase deficiency a useful clue to the diagnosis is a very high plasma concentration of 17-hydroxyprogesterone. A male baby without the salt-losing tendency may not be diagnosed until later childhood when he is tall, growing abnormally rapidly and showing signs of precocious sexual development. His ultimate height prognosis is, by then, very poor. It is possible to screen for the 21-hydroxylase deficient form of CAH by measuring 17-hydroxyprogesterone levels on the Guthrie test card blood spots.

This would both prevent this problem and give advance warning of an affected male baby who might develop a salt-losing crisis.

Partially virilized female infants usually require surgery to reduce the size of the clitoris, while retaining the nerve and blood supply to the glans, during the first year of life.

Rarer forms of CAH may present with inadequate virilization in male babies, or with hypertension – the chromosomes should always be checked in any baby with ambiguous genitalia as it is usually not possible by clinical examination to tell the genotypic sex of the baby. To make a definite diagnosis and to provide proper management, these babies must be referred to a centre of paediatric endocrinology.

Groin and scrotal swellings

1 *Inguinal hernias* are common in the preterm baby, particularly males. They seldom strangulate during the first few weeks of life,

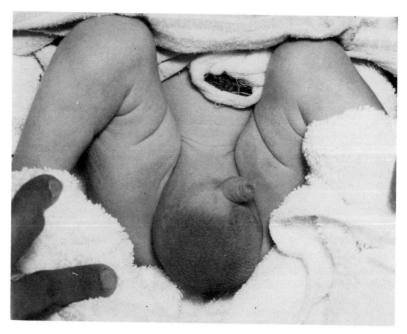

Fig. 10.24 Bilateral hydroceles

but almost never disappear spontaneously. They are best treated electively by herniotomy before the baby is discharged home.

2 *Hydrocele* (Fig. 10.24) (which, unlike an inguinal hernia, cannot be reduced and which transilluminates), almost never needs treatment and resolves spontaneously over the succeeding months.

3 *Undescended testes* may cause a swelling in the groin (see p. 82).

Torsion of the testis

A testis may twist at any time during life, including the antenatal period. Acute torsion may be suspected when there is a red, swollen and tender scrotum. The testis is enlarged and feels unusually firm or hard. It can be difficult to differentiate this from epididymitis. When torsion is suspected, a surgical opinion must be obtained at once, since viability of the testis can only be ensured by surgery. A hard, non-tender testis may indicate a previous torsion; ultrasound examination will help to differentiate this from other testicular swellings such as tumours. If torsion occurs in one testis, the other testis should be secured surgically since there is a higher risk of torsion on that side as well.

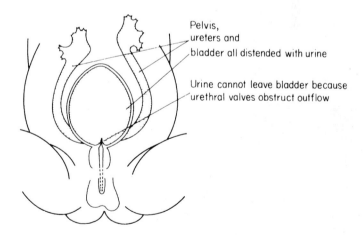

Pelvis, ureters and bladder all distended with urine

Urine cannot leave bladder because urethral valves obstruct outflow

Fig. 10.25 Urethral valves, an important cause of hydronephrosis in boys. Note the distended bladder, ureters and kidney pelvices. From S. Wallis & D. Harvey (1979) (*Nursing Times*) by permission of the authors and editor

Urethral valves

These valves occur nearly always in male infants. They obstruct the outflow of urine from the bladder causing bladder, and sometimes renal, enlargement at birth (Fig. 10.25). For this reason it is always important to palpate these organs at the routine postnatal examination. The baby has a poor stream (dribbling) or may develop urinary tract infections. The diagnosis may be investigated by ultrasound or cystography. Rather as in cystic fibrosis, the earlier the presentation the worse the prognosis, but the obstruction should be relieved surgically as soon as the diagnosis is made so as to minimize renal damage from infections and back pressure. If they are discovered during the pregnancy prenatal surgery may be carried out. A pig-tailed catheter is inserted from the bladder to the amniotic fluid, bypassing the valve (Kullendorff *et al.*, 1984).

Phimosis

Phimosis seems to be an imaginary congenital abnormality. There are no surgical, as opposed to social and religious, indications for circumcision in the newborn period. Unless parents hold strong

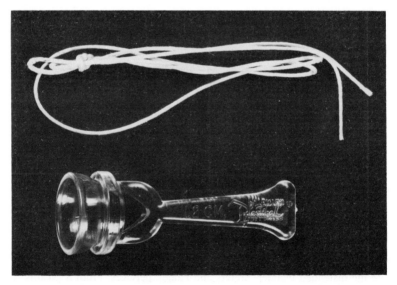

Fig. 10.26 The Plastibell for neonatal circumcision (*Hollister*)

religious convictions, it is worthwhile taking time to try and dissuade them from inflicting an unnecessary operation on their son. The operation carries a definite, although small, morbidity and mortality from anaesthesia, haemorrhage or infection.

Circumcision was often carried out without anaesthetic in the first two weeks of life using the plastic bell technique (Fig. 10.26) which reduces risks of haemorrhage. The baby, however, experiences considerable pain during the procedure so, at the very least, local anaesthesia is essential. After the neonatal period the operation is best delayed at least until two years of age when the risks from general anaesthesia are extremely small.

Chromosomal Abnormalities

Down syndrome

Down syndrome is associated with an extra chromosome 21 (see Fig. 2.7). It occurs in nearly 2 per 1000 live births and is the commonest cause of learning difficulties (IQ 50 or less) in the UK, accounting for about one-third of such children.

The incidence of the condition seems to be related to ageing of the maternal oocyte. Thus a woman below the age of 25 years has less than a 1 in 2000 chance of giving birth to a baby with Down syndrome whereas a woman over 45 years has about a 1 in 50 chance (Fig. 10.27).

The physical features of babies with Down syndrome are very characteristic so that the mother may sometimes make the diagnosis at the delivery. The name mongolism was given to these babies because of the superficial resemblance that they have to oriental people, with almond-shaped eyes that slant upwards and outwards and inner epicanthic folds (Fig. 10.28). The term is offensive and should not be used. Down syndrome babies from oriental races look very similar to those in the West. Some oriental paediatricians have even called them 'international children' because they are the same in all parts of the world.

Other features of babies with Down syndrome include: marked hypotonia, which is in many ways the most characteristic feature; a skull flattened from front to back (brachycephaly) with a particularly flat occiput and a thin neck; a small mouth with a tongue that commonly protrudes (the tongue is of normal size, unlike the large tongue of the cretin, and protrudes because the mouth is small); the

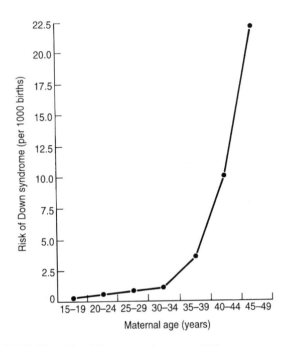

Fig. 10.27 The risk of Down syndrome at different maternal ages

eyes commonly show speckling of the iris (Brushfield spots); broad hands with short fingers and a particularly short incurving little finger (clinodactyly); classically the palm shows a single (simian) crease and abnormalities of the dermal ridge patterns; and a wide fissure between the first and second toes (Fig. 10.29). Associated features include congenital heart disease, particularly ostium primum atrial septal defect and ventricular septal defect, and also gastrointestinal anomalies such as oesophageal atresia, duodenal atresia or imperforate anus.

Most babies with Down syndrome have a triradius in the middle of the palm instead of the base of the hand. An auriscope is the best instrument for inspecting the hand.

It may be difficult to make an accurate clinical diagnosis in the first week. A chromosomal analysis must always be performed. Although children with Down syndrome are usually mentally handicapped, they are generally happy and affectionate children. They may, however, place a considerable burden on their parents, particularly once

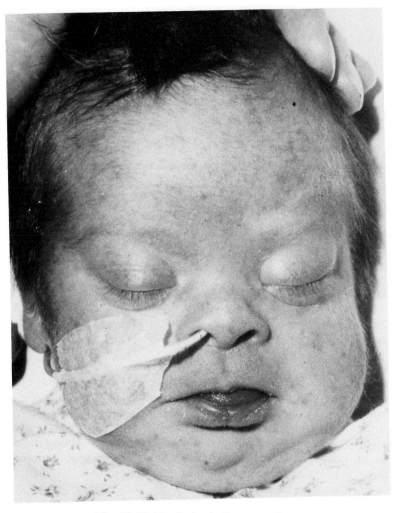

Fig. 10.28 The facies in Down syndrome

they progress from the baby stage. The timing of telling the parents of the diagnosis and its implications cannot be rigidly laid down. In general, it is best to tell them early, and both together if possible.

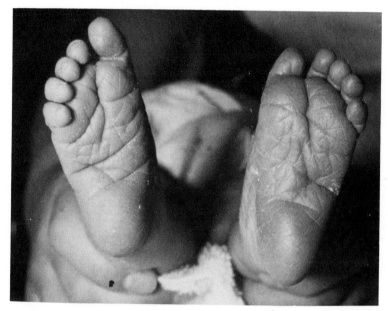

Fig. 10.29 The feet in Down syndrome

Other trisomies

Trisomy 18 (Edwards syndrome)

In this syndrome, the extra chromosome is number 18 (Fig. 10.30). It is much less common than trisomy 21 and the condition is often lethal during the early weeks of life. Characteristic features include a long narrow skull, low and malformed ears, prominent heels giving rise to the 'rocker-bottom' feet, and a short chest with broad spaced nipples (Fig. 10.31). Congenital heart disease is almost universal and is usually the immediate cause of death.

Trisomy 13 (Patau syndrome)

The extra chromosome is chromosome 13. The head is abnormal, with low-set malformed ears, and there are cardiac anomalies. A characteristic feature is the cleft lip and palate. There may also be extra digits. Severe mental retardation is universal.

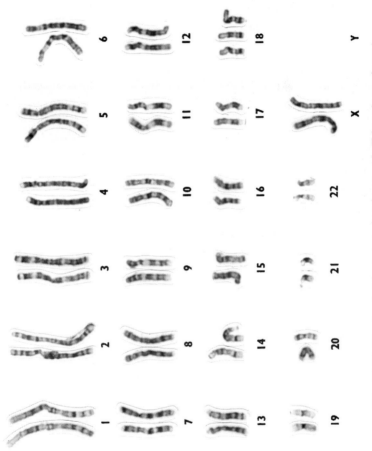

Fig. 10.30 The banded karyotype in trisomy 18 (Edwards syndrome)

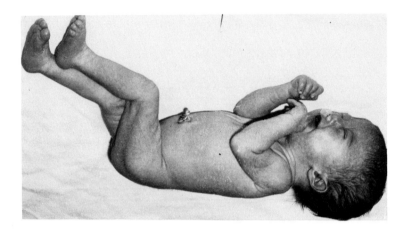

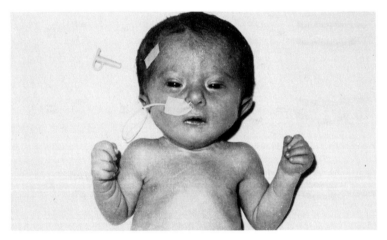

Fig. 10.31 A baby with trisomy 18 (Edwards syndrome)

Cri-du-chat syndrome

This is due to a partial deletion of the short arm of chromosome 5. The name derives from the kitten-like cry which these babies have during the newborn period. They may lose this feature as they get older. They usually have small heads (microcephaly) and congenital heart defects. A related condition due to partial deletion of the short arm of chromosome 4, is known as Wolf syndrome. These two syndromes have many features in common but in Wolf syndrome convulsions are a particular feature and may be very resistant to treatment with anticonvulsants.

Sex chromosome abnormalities

The sex chromosome anomaly which may be diagnosed in the newborn period is Turner syndrome: in this condition, which is confined to females, there is only one female sex chromosome. This usually results in streak ovaries and infertility. Diagnostic features in the newborn period include congenital lymphoedema of the extremities, redundant skin around the neck, and a low birth weight for the baby's gestational age.

References and Further Reading

See also References and Further Reading in Chapter 9.

Campbell, S. & Pearce, J.M. (1983) Ultrasound visualisation of structural anomolies. *Brit. Med. Bull.*, *39*, 322.

Chittmittrapap, S., Spitz, L., Kiely, E.M. *et al.* (1989) Oesophageal atresia and associated anomolies. *Arch. Dis. Child.*, *64*, 364.

Cunningham, C. (1982) *Down's Syndrome: an Introduction for Parents.* London: Souvenir Press.

Kenner, C.A. *et al.* (1988) *Neonatal Surgery: A Nursing Perspective.* Grune & Stratton.

Kullendorff, C.M., Larsson, L.T. & Jorgensen, C. (1984) Advantages of antenatal diagnosis of intestinal and urinary malformations. *Brit. J. Obstet. Gynaecol.*, *91*, 144–147.

Lafferty, P.M., Emmerson, A.J., Fleming, P.J. *et al.* (1989) Anterior abdominal wall defects. *Arch. Dis. Child.*, *64*, 1029–1031.

Lorber, J. (1971) Results of treatment of meningomyelocele. *Developmental Medicine and Child Neurology*, *13*, 279.

Manchester, D., Stewart, J. & Sujansky, E. (1991) Genetics and dysmorphology. In *Current Pediatric Diagnosis and Treatment*, 10th ed., pp. 1016–1049, ed. Hathaway, W., Groothius, J., Hay, W. & Paisley, J. Norwalk: Appleton & Lange.

Millard, D.M. (1984) *Daily Living with a Handicapped Child.* London: Croom Helm.

Moore, K.L. (1988) *The Developing Human: Clinically Orientated Embryology.* Philadelphia: W.B. Saunders.

Morgan, B. & Wright, M. (1986) *Essentials of Plastic and Reconstructive Surgery.* Mosby.

Smith, J.E., Christoff, B. & Zukowsky, K. (1993) Congenital abnormalities. In *Core Curriculum for Maternal–Newborn Nursing*, pp. 744–778, ed. Mattson, S. & Smith, J.E. Philadelphia: W.B. Saunders.

Stoodley, N., Sharma, A., Noblett, H. *et al.* (1993) Influence of place of delivery on outcome in babies with gastroschisis. *Arch. Dis. Child.*, *68*, 321–323.

Thomas, R. & Harvey, D. (1992) *Neoenatology*. Colour Guide Series. Edinburgh: Churchill Livingstone.

Torfs, C., Curry, C. & Roeper, P. (1990) Gastroschisis. *J. Pediatr.*, *116*, 1–6.

Weston, M.J., Andrews, H.S., Smoleniec, J.S. *et al.* (1991) Multidisciplinary approach to the management of fetal anomalies. In *Proceedings of the Annual Meeting of RCR*, p. 102. Dublin.

Whittle, M.J. & Connor, J.M. (1990) *Prenatal Diagnosis in Obstetric Practice*. Oxford: Blackwell Scientific.

—11

Congenital Heart Disease

Babies with heart disease may present difficult clinical problems during the first week of life. A deeply blue baby may have cyanotic congenital heart disease, but this is often difficult to distinguish from a lung problem such as meconium aspiration with persistence of the fetal circulation. Some remarkable circulatory changes occur normally at birth and it is important to understand these changes if one is to attempt a diagnostic approach to congenital heart disease.

Changes in the Circulation at Birth

A large part of cardiac output *in utero* (Fig. 11.1) is directed towards the placenta to allow gas exchange. The two umbilical arteries come from the internal iliac arteries, pass around the pelvis and up the abdominal wall to the umbilicus where they spiral through the umbilical cord to the placenta. Carbon dioxide is excreted across the placenta into the mother where her respiration holds the partial pressure of carbon dioxide (P_{CO_2}) at the same level in both the fetus' blood and her own blood; the value is around 5.5 kPa (40 mmHg). Oxygen passes across the placenta from the mother into the fetus. The mother's blood supply to the uterus flows into a lake of blood in the deciduum of the uterus with villi from the placenta in this lake. The oxygen passes across the placental membranes into capillaries and thence into the umbilical vein. This vein is, therefore, one of the few in the body that contains oxygenated blood. The vein spirals with the arteries in the umbilical cord and from the umbilicus passes upwards and backwards to join the portal vein underneath the liver. In adult life, the portal vein flows to the liver, but this organ can be bypassed in fetal life by a vein known as the ductus venosus, which connects the portal vein to the inferior vena cava. Therefore, most oxygenated blood passes direct from the placenta into the inferior vena cava and subsequently into the right atrium of the heart.

In the right side of the heart there is a fascinating mechanism for separating this stream of blood from the blood coming down the superior vena cava. A crescent-shaped hood directs the flow from

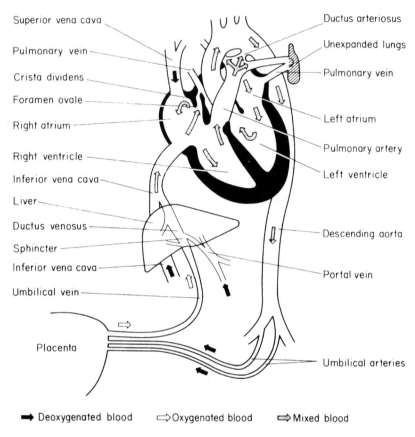

Deoxygenated blood   Oxygenated blood   Mixed blood

Fig. 11.1 The fetal circulation. Arrows indicate the direction of the blood flow. Adapted from Langman (1969)

the inferior vena cava through the foramen ovale into the left atrium. The foramen ovale is an opening in the wall between the two atria and has a valve which can be closed only from the left side of the heart. This mechanism allows oxygenated blood to pass directly into the left atrium and thence into the left ventricle and out into the body.

Blood from the superior vena cava passes into the right atrium and then into the right ventricle and out into the pulmonary artery. In postnatal life it would then flow to the capillaries in the lungs to take up oxygen and excrete carbon dioxide. However, this mechanism is not available in the fetus and the amount of blood flowing to the lungs is very small, mainly because there is constriction of the pulmonary arteries. A channel called the ductus arteriosus connects the pulmonary artery with the aorta. Therefore, in the fetus, the lungs are bypassed because blood flows through this ductus into the aorta and to the lower part of the body where much of it flows to the placenta through the umbilical arteries.

Oxygenated blood flowing into the heart through the inferior vena cava is thus partially mixed with deoxygenated blood which reduces the partial pressure of oxygen (Po_2). Blood in the aorta is also a mixture of oxygenated blood flowing out of the left ventricle and deoxygenated blood flowing through the ductus arteriosus. The Po_2 in the fetus is much lower than that in later life, about 3 kPa (20–25 mmHg). This low Po_2 is appropriate to the fetus because the oxygen dissociation curve of fetal haemoglobin (HbF) is to the left of adult haemoglobin (Fig. 11.2). This allows more oxygen to be carried by the blood at low tensions than in an adult who has haemoglobin A in his or her red cells. Factors such as acidaemia shift the curve to the right thus reducing the percentage saturation for a given Pao_2. During labour, the blood gases and pH are relatively stable although there is a tendency for the pH to fall gradually from 7.4 to about 7.3; this is partly due to an accumulation of lactic acid due to the interruption of

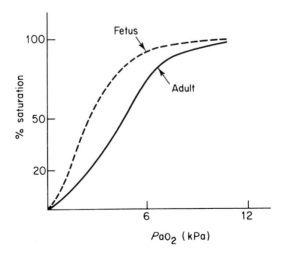

Fig. 11.2 The oxygen dissociation curve

blood supply to the placenta during uterine contractions. At birth, there is often marked acidaemia, which is partly respiratory, because CO_2 cannot escape from the baby when the umbilical cord is compressed, and partly metabolic as a result of accumulation of lactic acid from hypoxia. The Po_2 values in cord blood are variable and may reflect a recent occlusion of the umbilical cord in a normal baby.

The first breath has always caused excitement in those present at a birth, or dismay if it does not occur. A number of stimuli produce the first breath. *In utero*, a baby produces movements of the thorax during rapid-eye-movement sleep; these movements can be seen by ultrasound between one-third and one-half of the time. At birth mild cooling, hypercarbia, hypoxia and physical stimuli probably combine together to start regular breathing (see Chapter 3).

As the lungs expand, there appears to be a mechanical effect on the pulmonary arterioles which dilate. This means that there is a flood of blood through the lungs; the pressure in the left atrium rises so that the valve of the foramen ovale closes. The wall of the ductus arteriosus is sensitive to the tension of oxygen in the blood; as this rises shortly after birth, the ductus closes. Interruption of the blood supply in the umbilical cord leads to closure of the ductus venosus. Eventually, the umbilical vein inside the body and the umbilical arteries become mere cords. These changes are shown in Fig. 11.3.

Shortly after birth the blood Pco_2 and pH return to normal newborn values shown in the appendix. However, there is a normal right-to-left shunt, mainly in the lung, during the first few days of life; the Po_2 does not therefore reach peak values (13 kPa or 100 mmHg) until the end of the first week.

All these anatomical changes do not occur immediately. For instance a preterm baby may have a patent ductus arteriosus for many weeks after birth.

Signs and Symptoms in the Newborn Period

There are several possible presenting features, one or more of which is usually present:

1 Tachypnoea.
2 Dyspnoea.
3 Cyanosis.
4 Tachycardia.

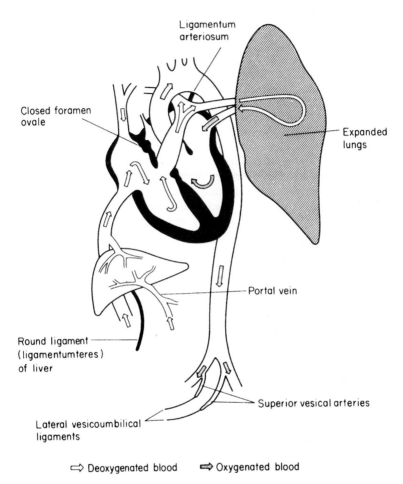

Ligamentum
arteriosum

Closed foramen
ovale

Expanded
lungs

Portal vein

Round ligament
(ligamentumteres)
of liver

Superior vesical arteries

Lateral vesicoumbilical
ligaments

⇨ Deoxygenated blood   ⇨ Oxygenated blood

Fig. 11.3 The circulation after birth. Adapted from Langman (1969)

5 Murmurs.
6 Deterioration in feeding or taking longer over feeds.
7 Grunting.
8 Peripheral oedema.

Infants with any of these features should have a full cardiovascular examination. Cardiac failure is not always easily diagnosed in a small baby. The following are the most important clinical signs: a pale, anxious baby; tachycardia (more than 160/min), marked tachypnoea, usually over 60/min; crepitations; an enlarged liver (this is usually best felt in the middle of the epigastrium not in the right midclavicular line as in childhood); peripheral oedema, seen in eyelids, hands or feet or presenting as excessive weight gain. The earliest sign of cardiac failure is often persisting unexplained tachypnoea. The causes and management of cardiac failure are described on p. 273.

Several types of congenital heart disease may be extremely difficult to diagnose in the neonatal period. For instance, a ventricular septal defect may show no abnormal physical signs and the murmur often appears only after several weeks. Coarctation of the aorta classically produces femoral pulses which are absent or very difficult to feel, but during the period when the ductus arteriosus is still open there are strong pulsations which disappear only after several days. Some babies with cyanotic congenital heart disease such as Fallot's tetralogy are not cyanosed early in life.

In examining a baby for heart disease it is important to look for all the features of cardiac failure and to examine the peripheral pulses, particularly the femoral pulses, very carefully and repeatedly.

Investigations

Some investigations may help:

Chest radiograph

It is difficult to take a chest radiograph in a standard way in the newborn period, so it is common to see radiographs that have not been centred properly or taken at the right distance. The breadth of the cardiac shadow in relation to the breadth of the thorax is rather greater than in an adult and is often a little over 50%. Although the heart may be large in a baby who has had asphyxia during birth, the films may be very useful if they show a very large heart (see Fig. 11.4) which gives a clue to the diagnosis. One can also assess the number of blood vessels in the lung fields (oligaemia or hyperaemia). Some conditions have a characteristic shape to the cardiac shadow.

Electrocardiogram (ECG)

The ECG is difficult to assess in neonatal life because it changes so rapidly with age and many of the features are very different from

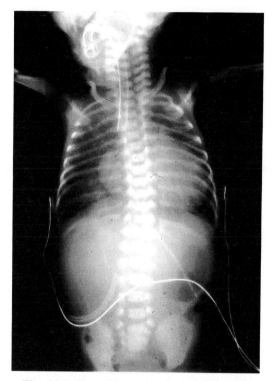

Fig. 11.4 Chest X-ray showing cardiomegaly

those seen in adults or older children. It is reasonable to record from standard leads (I, II, III, AVR, AVL and AVF) and a selection of chest leads; those often chosen are V4R, V1, V3 and V6. Without very small electrodes one cannot obtain intermediate chest leads.

Axis on standard leads.   There is a marked right axis in normal babies. The axis is obtained in the same way as in older children; Figure 11.5 demonstrates the axes in relation to the standard leads showing that lead I is 0°, lead III is $+ 120^\circ$ and so on. A quick way of finding the approximate QRS axis is to look at the standard and V leads to find which one has R and S deflections which are almost equal. The QRS axis will then be 90° clockwise to that lead.

The mean QRS axis is about $+ 135^\circ$ at birth and decreases to a

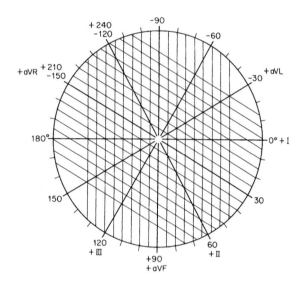

Fig. 11.5 ECG axes

mean of + 110º by the fourth week of life. There is further left axis deviation through infancy and early childhood (Fig. 11.6).

At birth left axis deviation is very abnormal and is often the result of a conduction defect in the left ventricle; it is found in atrioventricular defects and tricuspid atresia.

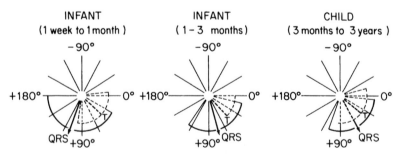

Fig. 11.6 Normal ECG axes in infants and young children

T wave. The T wave is normally upright in the right precordial leads (V4R and V1) for at least 72 hours. A useful rule is that an upright T wave after that time is abnormal.

Right ventricular hypertrophy. The single most useful ECG sign is the upright T wave seen in right ventricular hypertrophy associated with an R/S ratio of greater than 1 in lead V1. Nevertheless it is sometimes difficult to be certain of right ventricular hypertrophy in the newborn period, and some other ECG features are summarized in Table 11.1.

Left ventricular hypertrophy occurs in conditions such as aortic stenosis. Criteria for its recognition are shown in Table 11.1.

Echocardiography

Echocardiography is now widely used (Rigby *et al.*, 1984). Advantages of the technique are that it can be done at the mother's bedside in the postnatal ward or in the special care nursery, and that the

Table 11.1 Criteria for evaluation of electrocardiograms in infants and children.

Right ventricular hypertrophy
1 R in V1 0–24 hours, 20 mm; 1–7 days, 29 mm; 8 days to 3 months, 20 mm
2 S in V6 0–7 days, 14 mm; 8–30 days, 10 mm
3 R/S ratio in V1 1–3 months, 7mm or more
4 S in V6 0–3 months, 6.5; 3–6 months, 4.0 or more

Left ventricular hypertrophy
1 S in V1, more than 20 mm at all ages
2 R in V6, 20 mm or more
3 Secondary T inversion in V5 or V6
4 Q 4 mm or more in V5, V6 or V7

Combined ventricular hypertrophy
Direct evidence of RVH + LVH
or RVH + Q of 2 mm or more in V5 or V6
or inverted T in V6 (after positive in right chest leads) + RVH

Right atrial hypertrophy
1 Peaked P waves, 3 mm or more in any one lead
2 Qr pattern in RV3 or V1

Left atrial hypertrophy
1 Bifid P in any lead
2 P duration of more than 0.09 seconds
3 Late inversion of P in V1 or more than 1.5 mm

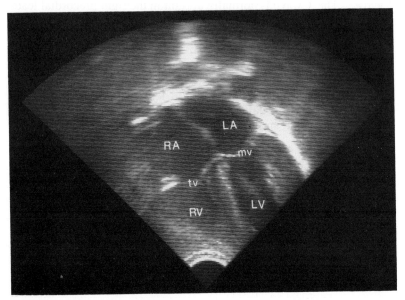

Fig. 11.7 A four-chamber echo of a normal heart (LA, left atrium; LV, left ventrical; RA, right atrium; RV, right ventricle; tv, tricuspid valve; mv, mitral valve)

technique is non-invasive. A clinician experienced in the technique will easily identify echoes from the various chambers and valves in the heart, to decide if the heart is structurally normal or, for example, to identify septal defects and pericardial effusion. A normal four-chamber echo is shown in Fig. 11.7. In many centres the majority of newborn babies now go to cardiac surgery without catheterization on the basis of the echo findings. However local expertise, experience and surgical practice will determine policy in individual centres.

Blood gases

An arterial sample (if possible from the right radial artery) from a baby breathing air and a further sample while breathing 100% oxygen for 10 minutes can provide very good evidence of a presence of a right-to-left shunt. In general, the arterial Po_2 in 100% oxygen rarely exceeds 25 kPa in cyanotic heart disease but may easily rise above that in lung disorders. The test is most useful from about 4 days of age, but may not be diagnostic earlier if the baby is very ill with lung disease. In addition, the test may be dangerous, as high concentrations of oxygen may cause the ductus to close. It should only be performed with careful monitoring and with prostaglandin immediately available, see p. 268.

Cardiac catheterization and angiocardiography

Complicated types of congenital heart disease may need further investigation before surgery is undertaken. These investigations must be performed in specialist units.

Types of Congenital Heart Disease

A useful distinction in considering congenital heart disease is between pink babies (acyanotic) and blue babies (cyanotic). In every case of central cyanosis there must be a right-to-left shunt, where some blood passes from the right to the left side of the heart without perfusing air-filled alveoli. In these situations, crying usually deepens the cyanosis. In acyanotic congenital heart disease there may be a left-to-right shunt, where blood passes back from the left to the right side of the heart and, therefore, passes through the heart twice during a single circulation; alternatively there may be a valvular abnormality. It is important to realize that any heart lesion may cause heart failure and this may lead to cyanosis even in 'acyanotic' heart disease. Newborn babies with cyanotic heart disease are particularly prone to, and vulnerable from, hypothermia. Their environmental temperature should be kept at the upper end of the neutral range (see Chapter 6).

Common congenital heart defects are:

1 *Left-to-right shunt*
   Ventricular septal defect
   Patent ductus arteriosus
   Atrial septal defect
2 *Right-to-left shunt*
   Transposition of the great arteries
   Tetralogy of Fallot
   Pulmonary atresia
   Total anomolous pulmonary venous drainage

3 *Obstructive*
  Aortic stenosis
  Pulmonary stenosis
  Coarctation of the aorta
  Hypoplastic left heart

During the newborn period, babies who develop signs of congenital heart disease often have severe lesions with very complicated anatomical defects. For instance, coarctation of the aorta, (although it theoretically has no shunt), is often associated with a ventricular septal defect. On the other hand, a ventricular septal defect may have no shunt at first as the right ventricular pressure is initially as high as that in the left ventricle (see below).

Left-to-right shunt

Ventricular septal defect (VSD)

This is the commonest congenital heart lesion. There is a window in the membranous or muscular septum between the two ventricles (see Fig. 11.3). It may be the only abnormality, but often accompanies other forms of congenital heart disease. Since the pulmonary artery resistance, and therefore right ventricular pressure, is much higher in the newborn than later in the first year of life, there may be very little shunt through the defect at first. The baby's heart sounds are usually quite normal in the newborn period and no murmur is heard.

As the pressure on the right side of the heart drops over the first few weeks, the characteristic pansystolic murmur is heard all over the praecordium. Large defects present, therefore, with cardiac failure around the second month of life. With a small defect the chest radiograph is normal; with large ones there may be cardiac and left atrial enlargement with pulmonary plethora. There may be evidence of right or biventricular hypertrophy on ECG. Eighty per cent of VSDs close completely and spontaneously before eight years of age.

Patent ductus arteriosus (PDA)

It is difficult to be certain whether persistent PDA is a congenital heart lesion in the newborn period since all babies have an open ductus at birth which may persist for many weeks in preterm babies, before closing spontaneously. PDA is twice as common in females as males (Wolfe & Wiggins, 1991). Characteristic signs are a continuous systolic and diastolic murmur below the left clavicle with left ventricular hypertrophy, a loud pulmonary second sound and a collapsing (bounding) pulse (check the systolic and diastolic blood pressures: the pulse pressure will be abnormally wide). The classical physical signs are often not present and only a systolic murmur may be heard. The chest radiograph and ECG are usually normal. In babies with rubella syndrome it is common for PDA to persist and for there to be an additional septal defect (Wolfe & Wiggins, 1991). In infants with respiratory distress syndrome, where oxygenation is variable and the Pao$_2$ is low, there is a tendency for the ductus to remain open. This may result in a right-to-left shunt if pulmonary resistance is high (especially if the baby is acidaemic), but more frequently a left-to-right shunt occurs and results in an increased cardiac output which can lead to cardiac failure. Cyanosis may appear when the baby cries as the pressure in the right heart then exceeds that in the left.

In the majority of preterm babies no treatment is required as the ductus closes spontaneously. As prostaglandins maintain the patency of the ductus, the prostaglandin synthetase inhibitor indomethacin has been used very successfully to obliterate the ductus in symptomatic babies with RDS (Gersony *et al.*, 1983; Peckham *et al.*, 1984). (See also Chapter 8.) Treatment with indomethacin is effective only in the preterm infant and not the full-term infant with PDA. Complications have included oliguria and displacement of bilirubin from albumin. The place for indomethacin, or surgical intervention, in sick babies is not yet established, and meticulous supportive treatment is very important. Indomethacin should be given orally, 0.1 mg/kg once; the same dose is repeated after eight hours and a third dose of 0.2 mg/kg given 24 hours after the first dose. If there is no effect, more should *not* be given. Fluid restriction and administration of frusemide may also be required, in the early stages of treatment, prior to indomethacin.

Atrial septal defect (ASD)

The common, less serious type of ASD in which there is a defect in the upper part of the septum (ostium secundum) presents only rarely in the newborn period. Babies with the more serious ostium primum defect in the lower portion of the septum often have associated abnormalities of the mitral valve or, more seriously, a common atrioventricular canal (endocardial cushion defects). Such babies may present in the early weeks of life with a harsh systolic murmur audible widely over the praecordium, often associated with a shrill and a loud and widely split second sound. Babies with a common atrioventricular canal may also show early cyanosis and tachypnoea with rapid onset of cardiac failure (thus mimicking transposition of the great arteries – see below).

Chest radiography shows general cardiomegaly and, in particular, left atrial enlargement, associated with increased pulmonary vascular markings (plethora). The ECG shows a characteristic pattern of left axis deviation with right ventricular hypertrophy and first degree heart block (prolonged P–R interval). Left atrial enlargement produces tall P waves.

There is a particular association between endocardial cushion defects and trisomy 21 where the incidence is about 20% (Wolfe & Wiggins, 1991). (See Chapter 10).

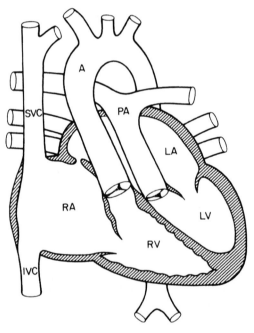

Fig. 11.8 Simple transposition of the great arteries (LV, left ventricle; LA, left atrium; RA, right atrium; IVC, inferior vena cava; SVC, superior vena cava; A, aorta; PA, pulmonary artery)

Right-to-left shunts

Transposition of the great arteries

Transposition is a common cause of right-to-left shunt in the newborn period. It can cause profound cyanosis and is important because urgent treatment is needed to save the baby's life. The major arteries are reversed so that the pulmonary artery leaves the left ventricle and the aorta leaves the right ventricle. There are therefore two separate circulations, since blood returns to the lungs from the left side of the heart and blood returns to the body from the right side of the heart (Fig. 11.8). During fetal life there is, of course, mixing through the ductus arteriosus and the foramen ovale. There is very commonly an associated septal defect (80%) (Wolfe & Wiggins, 1991), for example at ventricular level (Fig. 11.9) so that mixing can still occur after birth. However, many babies do not have any septal defect and mixing occurs only through the ductus arteriosus. When this closes, several days after birth, the baby may suddenly become deeply

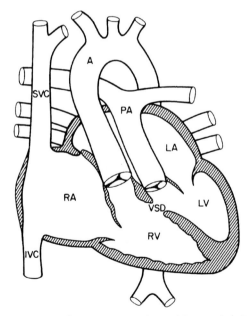

Fig. 11.9 Transposition of the great arteries, with associated ventricular septal defect (VSD) (for key see Fig. 11.8)

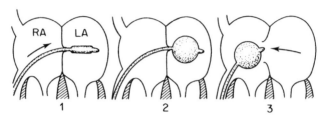

Fig. 11.10 Rashkind's atrial septostomy. 1, A catheter is passed into the right atrium (RA) and pushed through the foramen ovale into the left atrium (LA). 2, A balloon at the tip of the catheter is inflated. 3, The catheter is withdrawn sharply so that the inflated balloon tears the atrial septum, allowing oxygenated blood to reach the systemic circulation. From S. Wallis & D. Harvey (1979) *Nursing Times*, by permission of the authors and editor

cyanosed characteristically, irreversible by 100% oxygen. Tachypnoea develops within a few days, followed by increasing heart failure, cyanosis, acidaemia and death if untreated. Apart from the cyanosis, there are often no physical signs initially, although an ejection systolic murmur may be present. The ECG is usually normal at first but may later show left ventricular hypertrophy. The chest radiograph is said classically to show an 'egg on the side' appearance of the heart but is more often normal. When suspected it is important to confirm the diagnosis by echocardiography, but cardiac catheterization is also necessary urgently because a balloon septostomy (Fig. 11.10) can be performed to provide mixing of the two circulations. A definitive operation can be done towards the end of the first year but the balloon septostomy will enable the baby to survive until then.

Oxygen causes the PDA to close. It is now usual to give a prostaglandin infusion to maintain an open ductus until the baby can be transferred to a neonatal cardiac unit. At present we recommend an intravenous infusion of prostaglandin E_1 (PGE_1), 0.1 µg/kg/ min.

Pulmonary atresia and other forms of obstruction of the right ventricle together with septal defects

Babies with classical Fallot's tetralogy often present as an apparently uncomplicated VSD and then later show cyanosis as the infundibular muscle proximal to the pulmonary valve becomes hypertrophied and obstructs the outflow to the right ventricle. The other features are an overriding aorta and right ventricular hypertrophy (Fig. 11.11). The

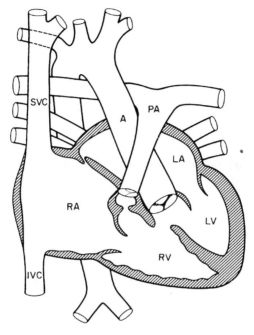

Fig. 11.11 Tetralogy of Fallot (for key see Fig. 11.8)

more severe types of right ventricular outflow obstruction may produce symptoms of cyanosis in the newborn period. Sometimes the pulmonary artery and valve are completely obliterated, so that the lungs are perfused only through the PDA (Fig. 11.12) and the baby becomes deeply cyanosed when this closes. If a baby becomes cyanosed, is given oxygen and then becomes even more deeply cyanosed, it is important to reduce the amount of inspired oxygen because this may be lifesaving. There is only a single second sound and a murmur may or may not be present. The baby is often very deeply cyanosed. The ECG shows marked right axis deviation, right ventricular and sometimes atrial hypertrophy. The chest radiograph shows a normally sized heart with a pulmonary artery 'bay' due to the small size of the main pulmonary artery; the apex of the heart is often said to be lifted up from the diaphragm. The lung fields are under-perfused (oligaemic) and therefore appear very translucent. A right-sided aortic arch is present in about 20% of cases.

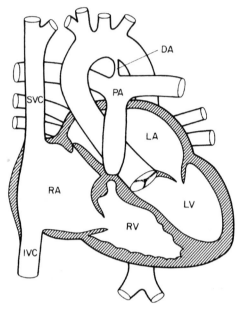

Fig. 11.12 Pulmonary atresia and patent ductus arteriosus (for key see Fig. 11.8)

Total anomalous pulmonary venous drainage (TAPVD)

In this condition the pulmonary veins empty into the right side of the heart and there is an additional right-to-left shunt at atrial or ventricular level, so that the mixed oxygenated and deoxygenated blood is perfused both to the lungs and to the body. There are various subgroups of the condition, but the most confusing and rarest is the type where the pulmonary veins empty into the inferior vena cava below the diaphragm, usually called the subdiaphragmatic type. There may be obstruction to the flow of these veins into the inferior vena cava. The ECG shows an axis to the right of normal and right ventricular hypertrophy.

Although much rarer, TAPVD is easily mistaken for RDS. In both cases there may be deep cyanosis, and a chest radiograph showing a small heart and over-filled plethoric lung fields with a ground-glass appearance. Giving 100% oxygen is a very important aid to differential diagnosis, as it hardly increases the arterial Po_2 in TAPVD.

Unfortunately, the worst forms of RDS have such a large right-to-left shunt that 100% oxygen may not alter the Po_2.

The mortality is still between 15 and 50%. The differential diagnosis of persistent cyanosis in the newborn is summarized in Table 11.2.

Obstructive lesions

Coarctation of the aorta

There may be only a small narrowing after the ductus, ('adult' type coarctation), or a much longer narrowing, often proximal to the ductus, ('infantile' type). The left ventricle is often much smaller than normal and at its most severe the condition may be called hypoplastic left heart syndrome (see below). A ventricular or atrial septal defect may be present as well. It is important to feel the

Table 11.2 Important causes of persistent cyanosis in the newborn period.

Pulmonary	Respiratory distress syndrome
	Pneumonia
	Pneumothorax
	Diaphragmatic hernia
	Tracheo-oesophageal fistula
	Lobar emphysema
	Wilson–Mikity syndrome
Cardiovascular	Severe cyanosis (usually the presenting feature)
	Transposition of the great arteries
	Pulmonary atresia or severe pulmonary stenosis
	Tetralogy of Fallot
	Total anomalous pulmonary venous drainage (with obstruction of venous return)
	Tricuspid atresia
	Ebstein's anomaly of the tricuspid valve
	Mild cyanosis initially
	Hypoplastic left heart syndrome including aortic or mitral atresia, preductal coarctation of the aorta
	Truncus arteriosus
Cerebral	Cerebral oedema
	Intracerebral haemorrhage
Miscellaneous	Congenital methaemoglobinaemia
	Bilateral choanal atresia
	Vasomotor instability (peripheral cyanosis only)
	Sepsis, especially septicaemia (peripheral cyanosis only)
	Traumatic cyanosis

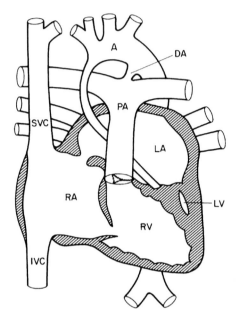

Fig. 11.13 Hypoplastic left heart syndrome with patent ductus arteriosus (for key see Fig. 11.8)

femoral pulses in every baby, particularly when one is specifically considering congenital heart disease. The femoral pulses may be easily palpable in a baby with coarctation if the aorta is well perfused through a PDA from the pulmonary artery. When the PDA closes, the femoral pulses may disappear quite suddenly. If the narrowed segment of the aorta is quite small, it is often possible to resect it and replace it with a graft. Unfortunately many babies have a very long segment of narrowed aorta with a very small left ventricle so their prognosis is, at present, very poor.

Hypoplastic left heart

In hypoplastic left heart syndrome there is a long segment of narrowed aorta and a very small left ventricle (Fig. 11.13). The baby is ductus dependent; thus when the duct closes there will be rapid deterioration over a few hours with a shock-like picture.

Table 11.3 Causes of cardiac failure in the newborn.

Volume or pressure overload of the myocardium
Large left-to-right shunts
Left or right ventricular outflow obstruction
Total anomalous pulmonary venous drainage (with or without pulmonary venous obstruction)
Coarctation of the aorta and hypoplastic left heart syndrome
Anaemia
Severe hypertension (rare)

Primary depression or failure of myocardial contractility
Hypoxaemia and acidaemia
Electrolyte abnormalities, e.g. hypocalcaemia or hypokalaemia
Hypoglycaemia
Myocarditis
Endocardial fibroelastosis
Coronary occlusive disease
Glycogen storage disease

Dysrhythmias with heart rate > 220/min or < 40/min

Valvular lesions

Many valvular lesions may be diagnosed in the neonatal period because they produce a murmur. Simple aortic or pulmonary stenosis produces an ejection systolic murmur. Luckily, these rarely produce cardiac failure in the newborn but it is important to follow up any baby who has had a loud murmur. A very soft ejection systolic murmur is heard in 95% of newborn babies.

Cardiac Failure

Causes of cardiac failure in the newborn are shown in Table 11.3. Babies with evidence of cardiac failure should be managed as follows:

1 Restrict fluid intake to 120–150 ml/kg/day.
2 Give frusemide 1–2 mg/kg once or twice daily.
3 Digitalize (Table 11.4).
4 Nurse in a neutral thermal environment (at the lower end for babies with acyanotic heart defects and large left-to-right shunts) with head elevated.
5 Give appropriate concentrations of added oxygen if necessary.
6 Consider sedation and ventilation.

Table 11.4 Digitalization in the event of cardiac failure.

Digitalization dose	Oral initially 20 µg/kg (0.02 mg/kg); then 10 µg/kg (0.01 mg/kg for 2 doses) Intramuscularly initially 15 µg/kg (0.015 mg/kg); then 8 µg/kg (0.008 mg/kg for 2 doses)
Maintenance dose	Oral 10 µg/kg/24 hours (0.01 mg/kg/24 h) Intramuscularly 8 µg/kg/24 hours (0.008 mg/kg/24 h) Give half maintenance dose every 12 hours Reduce dose slightly for infants < 2 kg

It is important to assess the effects of digoxin on the individual baby and to adjust the dose according to clinical response and plasma levels, to avoid digoxin toxicity. In those on long-term therapy, remember to increase dosage according to weight.

Check electrolytes and urea initially and regularly and give potassium supplements if needed.

Arrhythmias

Arrhythmias may cause cardiac failure in newborn babies.

Paroxysmal atrial tachycardia (PAT)

Many normal newborn babies achieve heart rates of 160–180/min or more when crying, but a persistent tachycardia of more than 180/min in a quiet or sleeping baby is an important clue to the diagnosis of PAT which may be confirmed by ECG. Often the rate may reach 300/min and congestive cardiac failure develops. Occasionally fetal tachycardia may cause intrauterine cardiac failure and the infant may then be born with peripheral oedema and hepatomegaly (hydrops fetalis, see pp. 68 and 296). During episodes of PAT lasting more than a few hours, the baby becomes very ill with pallor, cyanosis, restlessness and irritability.

An episode may be aborted by vagal stimulation, for example by massage over one carotid sinus in the neck, but the infant usually requires to be digitalized (see Table 11.4 for dose regimen) as recurrence is otherwise common. Therapy should be continued for about one year. In rare cases, or if there is severe circulatory failure, cardioversion (DC shock) may be necessary to abolish episodes. There is seldom any underlying structural heart disease in PAT.

Congenital complete atrioventricular block (congenital heart block)

Fetal bradycardia is usually a sign of hypoxia but occasionally the neonate is found to have a persisting slow heart rate (often less than 60/min). This is due to a congenital defect in the main conducting system of the heart (bundle of His). The ventricles do not keep pace with the contraction rate of the atria and there is complete dissociation of the P waves and QRS complexes on the ECG.

About 30% of such babies have other associated structural heart defects, especially single ventricle, transposition of the great arteries or PDA, so that the prognosis depends on the severity of the associated lesion.

In the 70% without other abnormalities, the prognosis is good without treatment, although some patients need permanent pacemakers to prevent episodes of dizziness or syncope in later life.

There appears to be an important association with systemic lupus erythematosus in the mothers of many babies with congenital heart block.

References and further reading

Berman, W. (1991) *Handbook of Pediatric ECG Interpretation* St Louis: Mosby.
Doyle, E.F., Engle, M.A., Gersony, W.M. *et al.* (eds) (1986) *Pediatric Cardiology.* New York: Springer-Verlag.
Gersony, W.M., Peckham, G.J., Ellison, R.C. *et al.* (1983) Effects of indomethacin in premature infants with patent ductus arteriosus: results of a national collaborative study. *J. Pediatr., 102*, 895–905.
Langman, J. (1969) *Medical Embryology*, 2nd ed. Baltimore: Williams & Wilkins.
Lehrer, S. (1992) *Understanding Pediatric Heart Sounds.* Philadelphia: W.B. Saunders.
Long, (1989) *Fetal and Neonatal Cardiology.* Philadelphia: W.B. Saunders.
Peckham, G.J., Miettinen, O.S., Ellison, R.C. *et al.* (1984) Clinical course to 1 year of age in premature infants with patent ductus arteriosus: results of a multicenter randomized trial of indomethacin. *J. Pediatr., 105*, 285.
Rigby, M.L., Pickering, D. & Wilkinson, A. (1984) Cross sectional echo-

cardiography in determining persistent patency of the ductus arteriosus in premature infants. *Arch. Dis. Child.* 59, 341–345.

Rowe, R.D., Freedom, R.M., Mehrizi, A. *et al. (1981) The Neonate with Congenital Heart Disease*, 2nd ed. Philadelphia: W.B. Saunders.

Wolfe, R. & Wiggins, J. (1991) Cardiovascular diseases. In *Current Pediatric Diagnosis and Treatment*, 10th ed., eds Hathaway, W., Groothuis, J., Hay, W. *et al.* pp. 412–469, Norwalk: Appleton & Lange.

—12

Jaundice

In the 1970 British Births survey, about one in five newborn babies developed jaundice. At present about 60% of babies of birthweight less than 2000 g have a peak plasma bilirubin over 170 μmol/l. To know why newborn babies become jaundiced and the particular importance of neonatal jaundice, it is necessary to understand how bilirubin is formed and excreted from the body.

Bilirubin Metabolism

Haemoglobin (Hb) is a constituent of red blood cells (RBC). Its most vital function is the transport of oxygen to the tissues. Preterm red blood cells have a life-span of approximately 40 days (Mollison, 1983), compared to 70 days in the term baby and 120 days in the adult. At the end of their life the enzyme systems start to deteriorate, and these aged cells are removed from the circulation by the reticuloendothelial (RE) system (specifically the liver and spleen). The contained haemoglobin is broken down into its two constituents: globin, a protein which is conserved and re-utilized by the body; and haem, which cannot be reused and is degraded by a number of steps so that it can be excreted (Figs 12.1 and 12.2). Bilirubin is a product of this degradation and its accumulation in the blood causes yellow staining of the skin and other tissues, thereby producing jaundice.

The first step in the conversion of haemoglobin (Fig. 12.1) also takes place in the RE system and forms bilirubin (35 mg from each gram of Hb – equivalent to 600 μmol) which is fat-soluble and water-insoluble; it therefore cannot be excreted in bile or urine, but has a high affinity for fatty tissue and the brain. On its way to the liver bilirubin does not travel free in plasma but is bound to the small protein albumin (16 mg bilirubin – approximately 300 μmol – to 1 g albumin), and in this form cannot leave the blood and enter the brain. It is also known as pre-hepatic or unconjugated bilirubin as it has not yet been conjugated in the liver. However, if there is too much unconjugated bilirubin in the plasma to be bound by albumin (i.e. the albumin-binding capacity of the plasma is exceeded), it may spill

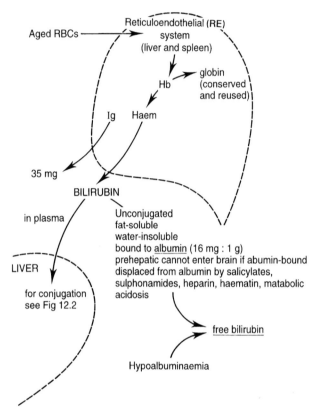

Fig. 12.1 The formation of bilirubin

over into the brain and other tissues. In full-term infants this does not usually occur at serum bilirubin levels under 340 μmol/l unless there are substances present which displace bilirubin from albumin (e.g. drugs such as salicylates, sulphonamides, heparin, haematin formed during haemolysis, or the baby has a metabolic acidosis or hypoalbuminaemia). Large amounts of bilirubin must be dealt with by the neonate's liver because during the early days of life there is a high rate of red cell destruction. This is related firstly to the shorter life of neonatal red cells and secondly to the high fetal and neonatal haemoglobin levels (18–19 g/dl) enabling the fetus to maintain an oxyhaemoglobin of 11 g/dl (see Chapter 6, the early anaemia of the

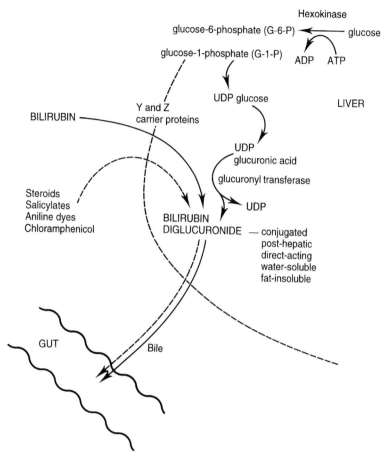

Fig. 12.2 The conjugation and excretion of bilirubin

preterm baby). Clearly, therefore, there will be a high bilirubin load to excrete. Late clamping of the cord leading to placental transfusion may exacerbate the problem, particularly in preterm and low birthweight babies.

The albumin-bound bilirubin enters the liver cells (Fig. 12.2) with the aid of two carrier proteins, Y and Z. Once in the cell, the molecule is converted by a series of enzyme reactions that require glucose and oxygen to form bilirubin diglucoronide. This last step, conjugation, is catalysed by the enzyme glucuronyl transferase.

Bilirubin diglucuronide is thus known as conjugated or post-hepatic bilirubin. Other substances are excreted by the same pathway as bilirubin (Fig. 12.2) and should normally not be given to the newborn baby, for example steroids, salicylates, and chloramphenicol (chloramphenicol may need to be used if the baby has meningitis). Thus hypoxia or hypoglycaemia in the perinatal period may compromise bilirubin conjugation. Bilirubin diglucuronide is water-soluble and fat-insoluble. It cannot therefore enter the brain and cause damage. It is excreted via the bile into the gut and, being water-soluble, can also be excreted in the urine.

The capacity of a normal newborn baby to excrete a given bilirubin load is only about one-fiftieth of that of an adult. In the fetus the bilirubin is excreted across the placenta in unconjugated form and conjugated bilirubin would not cross. At birth, therefore, major changes in metabolic mechanisms are necessary to excrete bilirubin. These changes are comparable in complexity to the circulatory changes from fetal to neonatal life. Thinking of the mechanisms in these terms helps to explain why so many normal babies become jaundiced. The preterm baby is even more likely to become jaundiced (see Chapter 6). Reasons include a relative glucuronyl transferase deficiency in the neonate's 'immature' liver, deficiencies in the Y and Z carrier proteins, and the relatively high bilirubin load to excrete.

All babies, therefore, have hyperbilirubinaemia by adult standards, and in many normal babies frank jaundice appears (for this to occur plasma bilirubin levels must exceed 80 μmol/l in Caucasian infants). Jaundice usually reaches a maximum at three to six days.

Further investigation and possibly treatment are necessary when:

1 Jaundice appears during the first 24 hours of life.
2 Jaundice persists after two weeks of age.
3 The bilirubin level is above 250 μmol/l (less in a preterm baby – see below).
4 There is a conjugated hyperbilirubinaemia (above 30 μmol/l).
5 Jaundice is present in an ill baby.

In all these situations, medical advice should be sought without delay and the baby examined and investigated.

Table 12.1 Some important causes of jaundice.

Pre-hepatic	Hepatic	Post-hepatic
Unconjugated bilirubin	**Unconjugated bilirubin**	**Mixed conjugated and**
Haemolytic disorders	Breast milk jaundice	**unconjugated bilirubin**
Rhesus isoimmunization	Congenital hypothyroidism	*Extrahepatic obstruction*
ABO incompatibility	Hereditary glucuronyl	Congenital biliary atresia
Red cell enzyme defects	transferase deficiency	Choledochal cyst
(e.g. glucose-6-phosphate		Bile plug syndrome
dehydrogenase deficiency	**Mixed conjugated and**	
and pyruvate kinase	**unconjugated bilirubin**	**Unconjugated bilirubin**
deficiency)	*Inborn errors of metabolism*	*Increased enterohepatic*
Hereditary spherocytosis	Cystic fibrosis	*circulation*
	Galactosaemia	Paralytic ileus
Infections	Tyrosinaemia	High intestinal obstruction
Septicaemia	Alpha-1-antitrypsin	(e.g. pyloric stenosis,
Urinary tract infections	deficiency	duodenal atresia)
Meningitis	Fructosaemia	
Bruising, haematomas	*Hepatitis*	
Cephalhaematoma	Rubella	
Bruising during	Cytomegalovirus	
delivery	Toxoplasmosis	
	Herpes simplex	
Polycythaemia	Syphilis	
Twin transfusion syndrome	Hepatitis B	
Maternofetal transfusion	Listeriosis	
Delayed clamping of cord	Coxsackie virus	
Infants of diabetic mothers		

Causes of Jaundice

The possible causes of neonatal jaundice classified according to aetiology are listed in Tables 12.1 and 12.2. Some of these conditions are discussed in detail below.

Apart from the physiological jaundice of many newborn babies (described above), the most important common causes of jaundice are:

1 *Red cell incompatibility*, usually due to either rhesus haemolytic disease or ABO incompatibility, where jaundice usually appears within the first 24 hours.

2 *Infections*, usually urinary tract or septicaemia, which seldom cause jaundice in the first 72 hours.

Table 12.2 Drugs and metabolic factors that increase the danger of neonatal jaundice.

Drugs that compete for albumin-binding sites
Sulphonamides
Salicylates
Heparin
Intravenous diazepam (the sodium benzoate carrier rather than the drug itself)

Reduced bilirubin binding capacity results from
Drugs, as above
Haematin (derived from haemolysis)
Acidosis
Hypoxia
Hypoglycaemia
Low albumin levels (preterm babies)

Drugs interfering with glucuronyl transferase
Novobiocin

3 *Breast milk*. It appears that there are three factors associated with breast milk jaundice. One is that breastfeeding appears to inhibit glucuronyl transferase, therefore the conjugation of bilirubin is diminished. Secondly, there is delayed passage of meconium compared to bottle fed babies, and this increases the entero-hepatic circulation: in other words there is more time in the gut for the conjugated bilirubin to be broken down and reabsorbed. The third factor is the presence of betaglucuronidase, which will split conjugated bilirubin and increase the reabsorption of unconjugated bilirubin. Jaundice due to breast milk is never a reason for stopping breastfeeding (see persistent jaundice).

There are a number of rarer causes of jaundice which it may be important to exclude. Some, such as hypothyroidism, galactosaemia, bile duct atresia or viral hepatitis, cause prolonged jaundice (see below).

Investigation of Jaundice

Bilirubin estimation

All babies who appear significantly jaundiced on clinical examination should have a plasma bilirubin estimation. Jaundice meters are now available, to determine whether a laboratory test is necessary.(Goldman *et al.*, 1982; Strange & Cassady, 1985). When pressed against the forehead, a beam of light is emitted from the meter. The reflection of this beam is interpreted as a measurement of the degree of yellowness, and displayed as a 'transcutaneous bilirubin index' (tcBI). This corresponds to the depth of skin jaundice, not the serum bilirubin. It is particularly useful when assessing non-Caucasian babies in whom observable jaundice may be minimal. Any baby who appears jaundiced during the first 24 hours of life must have an urgent bilirubin estimation.

Estimation of conjugated bilirubin

This must be done at least once during the course of jaundice in any baby who needs bilirubin estimations. If the conjugated bilirubin is more than 30 μmol/l a search should be made for the cause. The most important causes are rhesus incompatibility, congenital bile duct obstruction, α_1-antitrypsin deficiency, cystic fibrosis, intrauterine viral infection or an inborn metabolic error such as galactosaemia.

Mother's blood group and tests for antibodies or haemolysins

The mother's notes must always be reviewed to ensure that a rhesus problem has not been overlooked. The tests are done routinely during the antenatal period, but may have been missed.

Baby's blood group and Coombs' antibody test

These tests should be carried out by the laboratory on any baby who is jaundiced (see p. 297).

Baby's haemoglobin

It may be necessary to check this on a severely jaundiced baby – if jaundice is due to haemolysis the baby may become anaemic.

Additional tests

Additional tests may be needed if there are clinical indications or if the bilirubin level is more than about 250 μmol/l and otherwise unexplained.

Check the notes to see if there is a possible cause for jaundice such as *cephalhaematoma*, *bruising* or a *preterm* or *difficult delivery*. Make certain the laboratory have looked for spherocytes and done a

reticulocyte count. Ask about a family history of spherocytosis. A reticulocyte count of more than 10% in the absence of blood group incompatibility should be repeated at one week and, if still more than 10%, should be investigated to be certain that there is no inherited haemolytic anaemia, for example pyruvate kinase deficiency.

Glucose-6-phosphate dehydrogenase (G-6-PD) assay should be requested for any baby with a bilirubin over 200 µmol/l whose parents originated from southern Europe, Asia or Africa. The assay should be done on any child whose mother is believed to be a carrier for G-6-PD deficiency or on any girl whose father has the condition.

The urine should be tested for *reducing substances* to exclude galactosaemia. If a reducing substance is present, its identity can be determined by sugar chromatography.

Urine for culture can be obtained from a clean catch or by suprapubic aspiration. *Blood culture* or *lumbar puncture* might be necessary in some cases where infection is suspected. *Swabs* from obviously infected areas are valuable, as is an ear swab after pro-longed rupture of membranes. Routine swabbing is not helpful as it can provide evidence only of colonization rather than infection.

IgM and cytomegalovirus (CMV), toxoplasma and rubella antibody titres should be estimated. A raised IgM (especially in cord blood) is valuable evidence of intrauterine infection. Jaundice, especially in a small-for-gestational-age (SFGA) infant with other stigmata, may be due to CMV, toxoplasmosis or congenital rubella.

T_4 *and TSH* estimations will exclude hypothyroidism (see below).

Albumin binding of bilirubin (ABB) may be measured. Unconjugated bilirubin is carried in the blood bound to albumin. When all the binding sites are saturated, the amount of free bilirubin increases and it is thought that kernicterus then occurs. If we could estimate the bilirubin level at which a baby's albumin were saturated, it would be possible to plan individual treatment for jaundice instead of relying on bilirubin levels. Unfortunately the present methods are complex and require several millilitres of blood; therefore the estimation cannot be done routinely. ABB measurements are available in certain specialist units; in some situations, e.g. cord blood from a rhesus baby or at the beginning of an exchange transfusion, they are particularly useful.

Persistent jaundice

Bilirubin levels above 150 µmol/l at two weeks of age should be investigated. It is important to determine whether the bilirubin is conjugated or unconjugated, as ordinary physiological jaundice may otherwise merge unnoticed into obstructive jaundice. In the latter situation there would be a history of pale stools and dark urine. The investigation of prolonged jaundice must include looking for evidence of intrauterine infection and of galactosaemia and haemolysis. Primary hypothyroidism will now be detected as it is routinely screened for in the UK. Check that the Guthrie test has been done and the TSH level is not raised (see Chapter 4). A not infrequent cause of prolonged jaundice is breastfeeding. It is likely that some mothers excrete an enzyme in their milk which unconjugates bilirubin in the gut. It is, of course, important to exclude the other serious causes listed above before making this diagnosis. Breast milk jaundice is generally harmless and is emphatically *not* a reason for stopping breastfeeding although a detailed explanation must be given to the parents. If breastfeeding is discontinued or interrupted for 48–72 hours, the serum bilirubin level falls immediately. On resuming breastfeeding, the rate of increase is much slower, and the levels subsequently decline to normal values (Gartner, 1983).

Management of Jaundice

General measures

There is good evidence that early feeding after birth will reduce the prevalence of jaundice. If there is marked loss of weight, high packed cell volume, signs of dehydration or poor milk intake the feeding regime should be reviewed. The baby can be put to the breast frequently or given three-hourly bottle feeds. There is no evidence that supplementing breastfeeding with water or dextrose solutions will prevent jaundice appearing or make it disappear quicker, and since this practice is detrimental to establishing lactation and breastfeeding, it should not be done.. Jaundice appearing in the first 24 hours is due to blood group incompatibility until proved otherwise and requires urgent investigation. An infection should be treated with antibiotics.

Plotting the level of jaundice

All babies with rhesus disease, jaundice in the first 24 hours or a plasma bilirubin over 250 µmol/l should have a bilirubin chart (Fig. 12.3). A horizontal line should be drawn on the chart at the plasma

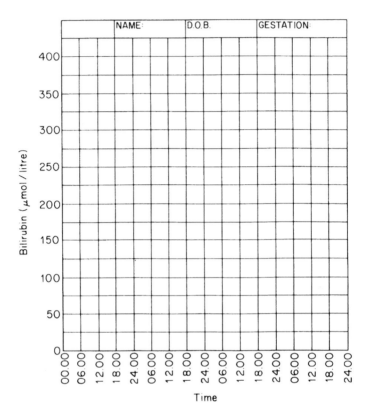

Fig. 12.3 A bilirubin chart

bilirubin which would be an indication for exchange transfusion (ET) in that baby, because of a danger of kernicterus (see below). Depending on the rate of rise, which is linear, you can decide when to do another bilirubin estimation or whether to do an ET. Remember that it generally takes about three hours to organize an exchange.

Techniques for lowering plasma bilirubin levels

In cases where bilirubin levels are rising rapidly or are already dangerously high, exchange transfusion is the treatment of choice (see below). In less urgent situations other techniques for lowering serum bilirubin have been employed.

Phenobarbitone

Phenobarbitone is metabolized by the liver. Its metabolism causes induction of many liver enzymes, including glucuronyl transferase essential for the conjugation of bilirubin. There is good evidence that phenobarbitone given to mothers from the 32nd week of pregnancy will result in infants who are less jaundiced. However, the development of severe neonatal jaundice is often not predictable, so that this is of little practical value. Treating the newborn baby with phenobarbitone from birth will reduce the bilirubin level at four days or later, but we do not recommend it as it makes the baby very sleepy and more effective techniques are now available (Wallin & Boreus, 1984).

Phototherapy

The chance observation in the pathology laboratory at Rochford Hospital, Essex, that jaundiced serum left in sunlight over the lunch hour was considerably paler led to the placing of babies in sunlight to reduce their jaundice; this was successful. It was found subsequently that the bilirubin molecule maximally absorbs light of wavelength 450 nm (the visible blue part of the spectrum) and in so doing is broken down to a number of non-toxic photodegradation products which the baby can easily excrete. It is possible that the light also has an effect on the excretion of bilirubin by the liver. In practice, blue light is not often used since it makes all babies look cyanosed and this prevents the recognition of cyanosis in a sick baby. Fluorescent lights have a high output at the visible blue part of the spectrum while giving the infant a relatively normal skin appearance. They are readily available commercially.

There is good evidence that phototherapy is effective in reducing jaundice (or slowing the rate of worsening in severely affected babies) by breaking down bilirubin in the skin and skin capillaries. There are side-effects, but these are not usually very serious: skin rashes and loose green stools (due to the excretion of biliverdin and other photodegradation products) are common. Because of the additional water lost in this way and through the skin, an extra fluid intake of 30 ml/kg/day should be given. Extra calories are needed to counteract intestinal hurry, and babies who are otherwise well will demand more frequent feeds to cope with this. Weight, urine output and osmolality or specific gravity should be checked and the fluid intake further increased if necessary. Conventionally, infants' eyes are protected during treatment – retinal damage has been reported in animals (Messner *et al.*, 1975). It is important to explain phototherapy to parents and warn them that their baby's eyes will be covered, otherwise needless anxiety will be caused. Phototherapy does not necessitate separating mother and baby; the phototherapy machine should be used alongside the mother's bed. She should feed and cuddle the baby in the normal way. It has been found that it is as effective to give phototherapy intermittently (say one hour in three) and this reduces the incidence and severity of side-effects (Lav & Fung, 1984). Other methods employed include 'extra strength' phototherapy units, and the use of a Bili blanket, which allows the parents to have greater access to their baby without needing to discontinue treatment. The baby's temperature should be recorded every three to four hours (small babies could become hypothermic without a heat shield; big babies could overheat unless the incubator thermostat is turned down to minimum or off altogether). The baby should be nursed naked and turned at intervals to allow maximal skin exposure to the light.

Any baby whose jaundice is not being adequately controlled by phototherapy will need an exchange transfusion. However, the use of phototherapy has reduced the frequency with which exchange transfusion need be performed. Our criteria for the use of phototherapy would be a bilirubin of 340 µmol/l in a term baby, with correspondingly lower thresholds in preterm, SFGA or sick infants, for example 150–180 µmol/l at 28 weeks and 200–240 µmol/l at 34 weeks gestation. It is sensible to treat rhesus babies with phototherapy from birth and it could also be used early for a preterm baby with bruising (Brown *et al.*, 1985).

Intravenous albumin

It may sometimes be useful to give a baby an intravenous albumin transfusion, especially if there is a delay in obtaining blood for exchange transfusion. It reduces the likelihood of kernicterus by increasing the bilirubin-binding capacity of the blood. It is confusing because its use *increases* the plasma bilirubin level as conventionally measured, although the baby is safer.

Exchange transfusion (ET)

Indications.   Estimate the danger level for kernicterus in the baby. The following are reasonable guidelines:

Gestation	Bilirubin (μmol/l)
39 weeks or more	380
35–38 weeks	350
31–34 weeks	280
30 weeks or less	240

The danger level may be lower if the baby is ill, is very acidaemic or has had a drug which competes with bilirubin for the albumin binding sites (see Table 12.2). Some other units use lower values because this will prevent kernicterus found at autopsy but there is no good evidence that lower values must be taken in order to prevent clinical kernicterus; indeed some would think these criteria overcautious. The indications in haemolytic disease are shown in Table 12.3.

Table 12.3 The management at birth of haemolytic disease (HDN).

Hb (g/dl)	Coombs'	Diagnosis	Procedure
Above 15	Negative	Unaffected	None
Below 15	Negative	Fetal haemorrhage	May need simple transfusion
14–16	+	Mild HDN	May need phototherapy. May need simple transfusion later
12–14	++	Moderate HDN	Phototherapy. Exchange transfusion if jaundice appears in first 24 hours and if bilirubin rises more than 80 μmol/l in 12 hours
7–11	++	Severe HDN	Early exchange transfusion. Phototherapy
Under 7	+/−	Hydrops	Immediate venesection to reduce venous pressure followed by extended controlled replacement with packed blood; treatment of cardiac failure and respiratory support

Technique.   Exchange transfusion is usually done in the special care baby unit. Exceptions include the infected baby or the hydropic infant requiring urgent transfusion in the labour ward. In most cases the need for exchange can be anticipated in good time to order fresh blood (see below), obtain a warm incubator or an overhead heater and set up the necessary equipment for monitoring ECG, temperature and blood pressure. Sterile techniques must be used. The baby must be kept warm and relatively immobile; gentle restraint of the hands and feet may be necessary to prevent catheters becoming dislodged. Before starting, the baby's stomach should be emptied and a nasogastric tube left in place.

Blood is taken from the first sample withdrawn and checked for Hb, PCV, ures and electrolytes, calcium, glucose and bilirubin. Bilirubin estimation is repeated at the halfway stage, and the full investigations repeated at the end.

Blood is always first removed from the baby before the same volume is transfused. In this way the baby's blood volume is always normal or 10–20 ml below normal (which is safer than being too high). In most babies 10 ml aliquots are used. In babies weighing 3 kg or more 20 ml aliquots may be used but 5 ml aliquots should be used for very small or sick babies. Donor blood should be Rh-negative and preferably of the same ABO group as the baby's (O rhesus-negative

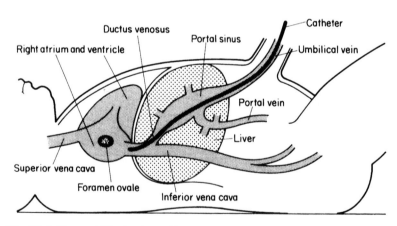

Fig. 12.4 The umbilical vein and its connections in the neonate. The position of the umbilical venous catheter is shown. Note how easy it would be to push it accidentally into the right atrium. From S. Wallis & D. Harvey (1979) *Nursing Times* by permission of the authors and editor

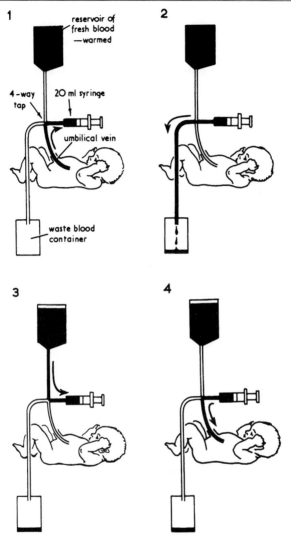

Fig. 12.5 Exchange transfusion. 1, Blood is drawn out into a syringe via an umbilical vein catheter. 2, This blood is discarded into a waste container. 3, blood warmed to body temperature is drawn into this syringe. The blood is crossmatched for compatibility with blood from the baby's mother. 4, This blood is injected slowly. The process is repeated until twice the baby's blood volume has been exchanged. From S. Wallis & D. Harvey (1979) *Nursing Times* by permission of the authors and editor

in extreme emergencies). It is essential that it is fresh (less than two days old) because the intrinsic rate of haemolysis is then less, and also the plasma potassium concentration is normal. It should be compatible with the mother's serum. The total volume of blood exchanged is 180 ml/kg body weight. The blood used must fit the following criteria:

1 Whole blood.
2 Less than two days old.
3 CMV negative.
4 HIV negative.
5 Hep B negative.
6 Hep C negative.
7 Rh negative.
8 HbS negative.
9 TPHA negative.
10 Low haemolysin titres.

Table 12.4 Exchange transfusion: materials and technique.

Materials needed

'Pharmaseal exchange transfusion tray	Blood bottles
Cut-down pack	Sequestrene × 2
Gown and gloves	Heparin 2 ml × 2
Ampoule of normal saline	Blood culture bottles × 2
Fine silk sutures on a cutting needle	
Chlorhexidine in spirit	
Antibiotic spray	
Large scalpel blade and handle	
Blood warmer and blood warming coil	

Technique
1 Place baby on Resuscitaire under heat-shield; connect skin temperature probe and turn to servo control; connect ECG monitor; gently restrain the limbs
2 Put on a gown, prepare tray, prime a suitable venous catheter with saline
3 Run the blood through the giving set. This is connected to the warming coil which in turn is attached to a four-way tap
4 Clean the umbilicus and cord clamp with chlorhexidine in spirit
5 Insert purse-string suture around base of cord (avoiding blood vessels and not piercing skin)
6 Cut cleanly through cord 1 cm above skin with a single slice of the scalpel blade. Pinch base to prevent blood loss
7 Identify vein and dilate gently
8 Insert the venous catheter; size FG 5 or FG 8. Stop as soon as there is a free flow of blood back from the vein (about 10 cm – see Fig. 12.4)
9 Tie catheter to the purse-string suture to prevent it falling out

The procedure is summarized in Fig. 12.5 and Tables 12.4 and 12.5. The purpose of the exchange is:

1 To correct anaemia.
2 To remove damaged and antibody-coated red cells.
3 To remove unfixed antibodies.
4 To remove bilirubin from plasma and tissues.

Dangers include:

1 Haemorrhage from disconnected tubing.
2 Thrombosis or embolism due to air or clots.
3 Infection leading to septicaemia.
4 Hypocalcaemia. This is because citrate is used to preserve blood. It binds calcium, thus lowering the amount of ionized calcium in the blood. In spite of this, calcium measured in the usual way will be normal. Some doctors inject 1 ml of 10% calcium gluconate intravenously after every 100 ml of blood exchanged although this is not necessary.
5 Hyperkalaemia is not a problem with fresh blood, but potassium leaks out of *old* red cells into the plasma.
6 Hypothermia. Infused blood should be warmed by passage through

Table 12.5 Exchange transfusion – method.

1 Slowly withdraw 20 ml blood from the baby (less in a preterm baby). Record records 20 ml 'blood out' on sheet; send samples for pre-exchange haemoglobin, plasma urea and electrolytes, calcium, bilirubin, sugar and blood culture
2 Draw up 10 ml (see text) of fresh blood and inject slowly into the baby, watching ECG monitor and baby's condition. Record '10 ml in' on sheet
3 Continue to exchange 10 ml blood at a time: the four-way tap is designed so that if properly connected you continue to turn it clockwise (from baby to waste to fresh blood and back to baby). Keep the baby in at least 10 ml deficit throughout. Each cycle should take about three minutes, depending on the baby's condition.
4 At the end of the exchange send samples of the last 'blood out' for post-exchange haemoglobin, plasma urea and electrolytes, calcium, bilirubin, blood culture and sugar. Then slowly restore the deficit until the total 'blood in' equals the total 'blood out'
5 Check the post-exchange bilirubin *before* removing the catheter: it may be necessary to continue the exchange transfusion
6 Check the blood gases and correct a severe metabolic acidaemia if necessary with intravenous sodium bicarbonate
7 Remove the catheter. Send the tip for culture. Pinch the base of the cord until there is no further bleeding. Put a *small* sterile gauze dressing on the umbilicus in such a way that any bleeding will be apparent. It is best to avoid stitching the stump unless *really* necessary

a heating coil in a water bath or preferably a proper blood warmer at body temperature. It is important to perform the procedure under a heater or with the baby covered in an incubator.

7 Cardiac arrhythmias associated with electrolyte disturbances or rapid injection or withdrawal of blood.

8 Hypoglycaemia.

9 Trauma or perforation of the umbilical vein at insertion of catheter.

10 Late portal hypertension due to venous thrombosis.

A complete cycle takes place as follows: 5, 10 or 20 ml of blood is slowly and gradually withdrawn from the baby; the syringe and four-way tap to which it is attached is turned through 90° clockwise so that the portal to the waste bag is open and the blood is rapidly ejected; the syringe is then turned clockwise through a further 90° and the same volume of donor blood is rapidly drawn up. The syringe is then turned clockwise through 180° and the donor blood slowly injected into the baby. The cycle is then repeated (see Table 12.5). The slower the exchange the more efficient the mixing of bloods and the more effective the procedure. For this reason, and to avoid cardiovascular disturbance, blood must be withdrawn from and injected into the baby slowly. It is useful to pause after injection and before withdrawal to allow further equilibration to take place. In practice, each cycle should take about three minutes.

Obviously, the earlier part of the exchange is more effective than later, by which time a high proportion of donor blood is being re-exchanged. There should therefore be no hesitation in stopping an exchange either temporarily or permanently if there is deterioration in the baby's condition.

Indications for stopping are:

1 Persistent or repeated bradycardia or tachycardia.

2 Cyanosis.

3 Arrhythmias.

At least one assistant is required to monitor the baby's temperature, pulse rate and general condition during each cycle, and keep a 'score' of volumes withdrawn and infused. After each withdrawal or infusion the operator calls, for example, '10 out' or '10 in'. The assistant totals these volumes as the exchange proceeds and is able to correct the doctor if there is confusion as to whether blood is due to be withdrawn or infused next. Such confusion is made less likely by the syringe always having to be turned clockwise, but it is easy to lose concentration during such a repetitive procedure. Following an ET the baby should be monitored carefully for at least four hours, in case of arrhythmias or hypoglycaemia. Bilirubin estimation should always be done two to four hours after an ET to be certain that it has not risen above the exchange indication level again, as in severely affected babies more than one exchange is sometimes necessary. As with the first exchange this is decided on the rate of bilirubin and total bilirubin level. However, there is always a sudden rapid rise after ET and so the rate of rise from the post-exchange specimen to one a few hours later is not a good indication of the subsequent rate of rise. Exchanged babies may become anaemic as transfusion may cause red cell production to be depressed for some weeks. A low platelet count is also common following an exchange transfusion. Babies who have had an exchange transfusion must have their haemoglobin levels checked weekly in the outpatient department and a simple top-up transfusion may be necessary.

The emergency treatment of hydrops fetalis by exchange transfusion is described in Chapter 3.

Conditions Causing Jaundice

Some conditions causing jaundice will now be discussed in greater detail.

Haemolytic disease

Excess haemolysis in the neonatal period may result from incompatibility between fetal and maternal blood groups. The incidence of the different types of disease varies in different parts of the world. In Britain, Rhesus incompatibility is common but becoming less so now that it can be prevented and ABO incompatibility is common, but often mild G-6-PD deficiency (an inherited red cell enzyme abnormality) is common in many parts of the world, for example east Asia and Greece.

Rhesus (Rh) incompatibility

Approximately 85% of Caucasians carry Rh antigen on their red cells and are therefore Rh+. The remainder have no Rh antigen and are therefore Rh−. If a Rh− mother gives birth to a Rh+ baby (the antigen coming from the Rh+ father), and if their ABO groups are similar, Rh+ fetal cells entering the mother's circulation during late pregnancy or parturition may sensitize her. She responds by forming Rh antibodies. When she is next pregnant with an Rh+ baby these antibodies, which are IgG immunoglobulins, are able to cross the placenta and destroy the fetal red cells. Initial sensitization usually occurs in this way but may occur during a miscarriage or if a Rh− woman is inadvertently transfused with Rh+ blood.

In fact there are three pairs of Rh genes, C, D and E. D is the most important and Rh+ means D+. A father may be Rh− or Rh+. If Rh+, he may be heterozygous (Dd) or homozygous (DD). If homozygous, all his children will be D+; if heterozygous, only half of them will be D+ and therefore at risk. Among Caucasians, one marriage in seven is between a Rh− woman and a Rh+ man, but only six babies in every 1000 born are affected by Rh disease. This is probably because many spouses are of unlike groups in the ABO system. This means that fetal red cells entering the maternal circulation are destroyed by naturally occurring haemolysins in the mother's blood, because of their ABO incompatibility with the mother, before they can cause sensitization. The disease is rare in east Asia because almost all the population are D+.

Problems can occasionally occur in D− women who have the C or E Rhesus antigen. On routine testing they are Rh− but sensitization may occur and may be all the more serious because diagnosis is delayed. C incompatibility can be severe, but E incompatibility is usually mild.

Fetuses are affected to different degrees depending on the strength of the maternal antibody response. Accordingly, there are different modes of presentation. In the most severe cases there is marked haemolysis *in utero* with fetal anaemia, cardiac failure and oedema. The liver and spleen, which are sites of fetal erythropoiesis, are considerably enlarged. Such babies are often stillborn or occasionally born preterm with signs of hydrops fetalis: pallor, gross oedema and hepatosplenomegaly. (The term hydrops is derived from the Greek *hydor* meaning water, and was used by Celsus in AD 30.) The prognosis is poor and immediate ET (see above) provides the only chance of survival. The emergency treatment of hydrops fetalis in the labour ward is discussed in Chapter 3. Less severely affected babies may look normal at birth, although liver and spleen may be palpable. However, within a few hours of birth they become clinically jaundiced with increasingly high levels of unconjugated bilirubin.

Table 12.6 Management of Rh disease.

1 Check Rh and ABO grouping at booking
2 If Rh-negative, measure Rh antibody titre and repeat throughout pregnancy
3 Check father's genotype if antibodies are present to see if he is homozygous or heterozygous
4 Amniocentesis by 20 weeks gestation if Coombs' antibody titre greater than 1 : 16. Spectrophotometry; repeated as indicated
5 Intrauterine transfusion, preterm elective delivery, exchange transfusion as indicated
6 *At birth.* Give 100 μg anti-D immunoglobulin intramuscularly to immunized Rh-negative mother within 48 hours of birth, miscarriage or abortion of a Rh-positive infant. Do Kleihauer test and give larger dose if there is a lot of fetal blood in the mother's circulation

Management.   This is summarized in Table 12.6.

Prevention is important. Red cells from the original Rh+ fetus which sensitizes the Rh− mother usually cross the placenta during labour or at birth and Rh antibodies take several weeks to develop. Sensitization is more likely if there has been a antepartum haemorrhage or in cases of retained placenta requiring manual removal. Antibody formation can be prevented if an intramuscular injection of 100 μg of anti-D immunoglobulin is given soon after the birth or miscarriage of a Rh+ fetus in order to destroy the Rh+ red cells. Thus, anti-D antibody both causes the illness and provides a means of preventing it.

All pregnant women must have their ABO and Rh blood groups determined early in pregnancy. If they are Rh−, their blood should be checked regularly throughout pregnancy for Rh antibodies. A rising antibody titre suggests that the fetus is Rh+ and is being increasingly affected.

If the Coombs' antibody titre rises above 1 : 8 the severity of the disease may also be monitored using a technique developed by Liley (1961). Amniotic fluid is obtained at amniocentesis by the 28th week of pregnancy and is examined spectrophotometrically. The bilirubin molecule absorbs light maximally if the light has a wavelength of 450 nm (this absorption is the optical density of bilirubin). If the optical density of normal bilirubin-free liquor is plotted on a logarithmic scale against wavelength, a straight line is obtained (Fig. 12.6). However, in the presence of bilirubin there is a 'hump' in the graph at 450 nm. The vertical height of the hump is proportional to the amount of bilirubin in the amniotic fluid and this indicates the severity of the disease. By plotting this difference in optical density

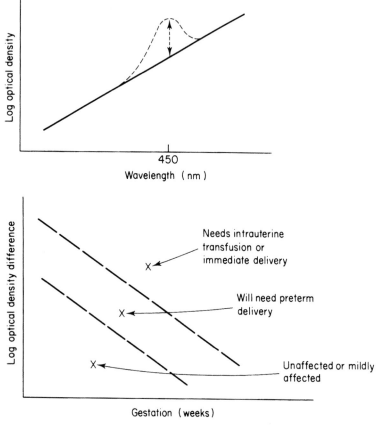

Fig. 12.6 Liley's charts (see text)

logarithmically against the gestational age of the fetus, Liley was able to determine how the pregnancy should be managed. He divided the graph into three zones. In the lower zone are mildly affected babies who may be allowed to go to term. In the middle are babies with moderately severe disease. The amniocentesis may be repeated at intervals to provide further guidance.

The moderately affected babies should be delivered at an optimal time which is a compromise between the complications and risks of preterm delivery, on the one hand, and those of haemolytic disease on the other. The usual time for delivery is between 34 and 37 weeks.

Severely affected babies may be delivered electively very early (28–33 weeks gestation) but the combination of haemolytic disease with extreme prematurity has a high morbidity and mortality. An alternative is to transfuse these babies *in utero* with Rh− blood compatible with that of the mother. This is possible because red cells are rapidly absorbed from the fetal peritoneal cavity. A cannula, aimed under radiographic control or ultrasonic screening, may be directed through the fetal abdominal wall and blood is then injected (Rodeck *et al.*, 1981). The transfusion temporarily corrects fetal anaemia by providing Rh− red cells which are not haemolysed. It may have to be repeated several times before delivery. The technique carries a risk for the fetus, particularly fetal bleeding which may result in intrauterine death. However, babies born alive are much less likely to be anaemic and have a better prognosis.

At birth, clamp the cord at once and cut it 5 cm from the umbilicus. Collect cord blood and arrange tests for blood group, direct Coombs' antiglobulin test (to detect the presence of antibody on the baby's red cells), bilirubin concentration, haemoglobin and packed cell volume. On the basis of these results a decision is made about further management (see Table 12.3). Mildly affected babies are placed under phototherapy (see above) and their bilirubin level checked four-hourly. Severely affected babies require early exchange transfusion.

It should be realized that a false-negative Coombs' test is found in some severely affected babies who have received several intrauterine transfusions. These babies' red cells have been largely replaced by transfused Rh− donor blood, hence the negative test result.

Phototherapy in a Rh-affected baby should be started at birth. There is good evidence that it will reduce the number of exchange transfusions.

ABO incompatibility

ABO incompatibility is common but usually mild. It frequently presents with jaundice within 24 hours of birth. Any baby jaundiced at this time must have blood group and Coombs' test checked. Classically the syndrome occurs in Group O mothers with Group A or B infants. Unlike in Rh disease, the Coombs' test is usually negative (although it may be positive in albumin), the anaemia is less severe and the antibodies that cause haemolysis occur naturally without previous sensitization. These antibodies are IgG immunoglobulins and are known as α- and β-haemolysins. They are able to cross the placenta from mother to baby and destroy group A or B cells respectively. They may be detected in maternal serum to confirm the diagnosis. Treatment is dependent on the rate of rise and absolute level of unconjugated bilirubin and is either by phototherapy or by exchange transfusion as described above. Some mothers have haemolysins which are IgM immunoglobulins. These cannot cross the placenta and therefore do not cause haemolysis in the baby.

Glucose-6-phosphate dehydrogenase (G-6-PD) deficiency

G-6-PD is an important enzyme in red cells as well as in leucocytes and other cells. A deficiency of the enzyme makes the red cells liable to haemolyse in certain situations, for example after taking some drugs (e.g. sulphonamides, primaquine, nitrofurantoin) or during an infection. Many Africans, West Indians and Black Americans have this enzyme defect; it is also common among inhabitants of Mediterranean countries who in addition may haemolyse if they eat broad beans, a condition known as favism. The condition is inherited as a sex-linked recessive, like haemophilia, thus males are usually affected while females are carriers. However, newborn babies who are G-6-PD-deficient may have spontaneous haemolysis (in the absence of an exogenous precipating factor). In addition, newborn baby girls may be affected, although not usually as severely as boys.

G-6-PD deficiency is the commonest indication for exchange transfusion in the Far East. In Britain, it must be considered in the differential diagnosis of neonatal jaundice in the above racial groups. G-6-PD may be checked easily in most laboratories.

Treatment is as for other causes of haemolysis and exchange transfusion is often necessary.

Many drugs that cause haemolysis in susceptible patients are excreted in breast milk and a mother who is breastfeeding must take care to avoid them. When the baby goes home, the parents should be given a list of drugs that the baby should avoid in the future and a copy should be sent to the family doctor with the discharge summary (Table 12.7). It is important to remember that babies with high reticulocyte counts may have falsely high G-6-PD levels as reticulocytes contain more G-6-PD than mature red cells. Even normal babies may have reticulocyte counts of up to 7% on the first postnatal day, while babies who are haemolysing may have considerably more. In such babies with G-6-PD deficiency, blood taken during the early days of life may not exclude the diagnosis; blood taken later will show low G-6-PD levels.

Table 12.7 Drugs that may cause haemolysis in G-6-PD-deficient subjects.

Aminoquinolines (antimalarials)	*Analgesics* Acetylsalicylic acid (aspirin)
Primaquine	Phenacetin (Acetophenetidin)
Pamaquin	Acetanilid
Chloroquine	Paracetamol
Pentaquine	
	Miscellaneous
Sulphones	Vitamin K (water-soluble analogues)
Dapsone	Napthalene (moth balls)
Sulphoxone	Probenecid
Thiazosulphone	Dimercaprol (BAL)
Diaminidiphenyl sulphone (DDS)	Methylene blue
	Acetylphenylhydrazine
Sulphonamides	Phenylhydrazine
Sulphanilamide	*p*-Aminosalicylic acid (PAS)
Sulphacetamide	Nalidixic acid
Sulphafurazole	Neoarsphenamine
Sulphisozaxole	Quinine
Sulphamethoxypyridazine	Quinidine
Salicylazosulphapyridine	Chloramphenicol
	Isoniazid
Nitrofurans	Trinitrotoluene
Nitrofurantoin	Broad beans (*Fava*)
Furaxolodine	
Nitrofurazone	

Others

Congenital spherocytosis, a hereditary disease in which red cells are small and spherical rather than disc-shaped, may sometimes present in the newborn period. There is usually a family history of jaundice or gall-stones. The neonatal jaundice which may result is generally mild but may need exchange transfusion.

Beta-thalassaemia hardly ever presents in the newborn as it is due to defective beta-chain haemoglobin production, and fetal haemoglobin (which makes up nearly all the baby's haemoglobin at birth) contains two alpha and two gamma (but no beta) chains. It is only when sufficient adult haemoglobin (alpha$_2$–beta$_2$) is produced during the second half of the first year of life that the condition may present.

In contrast, the less common *alpha-thalassaemia*, in which alpha chains are synthesized abnormally, produces abnormalities both in fetal life and later. If a fetus inherits the alpha-thalassaemia gene from both parents and is thus homozygous severe hydrops develops *in utero*. Its haemoglobin is made up entirely of gamma chains and is known as haemoglobin Bart's. Such babies often die *in utero*; a few reach term and may survive for a short time.

Obstructive jaundice

Obstructive jaundice is much less common than non-obstructive jaundice in the neonatal period. The differentiation between the two usual causes, hepatitis and biliary atresia, is frequently impossible without the use of special tests at specialist units, including the use of ultrasound and liver biopsy. Obstructive jaundice is characterized by a high level of conjugated bilirubin, pale stools and dark urine due to the presence of bile.

Biliary atresia

Biliary atresia may be either extrahepatic or intrahepatic (possibly secondary to hepatitis in some cases). Infants present with increasingly severe jaundice, which may, however, vary in intensity. The liver is enlarged and firm. Tests show that the bilirubin is conjugated and that the urine contains bilirubin but no urobilinogen. Distinction from hepatitis is often difficult. The prognosis is poor as only a small number prove to be operable. In the few infants in whom corrective surgery is possible it is important that the diagnosis is made before liver damage has taken place (by about two months of age).

Hepatitis

Hepatitis may be due to one of several organisms in the newborn, for example the viruses of hepatitis A and B, cytomegalovirus, herpes simplex, rubella or toxoplasmosis. Many of these are transplacentally acquired. In some cases the jaundice is part of a wider syndrome of disease more or less specific to the infecting organism. In the majority of cases, however, no cause is found. About 70% recover spontaneously. Results indicating severe hepatitis include markedly abnormal liver function tests. High IgM levels in cord blood or blood taken shortly after birth are good non-specific evidence of intrauterine infection. (IgM levels greater than 20 mg/100 ml are abnormal.) Compliment-fixation tests showing a rise in antibody titre to a specific organism may also be significant. In some cases, where there are low levels of α_1-antitrypsin in the blood, the hepatitis may progress irreversibly to cirrhosis and hepatic failure (see below).

α_1-Antitrypsin deficiency

Deficiency of α_1-antitrypsin is responsible for a significant proportion of cholestatic jaundice in infants, perhaps 5–30%. It is an autosomal recessively inherited condition although not all affected individuals will show clinical manifestations. Many different genetic variants exist. α_1-Antitrypsin is a glycoprotein synthesized in the liver which normally inhibits many enzymes which break down protein. It is thought that its lack allows a damaging process in the liver (however initiated) to continue unchecked.

Some infants deteriorate rapidly with ascites and hepatic failure within months. In others the course is more chronic with persisting conjugated hyperbilirubinaemia and, usually, cirrhosis by adolescence. Diagnosis is by finding low α_1-antitrypsin levels in serum and tissue fluids. Electron microscopy shows amorphous cytoplasmic granules in the liver cells.

The variety of clinical associations with the homozygous state makes genetic counselling difficult but the severity of the disease tends to be consistent in an individual family. It is now possible, using fetal blood sampling techniques, to identify the protease inhibitor phenotype sufficiently early in pregnancy to offer termination to parents who have already had a severely affected infant.

Hypothyroidism

This condition is discussed in Chapter 4.

Galactosaemia

Prolonged neonatal jaundice with predominantly conjugated hyperbilirubinaemia may be a presenting feature of galactosaemia. There may also be hepatomegaly and cataracts with poor feeding or vomiting and failure to thrive. The condition is due to the absence of the enzyme galactose-1-phosphate uridyl transferase which converts galactose to glucose. This causes toxic galactose to accumulate in the blood and damage the liver (sometimes causing haemorrhages as well as jaundice), and central nervous system leading to blindness and mental retardation. The galactose is excreted in the urine where it is detected by a positive Clinitest (Clinistix, which detect glucose, will be negative) and by sugar chromatography. There will also be proteinuria and abnormal aminoaciduria. The diagnosis is confirmed by finding a deficiency of the enzyme in red cells. Treatment is by excluding the lactose in milk from the diet (lactose is made up of galactose and glucose) by feeding with a proprietary low-lactose milk. Growth and development then take place normally. Vitamin supplements are necessary and the parents must subsequently be given a diet sheet telling them which foods must not be given to their baby. Galactosaemia is inherited as an autosomal recessive condition and the recurrence rate in subsequent pregnancies is one in four. The diagnosis can now be made antenatally by culturing amniotic cells (see Chapter 2). When there is a family history, cord blood should always be tested.

Fructosaemia

This rare inborn error of metabolism appears when fructose or sucrose, from which it is derived, are included in the baby's diet. It can present with neonatal jaundice and bleeding. Today it is likely to present later because sucrose is less used in artificial milk formulae. The urine contains reducing substances and hypoglucosaemia is common.

Kernicterus

It has been said that high unconjugated levels of bilirubin which exceed the albumin-binding capacity of the baby's plasma are dangerous, as bilirubin is able to enter the brain and cause damage. This condition is known as kernicterus. There is no unequivocally safe level of serum bilirubin. Levels of 380 μmol/l are usually safe in term babies; levels of 180 μmol/l could damage an ill baby of 28 weeks gestation. One of the problems is that kernicterus is sometimes seen as post-mortem when only very mild jaundice was present in life (serum bilirubin as low as 100 μmol/l). It is known that this post-mortem kernicterus can be prevented by treating jaundice at very low levels of bilirubin, but we do not know how important this is. Bilirubin is an antioxidant, and it is now thought that some bilirubin may serve a physiologically useful purpose. It is important to check bilirubin levels and relate them to the gestational and chronological ages and to the general condition of the baby. Plotting levels graphically is useful. Logically, the albumin-binding capacity of a baby's blood would be the most helpful measurement, but it is difficult to do in practice (see above).

Free unconjugated bilirubin enters the brain and causes damage by interfering with specific neuronal enzyme activities, particularly in the basal ganglia, corpus striatum and thalamus. Liver conjugation of bilirubin with glucuronic acid renders it fat-insoluble, unable to enter the brain and therefore non-toxic.

Clinically, affected babies are lethargic and poor feeders. They may subsequently become floppy or hypertonic, with head retraction and convulsions. The Moro reflex is abnormally stereotyped with only extension and no adduction. If the infant survives, there may be mental handicap, convulsions and, by two years of age, the signs of athetoid cerebral palsy with high-tone deafness.

The appearance of neurological signs in a deeply jaundiced baby is an indication for immediate exchange transfusion, with Group O rhesus-negative blood if necessary. Kernicterus should be exceedingly rare in properly organized neonatal units.

References and Further Reading

Brown, K.A., Kim, M.H., Wu, P. *et al.* (1985) Efficacy of phototherapy in prevention and management of neonatal hyperbilirubinaemia. *Pediatrics*, 75 (Suppl.), 393–400.

Gartner, L.M. (1983) Breast milk jaundice. In *Hyperbilirubinaemia in the Newborn: Report of the Eighty-fifth Ross Conference on Pediatric Research* eds Levine, R.L. & Maisels, M.J. Columbus, OH: Ross Laboratories.

Goldman, S.L., Penalver, A. & Penaranda, R. (1982) Jaundice meter: evaluation of new guidelines. *J. Pediatr., 101*, 253.

Lav, S.P. & Fung, K.R. (1984) Serum bilirubin kinetics in intermittent phototherapy of physiological jaundice. *Arch. Dis. Child., 59*, 892–894.

Liley, A.W. (1961) Liquor amnii analysis in management of pregnancy complicated by rhesus sensitisation. *Am. J. Obstet. Gynecol., 82*, 1359.

Maisels, M.J. (1992) Neonatal Jaundice. In *Effective Care of the Newborn Infant*, pp. 507–561, eds Sinclair, J.C. and Bracken, M.B.

Messner, K.H., Leure-Dupree, A.E. & Maisels, M.J. (1975) The effects of continuous prolonged illumination on the newborn primate retina (abstr). *Pediatr. Res, 9*, 368.

Modi, N. (1989) Jaundice. In *The Baby under 1000 g*, eds Harvey, D., Cooke, R.W.I. and Levitt, G.A. London: Wright.

Mollison, P.L. (1983) In *Blood Transfusion in Clinical Medicine*, 7th ed., p. 105. Oxford: Blackwell Scientific.

Rodeck, C.H., Holman, C.A., Karnicki, J. *et al.* (1981) Direct intravascular fetal blood transfusion by fetoscopy in severe Rhesus isoimmunisation. *Lancet, i*, 625–627.

Strange, M. & Cassady, G. (1985) Neonatal transcutaneous bilirubinometry. *Clin. Perinatol, 12,* 51.

Wallin, A. & Boreus, L.O. (1984) Phenobarbitol prophylaxis for hyper-bilirubinaemia in preterm infants. A controlled study of bilirubin disappearance and infant behaviour. *Acta Paediatr. Scand., 73,* 488–497.

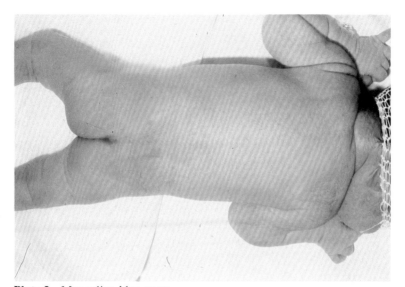

Plate I Mongolian blue spots.

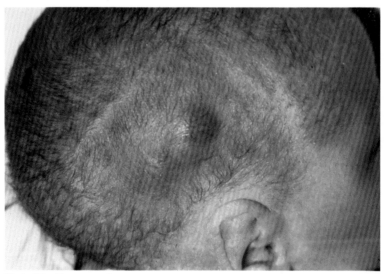

Plate II Fat necrosis.

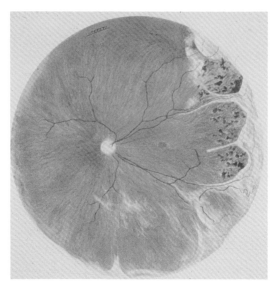

Plate III Retinal detachment in retrolental fibroplasia.

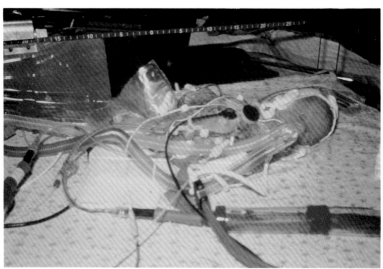

Plate IV Ventilated baby with several pneumothoraces. Heimlich flutter valves in use.

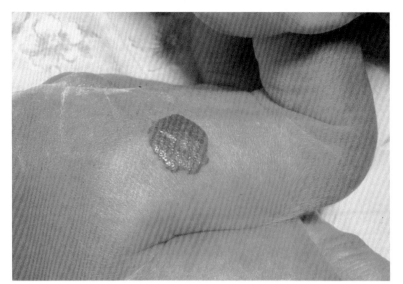

Plate V   Strawberry naevus.

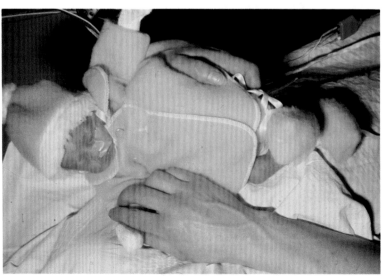

Plate VI   Baby dressed in own clothes.

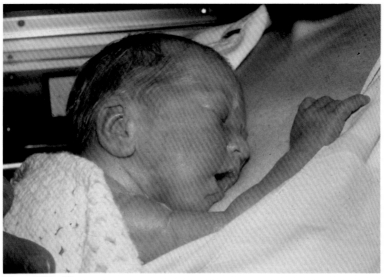

Plate VII Kangaroo care.

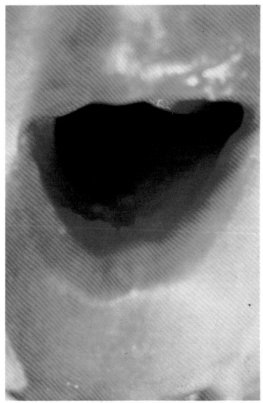

Plate VIII Cleft palate.

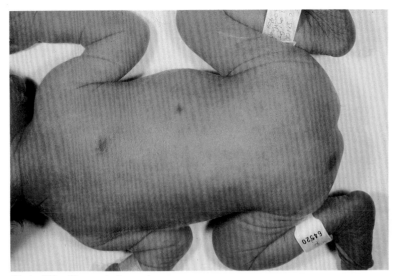

Plate IX   Pigmented naevi.

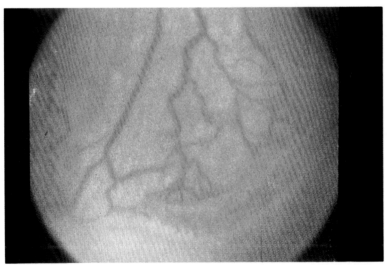

Plate X   Retinal changes in retinopathy of prematurity.

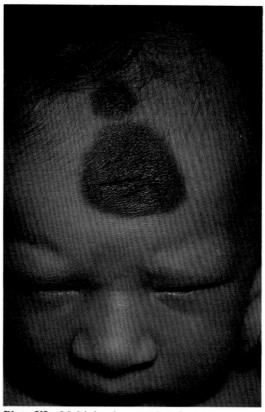

Plate XI Multiple pigmented moles.

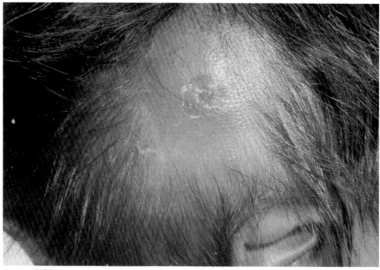

Plate XII Wound from scalp electrode.

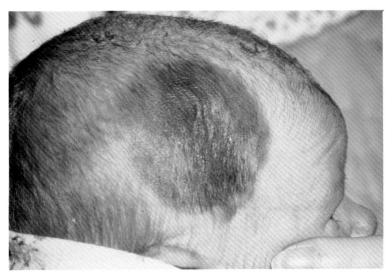

Plate XIII Severe bruising from ventouse extraction cap.

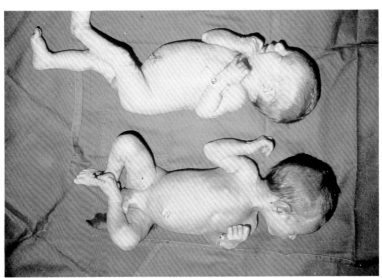

Plate XIV Twin to twin transfusion.

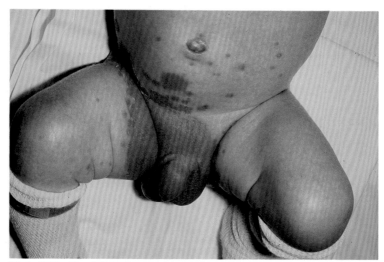

Plate XV   Candida infection.

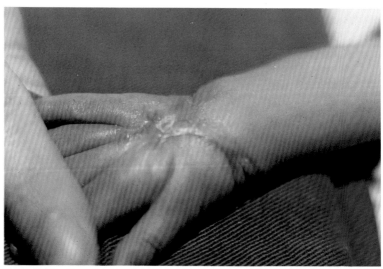

Plate XVI   Scarring at site of tissued intravenous infusion.

—13

Bleeding Disorders

Bleeding in the newborn infant may be due to local causes including trauma, asphyxia or infection or may result from failure of haemostatic mechanisms. Local haemorrhages may be due to local causes or they may occur secondarily to general haemostatic failure. The newborn infant has two mechanisms in the blood for preventing bleeding: platelets and coagulation factors. In the healthy full-term newborn baby the platelet count is usually above $100\ 000 \times 10^9/l$. Around one-third of babies on an intensive care unit will have platelet counts below this level, but they do not usually fall to a level where haemorrhage occurs – below $20\ 000 \times 10^9/l$. Some factors (V, VIII and fibrinogen) are low compared to older infants. Factor VIII: C levels are 30–50% higher in vaginally delivered babies, than those delivered by caesarian section. Factors synthesized in the baby's liver, which depend on adequate levels of vitamin K, are low at birth and drop even further during the first few days of life. Vitamin K is made by bacteria in the gut; at birth the gut is sterile and only gradually becomes colonized with bacteria during feeding. This process takes longer in breastfed than bottle-fed babies, and therefore vitamin K supplementation may be particularly important in breastfed babies. The normal postnatal drop in these factors (II, VII, IX and X) can be prevented by giving vitamin K to newborn babies. Preterm babies have low levels of nearly all clotting factors and their platelet count is relatively low until they reach the equivalent of about 30 weeks gestation. In addition, their blood vessels are fragile and easily damaged so they bleed and bruise easily.

Causes of Neonatal Bleeding

The conditions that cause bleeding in the newborn infant may be classified as follows:

Generalized bleeding tendency

Deficiency of coagulation factors may result from:

1 Exaggeration of the temporary drop in vitamin K dependent factors which occurs after birth. This is *haemorrhagic disease of the newborn* (HDN) and responds to the administration of vitamin K. It is most common in breastfed babies or those not given vitamin K as a routine. It is now less common in the neonatal period but may be seen later following gastrointestinal upset with or without antibiotic treatment.
2 Failure of synthesis in the liver. Bleeding due to hepatic disorders does not improve with vitamin K but is usually temporary.
3 Congenital disorders of coagulation factor synthesis, e.g. haemophilia (Factor VIII) or Christmas disease (Factor IX). These conditions are permanent but do not often present in the newborn period, except after circumcision.

Deficiency of platelets may be due to:

1 Impaired production, often associated with skeletal abnormalities. Fanconi's anaemia may present as isolated thrombocytopenic purpura at this age.
2 Excessive destruction. This may be secondary to maternal drugs, such as the thiazide diurectics, to maternal idiopathic thrombocytopenic purpura, when maternal antibodies cross the placenta, to maternal systemic lupus erythematosus or to intrauterine infection (e.g. toxoplasmosis or rubella). Platelet antigen incompatibility is being increasingly recognized; 98% of the population are antigen (PLA_1) positive, 2% negative. An allo-immune response may occur in the PLA_1 positive offspring of PLA_1 negative mothers – an analogous situation to rhesus disease (Daffos *et al.*, 1984). Isolated thrombocytopenic purpura may be seen with serious infection e.g. intrapartum acquisition of β-haemolytic streptococci.

Combined deficiencies, with low levels of both platelets and coagulation factors, are found when both are consumed in the process of disseminated intravascular coagulation (DIC). This almost always occurs in infants who are already extremely unwell with infection, hypoxia, hypothermia or severe rhesus disease. Clots may then form within the circulation in these very ill babies and the platelets and clotting factors cannot then be replaced quickly enough to prevent profuse bleeding into the tissues.

Local causes

Local causes of bleeding include:

1 Loose clamp or ligature on umbilical cord, or premature attempts to dislodge the cord remnant.
2 Birth trauma causing, for example, cephalhaematoma or subcapsular liver haematoma.
3 Subaponeurotic haemorrhage.
4 Gastrointestinal bleeding due to volvulus, fissure or polyp.
5 Intraventricular haemorrhage in hypoxaemia.
6 Intrapulmonary haemorrhage in hypothermia.

The commonest cause of bleeding in an otherwise well infant is haemorrhagic disease of the newborn. In the sick infant it is probably DIC.

The causes of local haemorrhage classified by site are summarized in Table 13.1.

There are three common clinical situations in which there is neonatal bleeding unassociated with haemostatic failure. *Vaginal bleeding* in newborn girls is common and is due to withdrawal from maternal circulating oestrogens. The mechanism is therefore analogous to the normal menses in the post-pubertal girl or withdrawal bleeding when coming off the contraceptive pill. Parents should be warned to expect this and reassured that it is harmless if it does occur.

Haemorrhage from the umbilical cord may be due to infection or to the cord ligature being too loose or having slipped. Most usually, however, it is due to fiddling with the partially separated cord, before it is ready to separate. *Haematemesis or melaena* in the neonate is most commonly due to swallowed maternal blood. This may have been swallowed either during delivery or from cracked nipples during breastfeeding. The blood can sometimes be shown to be of maternal origin if the haemoglobin is denatured by alkali (Apt's test, Table 13.2). Do *not* assume that swallowed blood is the cause; examine the baby carefully.

Blood Loss Before Birth

Causes of fetal haemorrhage include caesarean section with an anterior placenta praevia, abruption with tearing of blood vessels on the fetal side of the placenta, transplacental fetomaternal transfusion and trauma at artificial rupture of membranes. It is thought that fetomaternal transfusion occurs in up to 50% of pregnancies. In 10% the loss to the fetus is between 0.5 ml and 40 ml, but it may be as high

Table 13.1 Causes of local bleeding according to site.

Site of bleeding	Possible clinical associations	Possible haemostatic deficiencies
Umbilicus	Trauma, infection, loose clamp or ligature	Haemorrhagic disease of the newborn (HDN); Factor VII or XIII; fibrinogen
Skin petechiae	Asphyxia (cord around neck, facial petechiae), intrauterine infection	Thrombocytopenia
Bruising	Trauma	Any coagulation deficiency
Gastrointestinal tract	Swallowed maternal blood, nasogastric tube trauma	HDN
Pulmonary	Kernicterus, SFGA, RDS	DIC
Intra-abdominal	Breech delivery causing ruptured liver or spleen	
Genito-urinary	Urinary tract infection, renal vein thrombosis	HDN
Scalp	Vacuum extraction, subaponeurotic haemorrhage in Afro-Caribbean babies	HDN
Intracranial subdural	Trauma	
Intracranial subarachnoid	Infection	DIC, any haemostatic defect
Intracranial periventricular	Preterm, RDS	
Circumcision	Bad surgical technique. Less common with Plastibell circumcision	Any haemostatic defect; for example haemophilia may present in this way

as 100 ml or more in 1%. Fetal haemorrhage should be suspected if there is loss of bright red blood from the mother's vagina before delivery. The diagnosis may be confirmed by Apt's test – see above. A similar principle is used in Kleihauer's test to search for fetal cells in the mother's blood. Fetal haemoglobin does not denature with alkali, and fetal red cells can be detected in a film of maternal blood. The fetal cells stand out against 'ghosts' of maternal cells, and this allows an estimate to be made of the size of the fetomaternal transfusion.

Treatment is urgent if the baby is pale or shocked at delivery; it involves early delivery and clamping of the cord, followed by blood

Table 13.2 Apt's test.

1 Dissolve two drops of adult blood in half a test tube of water
2 Dissolve sufficient of the specimen to be tested in the same volume of water so that the colour obtained matches
3 Dissolve two drops of baby's blood in the same volume of water
4 Increase the volume of each solution by about one-fifth by adding 1% sodium hydroxide (NaOH)
5 Wait for one or two minutes
6 Within this time the tube containing adult blood changes from pink to yellow–brown as the alkali denatures the adult haemoglobin. Fetal blood remains pink
7 Compare the colour of the specimen tube and identify the specimen as of fetal or maternal origin

transfusion, with Group O rhesus negative blood if necessary. Initially 10–15 ml/kg should be given, and further transfusion carried out if the baby remains shocked, with a low blood pressure and poor peripheral perfusion.

History and Examination

In all cases, a careful history must be taken from the mother. A note should be made of her general health, anticoagulant therapy given, or other drugs taken during pregnancy, such as aspirin or phenytoin, which may increase the risk of bleeding disorders in the newborn. The birth history should be checked for evidence of trauma. The mother should be asked specifically about contact with rubella or other infections; whether there is a family history of bleeding tendency; about the infant's progress from birth; whether the baby is breast fed; and if vitamin K has been given.

The baby should be examined carefully. First the general circulatory state must be assessed; skin colour should be observed, and pulse, respiration rate and blood pressure measured. This examination must include palpatation of the liver and spleen to detect any enlargement, a search for congenital abnormalities, bruising and petechial haemorrhages. If localized bleeding has occurred from the umbilicus, the cord clamp should be checked, as sometimes this becomes loose as the cord shrinks after birth.

If there is bleeding beneath the scalp the head develops a generalized boggy swelling. Measurement of the head circumference is useful because the difference between the head circumference at birth and later will give an indication of the amount of blood lost into the scalp. Check that the baby has not had heparin, for example, in a blood transfusion.

Investigations

1 *Group and crossmatch* blood in case transfusion is required.
2 *Haemoglobin (Hb) and packed cell volume* to help assess severity of blood loss.
3 *Platelet count.* A count below 80–100 × 10^9/l is abnormal in the newborn. If the count is below 20 × 10^9/l there is a risk of bleeding.
4 *Clotting studies.* Thrombotest measures factors II (prothrombin), VII, IX, and X – the vitamin K dependent clotting factors. Prothrombin time tests for deficiencies of factors II, V, VII and X. Partial thromboplastin time tests for deficiencies of factors VIII (low in haemophilia), IX (Christmas factor), XI and XII. It will be prolonged if the prothrombin time or the thrombotest is abnormal; specific assays of individual factors may be necessary. Fibrinogen degradation products are elevated when fibrin clots formed in the circulation are broken down. They are usually raised when there is DIC.
5 *Apt's test* (see Table 13.2).

Management

Local bleeding

Any obvious local cause of bleeding from, for example, the umbilicus should be stopped with firm pressure and then a cord clamp or suture applied.

Transfusion

A baby who is pale and shocked, needs urgent transfusion. Blood should be taken for investigation but treatment should proceed before the results are obtained. An intravenous transfusion of Group O rhesus-negative blood is set up immediately (plasma can be used if blood is not readily available). Shock is corrected by giving 10–15 ml/kg over the first 10 minutes. The baby is then reassessed and more blood given as necessary.

Repeated estimates of haemoglobin and packed cell volume should be made to assess the baby's progress.

A pale baby who is not shocked should be observed carefully with half-hourly pulse, respiration, and blood pressure measurements. If bleeding is continuing internally there may be a sudden deterioration.

Most babies with a haemoglobin of less than 10 g/dl at birth will need a transfusion.

Emergency blood donation from walking donors is now considered unsafe. Whole blood and blood products obtained from the transfusion centre would have been screened for infections such as syphilis, hepatitis, CMV and HIV.

Vitamin K

In many countries such as the USA, vitamin K is given routinely. In the UK practice has varied over the past few decades. When vitamin K was introduced it was thought there was an increased risk of kernicterus. Vitamin K (Konakion) was introduced but many centres ceased to use routine prophylaxis.

Recently, there has been a resurgence of haemorrhagic disease of the newborn (HDN), particularly of the late onset variety, which occurs between seven days and six weeks. Despite this increase it is still quite a rare condition (McNinch & Tripp, 1991) but the prognosis is not good. Thirty to fifty per cent of babies with late-onset HDN will suffer severe brain damage or die. There has therefore been a return to routine prophylaxis. Intramuscular and intravenous administration of vitamin K_1 produce higher levels than its oral use, but many professionals and parents prefer the baby not to have an injection. The route of administration therefore varies between units.

Two studies have now reported an increased risk of childhood cancer with the use of vitamin K after birth (Golding *et al.*, 1992; Draper & Stiller, 1992). The second report suggests that the risk is related to injected vitamin K rather than its oral use. These were not controlled trials and the data were not complete, therefore there is some doubt over the relevance of these studies (Hull, 1992).

This leaves us with a problem in recommending routine clinical practice. Until further work has been done on the effects of injected vitamin K, it has been recommended that all babies receive an oral dose of 0.5 mg after the first feed, with two subsequent doses of 0.5 mg being given to breast-fed babies at seven days and six weeks. When an oral route is not possible, an intramuscular or intravenous dose of 0.1 mg may be given on the instructions of a paediatrician (Report of an Expert Committee, 1992).

There is at present the problem that Konakion has not been licensed for oral administration. Department of Health guidelines suggest that it must be properly prescribed by a doctor before being given.

If the platelet count is less than $100 \times 10^9/l$

Check whether the mother has been unwell or her platelet count is low. A mother who has systemic lupus erythematosus or thrombocytopenic purpura may produce a transient secondary thrombocytopenia in her baby. Healthy mothers may also pass antiplatelet antibodies across the placenta, resulting in transient thrombocytopenia. These babies are usually well apart from petechial haemorrhages in the skin or mucosae. If the platelet count remains low the bone marrow should be examined.

Examine the infant carefully. Congenital malformations are sometimes associated with bone marrow abnormalities, for example Fanconi's anaemia, where there is pancytopenia associated with upper limb malformation, and the radial aplasia thrombocytopenia syndrome. These diagnoses are confirmed by bone marrow examination. Enlargement of the liver and spleen with thrombocytopenia occurs with intrauterine infection; thus the baby should be screened for rubella, cytomegalovirus, toxoplasmosis and syphilis. Thrombocytopenia is usually transient in these conditions.

Sick preterm infants are most likely to develop DIC, particularly those with septicaemia or hypoxia and acidosis secondary to RDS or rhesus disease. The platelet count is low, the prothrombin and partial thromboplastin times are prolonged and fibrinogen degradation products elevated. It is most important to treat the precipitating illness vigorously with antibiotics, artificial ventilation and oxygen or exchange transfusion as indicated. The coagulation disorder is treated with transfusions of fresh plasma containing clotting factors and platelets. Fresh blood can be used if the haemoglobin level has dropped. If fibrinogen levels have dropped (below 1 g), cryoprecipitate is useful.

Platelet transfusions also have an important place in the treatment, but are usually reserved for those babies with severe haemorrhage, or platelet counts below $10 \times 10^9/l$. Coagulation studies must be repeated one to two hours after all products have been infused.

If the platelet count is normal but clotting times abnormal

In a baby who is bleeding, a prolonged prothrombin time or thrombotest less than 10% of normal is probably due to haemorrhagic disease of the newborn. This temporary deficiency of vitamin K dependent clotting factors should be treated by vitamin K_1 (Konakion) 1 mg intramuscularly or intravenously. The diagnosis is confirmed if the prothrombin time or thrombotest returns to normal within 12 hours. A prothrombin time or thrombotest remaining abnormal after an injection of vitamin K_1 indicates a deficiency of clotting factors. If the infant is well it is probably due to an inherited deficiency of a clotting factor and so the family history should be checked. The partial thromboplastin time will be prolonged and by repeating this test after adding small amounts of different clotting factors, the specific deficiency can be discovered. If the infant is sick a reduction of clotting factors may be due to severe liver disease, for example secondary to fructosaemia or galactosaemia, and the urine can be checked for reducing substances.

The mother should always be asked if she has taken anticoagulants or any other drugs which could interfere with the production of clotting factors in the baby. During the last few weeks of pregnancy most mothers taking anticoagulants are changed from a coumarin type drug, for example warfarin, to heparin which does not affect the fetus. Mothers on anticonvulsants should be given vitamin K at the onset of labour.

The baby may have had too much heparin during a blood transfusion or from heparinized saline in an umbilical arterial catheter. This can be reversed using protamine (1 mg for each 100 units of heparin, maximum 50 mg).

References and Further Reading

Daffos, F., Forestier, F., Muller, J.Y. *et al.* (1984) Prenatal treatment of alloimmune thrombocytopenia. Lancet, ii, 632.

Draper, G.J. & Stiller, C.A. (1992) Intramuscular vitamin K and childhood cancer. *BMJ, 305*, 709.

Golding, J., Birmingham, K., Greenwood, R. *et al.* (1992) Childhood cancer, intramuscular vitamin K and pethidine given during labour *BMJ, 305*, 341–346.

Hann, I.M., Gibson, B.E.S. & Letsky, E.A. (eds) (1991) *Fetal and Neonatal Haematology*. London: Ballière Tindall.

Hinchcliffe, R.F. & Lilleyman, J.S. (eds) (1987) *Practical Paediatric Haematology*. Chichester: John Wiley.

Hull, D. (1992) Vitamin K and childhood cancer. The risk of haemorrhagic disease is certain; that of cancer is not. *BMJ, 305*, 326–327.

—14

Neurological Disorders

Neurological disorders remain an important problem in the preterm baby. As many as 50% of those less than 30 weeks gestation will have evidence of periventricular haemorrhage (PVH) or germinal matrix haemorrhage (GMH). None the less, around 95% of preterm babies will attend normal schools. The price for very many more normal survivors is a few more surviving with disability. It seems that there is not a particularly high risk of serious sequalae for those of very low gestation, but this will need close monitoring.

Neurological disorders may be conveniently categorized as shown in Table 14.1. They may be considered as primary malformations (e.g. aqueduct stenosis) or as secondary deformations (destruction of

Table 14.1 Neurological abnormalities

Structural Central Nervous System (CNS) abnormalities
Hydrocephalus (see Chapter 10)
Microcephaly (see Chapter 10)
Hydranencephaly
Anencephaly (see Chapter 10)
Myelomeningocele (see Chapter 10)
Other midline abnormalities
    Dermal sinus
    Hairy patch
    Naevus
Degenerative diseases

Abnormal neurological behaviour unassociated with overt structural abnormalities
Cerebral irritation
Cerebral depression ± respiratory failure
Fits
Hypotonic baby
Kernicterus (see Chapter 12)
Meningitis (see Chapter 16)
Subarachnoid haemorrhage
Babies born to drug-dependent mothers

Traumatic lesions
Peripheral nerve palsy (see Chapter 5)
Brachial plexus palsy (see Chapter 5)

structures already formed). Some conditions are described in other chapters.

Hydrocephalus

Hydrocephalus (Fig. 14.1) has already been mentioned as a common association with myelomeningocele. It may also occur separately, due either to primary structural abnormalities (such as aqueduct atresia or stenosis) or to blockage secondary to infection (such as toxoplasmosis or meningitis) or intraventricular haemorrhage (Fig. 14.2). Hydrocephalus may only be discovered by measuring the head circumference regularly, but may now more commonly be detected by ultrasound scanning of the brain in the fetal or newborn period, and palliative

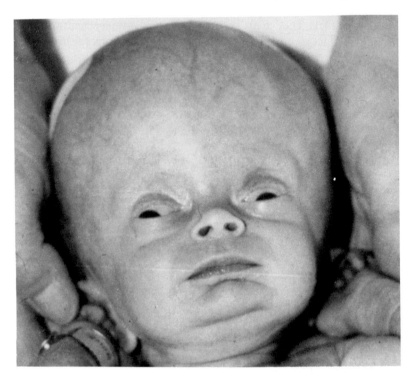

Fig. 14.1 Hydrocephalus

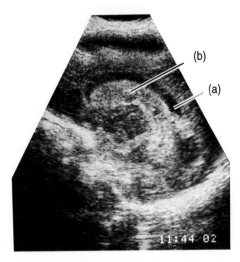

Fig. 14.2 Parasagittal cranial ultrasound scan showing intraventricular haemorrhage in the third ventricle. See page 332.

treatment undertaken if necessary (Clewell *et al.*, 1982). Every baby in a special care baby unit should be measured once weekly and the result plotted on a head circumference against gestational age chart (see p. 76). If the baby's head is enlarging too rapidly, the plot will gradually cross the centiles for the normal population. It is the abnormally fast rate of rise that is crucial for the diagnosis. A large, but normal, baby may have a head circumference above the 90th centile for age, but the head should grow parallel to that centile.

The head enlarges too quickly because the cerebrospinal fluid (CSF) is accumulating under increased pressure. Associated findings therefore include palpable separation of the skull sutures, a bulging anterior fontanelle and prominent scalp veins. A confirmation of hydrocephalus can be obtained by ultrasound scanning to measure the size of the lateral ventricles (Fig. 14.3). If the ventricles continue to enlarge too rapidly, the brain substance will be stretched and damaged (Fig. 14.4). To prevent this fluid must be removed from the lateral ventricles. Initially this may be done by ventricular taps, but if the hydrocephalus worsens a shunt operation is performed. This allows the CSF under raised pressure to drain into the baby's

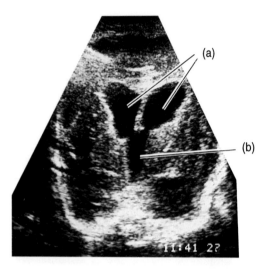

(a)

(b)

Fig. 14.3 Coronal cranial ultrasound scan showing dilatation of lateral ventricles and third ventricle. See page 332.

right atrium or peritoneal cavity (Clewell *et al.*, 1982; Cooke, 1986). A one-way valve prevents blood from entering the ventricle. Unfortunately, such shunts need revising as the baby grows or if they become blocked or infected. Low-grade infection by such organisms as *Staph. epidermidis* are common. For these reasons shunt operations should not be performed unless absolutely essential. Spontaneous arrest of hydrocephalus sometimes occurs, thus obviating the need for surgery.

Microcephaly

A very small head circumference is associated with mental handicap. Antenatal ultrasound scanning may warn the paediatrician by showing a small and slowly growing fetal head. Some babies with perinatal or postnatal brain damage, due for example to asphyxia or cytomegalovirus (CMV) infection, may have a normal head circumference at birth but the brain, and therefore the skull, does not grow postnatally. A measurement of the occipitofrontal circumference during the first week of life is therefore essential to provide a base-line measurement

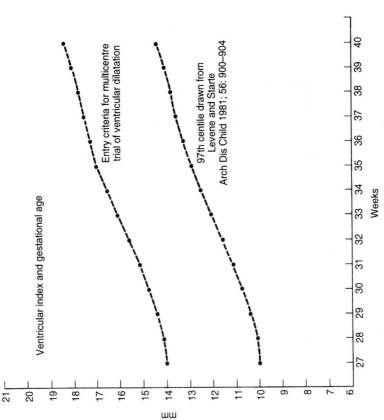

Fig. 14.4 Ventricular index and gestational age

and to identify babies whose heads are already small. A number of insults to the brain can cause microcephaly, particularly a large dose of radiation in the second trimester or intrauterine infections such as rubella or CMV. Sometimes the problem runs in families, but a number of cases cannot be explained.

Hydranencephaly

In this condition the cerebral hemispheres are largely absent and the skull vault contains a watery fluid. The diagnosis may already have been made by fetal ultrasound, but should be considered in a baby with a large or abnormally shaped head or who is exhibiting abnormal behaviour. It may be recognized by transilluminating the head in a darkened room when it will glow brightly. The diagnosis is confirmed by ultrasound. The condition is thought to be due sometimes to severe posthaemorrhagic hydrocephalus and sometimes to infarction or malformation.

The prognosis is usually hopeless, but the extent to which these babies are able to perform basic functions, such as suckling, is surprising and instructive (Cooke, 1987). A few of the post-hydrocephalus group do relatively well. The decision whether to shunt such babies is sometimes a difficult one (Cooke, 1986).

Midline Abnormalities Over the Spine

A naevus or hairy patch over the spine may cover an underlying spinal cord anbormality (e.g. meningocele) or an abnormality of the vertebrae (spina bifida occulta). It is important to perform a detailed examination of the lower limbs and bladder and anal sphincter function. Occasionally, a plain radiograph will reveal diastematomyelia in which a bony spur bisects the spinal cord.

It is common to find shallow coccygeal pits, which are harmless. Sacral or higher pits should be investigated. Rarely a deep pin-sized hole is found which communicates with the theca and is therefore a portal of entry for bacteria that will cause meningitis. These lesions should be sought at the routine postnatal examination and the baby referred urgently to a neurosurgeon.

A pit can be examined with an auriscope which will often enable the floor to be seen and a sinus to be excluded.

Progressive Degenerative Diseases

Most of these conditions do not present in the newborn period, but Werdnig–Hoffmann progressive spinal paralysis (see below) may appear at or within a few weeks of birth.

Cerebral Irritation

It is often difficult to know the significance of findings such as hypertonia, exaggerated tendon jerks, tremor or a high-pitched cry. They may be associated with perinatal hypoxaemia, with or without intracranial haemorrhage or kernicterus. They often seem to have a good prognosis and some of them may be due to headache. Serious signs include poor sucking, convulsions and apnoeic attacks. New neurological examinations and investigations are being developed as a guide to prognosis (Dubowitz *et al.*, 1985). Particular attention is being paid to the baby's ability to look at objects. It is helpful to distinguish between the irritable, bad tempered, inconsolable baby who does not like to be cuddled or handled (because of headache or other pain), who may have a cerebral cry and has a good prognosis, from the baby who may exhibit jaw, ankle, finger or hamstring clonus. The second group of babies may have metabolic upset (hypocalcaemia, hypomagnesaemia, hypernatraemia with thirst), may have drug withdrawal or may have a thyrotoxic mother.

Cyanotic attacks with apnoea carry a bad prognosis as does the need for tube feeding for more than about four days in a term baby. Many apnoeic attacks in such babies are in fact convulsions.

Ultrasound examination is extremely useful in showing structural abnormalities of the brain, such as hydrocephalus and haemorrhage or infarction around the ventricles. Magnetic resonance imaging (MRI) is being used more frequently than in the past and can produce spectacularly good imaging. Magnetic resonance spectroscopy is being developed to examine the chemical changes in the brain, particularly phosphates and protons. This may give an indication of irreparable brain damage. Near infra red spectroscopy (NIRS) can provide information about changes in the blood flow in the brain and intracellular oxygenation. Whilst ultrasound is now well established, the other technological advances are in the research phase of development.

Cerebral Depression

Diminished spontaneous movements, unconsciousness, hypotonia, depressed reflexes and convulsions, may carry a serious prognosis if the signs are prolonged. Brief periods may follow a very difficult or traumatic delivery. Hypotonia may occur in kernicterus.

Fits

Fits are common in newborn babies and are a great source of anxiety both to parents and medical and nursing staff. There are many causes, some peculiar to the newborn, but very often a clinical diagnosis can be made, baseline investigations ordered and appropriate treatment started before the results are available. It is a mistake to expect newborn babies to have grand mal fits of the kind that occur in adults, with an aura, tonic and clonic phases associated with incontinence or tongue-biting. It may be difficult to recognize fits, particularly in the preterm infant, in whom cycling movements, paroxysmal sucking, apnoeic attacks, jitteriness or athetoid movements may be considered normal. Fits are most commonly recognized by clonic movements of one limb, but these may again be difficult to differentiate from clonic movements of a preterm baby which may be normal. Movements that are associated with an apnoeic attack or are prolonged may be abnormal. EEG recordings have shown that many convulsions in preterm babies do not produce clinical signs. Some sick or preterm babies may show abnormal behaviour which is a manifestation of prolonged convulsions. Asphyxia is still a very common cause of fits and can itself lead to biochemical abnormality, for instance hypoglycaemia or hypocalcaemia.

In general there are three types of convulsions in the newborn baby. *Tonic or major fits* occur at any gestational age, including the preterm baby usually in the first 24 hours of life. They often represent severe brain damage and may be found following severe asphyxia, intracranial haemorrhage, kernicterus and some metabolic disorders. The baby lies rigidly and is hypertonic. There is usually no clonus but sometimes it may be present and sustained. The prognosis is poor.

Many *clonic fits* start focally with the baby fully conscious, but they may gradually become generalized and the baby may lose consciousness or become cyanosed. Such fits are rare in the preterm baby. The focal fits may represent a localized response to asphyxia or birth trauma, while generalized clonic convulsions are often seen in

biochemical disorders, for example hypoglycaemia or hypocalcaemia. These fits often start between 24 and 48 hours of life and have
a better prognosis.

Subtle fits are the most easily missed. These manifest themselves
by such things as cycling leg movements, recurrent apnoeic attacks
and nystagmus.

The distinction between jitteriness and true convulsions is sometimes thought to be blurred. In practice, they can usually be differ-
entiated; in jitteriness there is tremor with rapid alternating
movements of equal rate in each direction, whereas fits are rapid
contractions of specific muscle groups followed by a period of slow
relaxation of others; they therefore have a jerky quality. Jitteriness
can be stopped if the limb is moved passively, but will start again
when the limb is released. This will help to differentiate such things
as slow hamstring clonus from a fit. It must be remembered, however,
that some causes are common to both. Modern methods of neonatal
intensive care may disguise fits, for example if a baby is being
paralysed for ventilation there may be no clinical evidence of fits
apart from hypotension or bradycardias. This is where a 24-hour EEG
recording may be critically important.

The major causes of neonatal convulsions are listed in Table 14.2.

In many cases the diagnosis may be suspected from a brief history
and examination. For example, in the SFGA baby, suspect hypoglycaemia; in the very jaundiced baby, suspect kernicterus; if there has
been heavy maternal sedation, suspect drug withdrawal. Fits associated with hypoglycaemia often occur in babies who are SFGA or
babies of diabetic mothers (LFGA). Such babies should have routine
monitoring of blood glucose by strips and should be fed early to
prevent such a situation developing (see Chapters 6 and 15). Hypoglycaemia is not a diagnosis in itself. If there is no obvious cause, a
blood sample during hypoglycaemia to measure insulin, lactate, ketone
bodies, branched chain amino acids, growth hormone and cortisol is
crucially important for diagnosis and in planning long-term treatment.

Hypocalcaemia used to be common around the end of the first week
of life in artificially fed babies given milk with a high phosphate load.
Currently available formulae are more physiological and this problem
is now seldom seen. Now, fits at the end of the first week are not
always accompanied by hypocalcaemia; when they are found there is
often no demonstrable cause. Hypocalcaemia is also seen during the
first few days of life in preterm babies, but is hardly ever associated
with convulsions. Low plasma calcium values in Asian babies often
indicate a significant degree of osteomalacia from vitamin D

Table 14.2 Important causes of convulsions in the newborn

Metabolic	Hypoxic ischaemic encephalopathy
	Hypocalcaemia
	Hypomagnesaemia
	Hyperbilirubinaemia
	Hyperammonaemia
	Hypernatraemia
	Hyponatraemia and water intoxication
	Pyridoxine dependency
	Organic acidurias
	Galactosaemia
	Aminoacidopathies
	Alkalaemia
Intracranial haemorrhage	PVH
	Trauma with subdural haemorrhage
	Haemorrhagic disease
	Non-accidental injury
	Platelet deficiency
	Subarachnoid haemorrhage
Infection	Intrauterine: cytomegalovirus, toxoplasmosis, rubella
	Meningitis/encephalitis
	Septicaemia
	Gastroenteritis
Genetic	Cerebral malformations and dysplasias
Drug withdrawal	

deficiency in their mothers; ask the obstetricians to check the mother's calcium, phosphate and alkaline phosphatase. Hypocalcaemia may follow exchange transfusions when the baby's calcium is bound by the anticoagulant in the transfused blood, so reducing the plasma ionized concentration. Hypocalcaemic fits are sometimes seen in the severely ill baby, for instance those with septicaemia.

The relationship between calcium and magnesium levels is very variable. Some babies with low plasma calcium levels also have low magnesium levels.

Either a high or a low plasma sodium (more than 150 mmol/l or less than 120 mmol/l) may be associated with fits. Hyponatraemia is often due to severe water loss through the skin in very preterm babies – less than 30 weeks gestation. Excess doses of sodium bicarbonate may also produce a high plasma sodium. A low plasma sodium occurs during the first day when the mother has been given intravenous dextrose with oxytocin. It also occurs in other situations, such as the inappropriate ADH syndrome in very sick babies, overuse of intravenous dextrose, or preterm babies who have lost large quantities of sodium in their urine.

A history of trauma or intrapartum asphyxia is a frequent finding in babies who convulse within the first few days of life. There are usually other associated neurological signs, such as coma or poor sucking.

Management

Review the history

Check the notes for evidence of maternal diabetes, endocrine disorders, osteomalacia, infection, hypertension or pre-eclampsia, and whether there was prolonged rupture of membranes, difficult labour, instrumental delivery or fetal hypoxia. Note the Apgar scores and the milk the baby has received.

Examine the baby

Observe the infant's behaviour and note abnormal posture or movements, tone, pattern of respiration and nature and frequency of the cry. Look for external evidence of difficult birth, such as conjunctival haemorrhages, chignon (from ventouse), forceps blade marks, cephalhaematoma or traumatic cyanosis. Note any infected areas or signs of infection. Feel the fontanelle to ensure that it is not full or bulging and measure the head circumference and compare it with previous measurements.

Examine the baby's eyes with an ophthalmoscope to exclude cataracts, choroidorentinitis or haemorrhages. Transilluminate the skull.

Investigations

1 Check the blood glucose with a monitoring strip and measure the true blood glucose level if it is low.
2 Take blood for a full blood count, platelet count, packed cell volume and blood culture. Blood should also be screened for antibodies to congenital infections such as cytomegalovirus, rubella and toxoplasmosis. Biochemical tests on blood include glucose, calcium, electrolytes and urea; magnesium, phorphorus and bilirubin may be measured in some cases. Blood gas studies should also be performed.

3 Urine must be taken for estimation of protein and reducing substances, amino acid chromatography, microscopy, culture and sensitivity and virus culture.

4 Swab obviously infected areas and send these for culture.

5 Examine the cerebrospinal fluid (CSF) by lumbar puncture to diagnose meningitis. Cisternal or ventricular taps are only very rarely necessary. Lumbar puncture to detect blood in the CSF is often of little practical help, because it is common for a traumatic tap to occur. Normal CSF in the newborn is yellow and therefore xanthochromia cannot be used as a sign of a previous subarachnoid haemorrhage; the range for protein, sugar or cells is wide in CSF. CSF protein concentrations in preterm babies may be very high.

6 Ultrasound examination will detect most intracranial haemorrhages, particularly periventricular haemorrhage (PVH) bleeding. computer-assisted tomography (CAT) scan, if available, is also useful. MRI scans are now better than CAT scans, producing excellent definition. The baby has to be moved to the scanner and therefore it is quite a complicated examination. An electroencephalograph (EEG) may be useful for prognosis and to see if paroxysmal behaviour is due to cerebral arrhythmia. Twenty-four-hour EEG monitoring is sometimes used in preterm babies but EEGs are difficult to interpret in this age group. EEG is now essential for diagnosis and will help with prognosis. The recordings are best taken over 24 hours onto a cassette tape; the signal can be analysed by computer. The results need expert interpretation, particularly as there are dramatic changes in the EEG patterns with increasing gestational age. These are due to rapid developmental changes in the brain tissues between 24 and 40 weeks gestation. Anticonvulsant drugs may alter the recording, and the EEG may need to be repeated once the drugs have been withdrawn.

Treatment

If a cause is found, it must be treated. If fits recur or continue, whether or not the underlying cause is found, anticonvulsants should be used. Ensure careful attention to nutrition, temperature control, respiratory status and metabolic balance.

Hypocalcaemia or hypomagnesaemia.   In an emergency give 10% calcium gluconate 0.2 ml/kg slowly intravenously. Watch for cardiac arrhythmias or bradycardia. In most cases oral correction is adequate and safer: 10% calcium gluconate 100 mg/kg (about 1 ml) before each feed. It is sometimes necessary to correct hypomagnesaemia before the hypocalcaemia becomes correctable; a suitable dose is 50% magnesium sulphate 0.2 mg/kg intramuscularly or intravenously in an emergency or magnesium sulphate or chloride by mouth.

Hypoglycaemia.   If symptomatic, give intravenous dextrose 0.5 g/kg in 10% solution. This should be given into a large vein to reduce the risk of thrombosis. If asymptomatic hypoglycaemia is found, early feeding usually raises the blood glucose before symptoms occur. Blood sugars should be checked with blood glucose monitoring strips.

Meningitis.   See Chapter 16.

Anticonvulsants.   To abort prolonged or recurrent fits a number of anticonvulsant drugs can be used. An initial intravenous dose of phenobarbitone 20 mg/kg, or phenytoin 20 mg/kg can be given (Whitelaw *et al.*, 1983). This must be done in an intensive care setting, and facilities must be available to monitor the drug plasma levels. Diazepam in the form of the emulsion, 'Diazemuls', (less damaging to veins), (intramuscular or intravenous) is also useful, but the dose that controls the fits may produce severe respiratory depression or apnoea. The use of intravenous diazepam also carries the theoretical risk of increasing hyperbilirubinaemia by displacing bilirubin from its binding sites by the sodium benzoate component of injectable diazepam. Paraldehyde is also a useful drug, 0.1 ml/kg may be given by deep intramuscular injection, or rectally, when mixed with an equal volume of a mineral oil. It is commonly said that paraldehyde must be drawn up in glass syringes. This is not true provided that the drug is used immediately – it is only if the drug is drawn up in a plastic syringe and allowed to stand for some time that a reaction with the syringe may take place.

For long-term control the drug of choice in the newborn baby is probably phenobarbitone, 3–4 mg/kg/day orally after one intramuscular loading dose of 20 mg/kg. A problem with the drug is that its half-life is extremely variable in the newborn baby, ranging between 72 and 400 hours, so that accumulation may occur. It is important, therefore, to measure blood levels and adjust the dose accordingly. Chloral hydrate (25–50 mg/kg, six-hourly orally) is probably best used for jitteriness rather than true convulsions. Sodium valproate (starting dose 20 mg/kg/day orally in three divided doses; maximum 40 mg/kg/day) has turned out to be a much less useful drug in the control of neonatal convulsions than had been hoped.

Cerebral oedema. It is wise to restrict fluids. Steroids have no effect, but mannitol (250 mg/kg/dose eight-hourly for three doses) may be useful.

Prognosis

Prognosis varies with the cause. Most convulsions in the newborn stop eventually with or without treatment, so this is no cause for optimism in itself.

Fits with hyperbilirubinaemia (kernicterus) may lead to deafness and choreoathetosis. Hypoglycaemia with fits, if prolonged, is associated with mental retardation and cerebral palsy, but early diagnosis and treatment will prevent this and prolonged hypoglycaemia rarely occurs today. Hypocalcaemic fits carry a very good prognosis.

Bad prognostic signs include tonic fits in the first 24 hours, prolonged or recurrent fits despite treatment, associated neurological abnormalities and marked diffuse EEG abnormalities. It is true to say that in the past many babies did surprisingly well, but, with hypocalcaemia excluded, many other babies who had convulsions as newborn babies died or showed later disability. Modern obstetric practice has reduced the incidence and severity of intrapartum hypoxia; this together with neonatal intensive care results in a much better outcome for babies with problems relating to birth injury or asphyxia. Long-term follow-up using ultrasound scanning now allows quite accurate prognosis of cognitive and neurological development (Papille *et al.*, 1983; de Vries *et al.*, 1985).

The pertussis component of the triple vaccine should not be omitted in babies who have had neonatal fits. In the past the very small risk of developing encephalitis following the vaccine was overemphasized, with the result that many babies were unprotected from this serious disease, with a subsequent increase in the incidence of pertussis.

The Hypotonic Baby

Hypotonia is a common finding in ill babies, for instance those with RDS, septicaemia or kernicterus, or for a short period after a difficult or traumatic delivery. It is a normal finding in extremely preterm babies.

Rarely, it is the presenting feature in an otherwise well baby. It is useful then to check whether there is weakness, shown by lack of movement, as well as flaccidity. The most likely cause of a flaccid paralysis is *Werdnig–Hoffmann disease* (spinal muscular atrophy or progressive spinal paralysis); in modern obstetric practice spinal cord injury or transection is very rare.

Werdnig–Hoffmann disease is inherited in an autosomal recessive manner and is due to loss of motor neurons in the spinal cord. The onset is often before birth and the mother may report poor fetal movements. The infant gradually loses the ability to suck and develops breathing difficulties as the muscles of respiration become affected. Signs in the newborn include absent deep reflexes with muscle and tongue fasciculation. The disease is progressive, leading to death within a few years. No specific treatment is possible, apart from physiotherapy, and considerable support must be given to the family. Muscle biopsy shows the atrophy of denervation. Genetic counselling is essential since 1 in 4 future babies will be affected.

The most important differential diagnosis is *benign congenital hypotonia*. The cause of this condition is unknown but, as the name implies, it gradually improves during the first years of life. Unlike Werdnig–Hoffmann disease, the deep reflexes are present and there is no fasciculation. Muscle biopsy is normal.

Rare causes of hypotonia in the newborn include *congenital myopathies* (chronic and non-progressive, diagnosable by muscle biopsy); *glycogen storage diseases* affecting the CNS (e.g. Type II, Pompe's disease, recessively inherited); *organic acidaemias* (in which signs of respiratory failure rapidly develop; such inborn errors are recessively inherited, and are diagnosable from plasma and urine amino acid chromatography). Two commonly missed causes are *dystrophia myotonica* in the mother (diagnosed by electromyography (EMG) of the mother's thenar eminence), and *Prader–Willi* syndrome (where there are pronounced neonatal feeding difficulties, and later obesity, cryptorchidism, hypogonadism, mental retardation and, sometimes, diabetes mellitus). One should always ask the mother to grasp your hand, and failure to release the grasp is typical of dystrophia myotonica.

Hypotonia is a particular characteristic of children with *Down syndrome* (see Chapter 10) but cases are usually recognized from their other features.

Some babies born to mothers with myasthenia gravis have temporary hypotonia with sucking and respiratory difficulties. The diagnosis is confirmed by the intravenous injection of edrophonium chloride 1 mg which leads to rapid improvement. Maintenance therapy with neostigmine or prostigmine (1–5 mg orally with feeds) is then

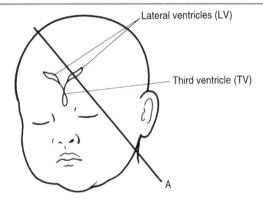

Fig. 14.5a Ultrasonography: Parasaggital plane

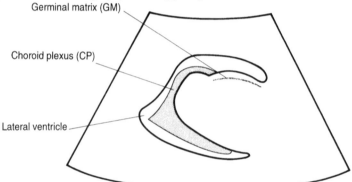

Fig. 14.5b Diagrammatic representation of parasagittal scan showing normal anatomy.

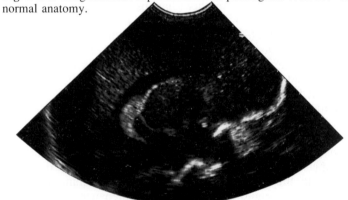

Fig. 14.5c Example of parasagittal scan

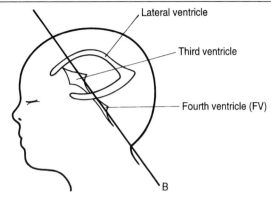

Fig. 14.5d Ultrasonography: Coronal Plane.

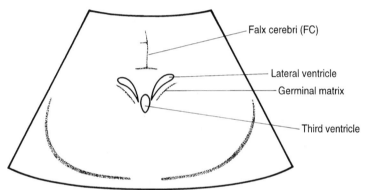

Fig. 14.5e Diagrammatic representation of coronal scan showing normal anatomy.

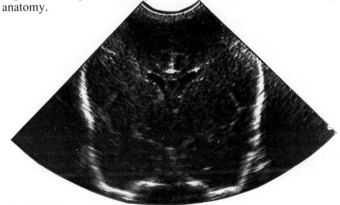

Fig 14.5f Example of coronal scan.

necessary and can be reduced gradually as improvement occurs (see also p. 189).

Intracranial Haemorrhage

There are many different possible sites of bleeding within or around the brain (see also Chapters 5 and 8). Prognosis will depend on time of onset, duration, site and severity (Papille *et al.*, 1983).

Periventricular haemorrhage (PVH). This is now known to be common in preterm babies under 32 weeks gestation and if severe may be fatal. PVH is also seen in term babies following asphyxia. Affected babies suddenly deteriorate and often become floppy with marked bradycardia, unresponsiveness and respiratory arrest. It seems that the haemorrhage starts from capillaries in the germinal layer in the lateral wall of the lateral ventricles (Fig. 14.6a) (Wigglesworth *et*

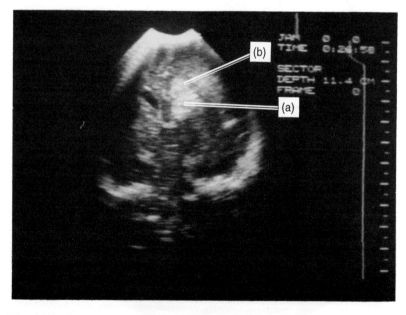

Fig. 14.6a Severe periventricular haemorrhage with blood in the ventricle and in the parenchyma of the brain. See page 332.

al., 1976). Such capillaries, already markedly dilated by hypoxia and hypercapnia, easily rupture during further engorgement as a result of hypertensive episodes from hypoxia or pneumothorax. The bleeding may extend into the ventricle, which can result in hydrocephalus from a blockage caused by thrombosis. Blood may plough into the cerebral matter, lateral to the ventricle, and this can lead to cerebral palsy, leaving porencephalic cysts in the brain. Some post-mortem appearances are shown in Fig. 14.6b.

Thus PVH is particularly likely to follow a hypoxic insult to the immature brain. Sequential ultrasound examinations of a sick baby will identify the haemorrhage in most cases, and may also be used to monitor any developing hydrocephalus.

Subarachnoid haemorrhage.   This is usually secondary to severe hypoxaemia and PVH but it may occur in an otherwise normal baby. Sometimes it is the result of an arterial malformation. There is a particular risk of hydrocephalus in survivors.

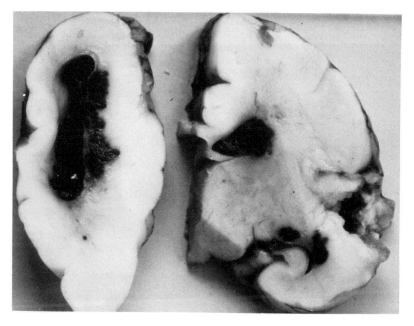

Fig. 14.6b The post-mortem appearances of periventricular haemorrhage.

Periventricular leucomalacia (PVL). This is now recognized to be an important form of damage to the neonatal brain. It is most common in the preterm baby where it is significantly associated with later cerebral palsy, and may follow a prolonged period of arterial hypotension. It also occurs after severe intrapartum hypoxia in term babies.

The periventricular region may be particularly vulnerable to circulatory impairment during hypotension because it is a boundary zone between different areas of blood supply. There is apparently some doubt about this.

It is now easier to recognize characteristic echo-dense areas by the use of serial ultrasound examination. Further ultrasound scanning can define the progression of the lesions to echo-free cystic areas, which need at least a week to develop. These cysts later disappear. (See Fig. 14.7.) As PVL involves destruction of tissue which would have become white matter it can prevent development of corticospinal motor pathways, resulting in spastic cerebral palsy or quadriplegia (de Vries *et al.*, 1985).

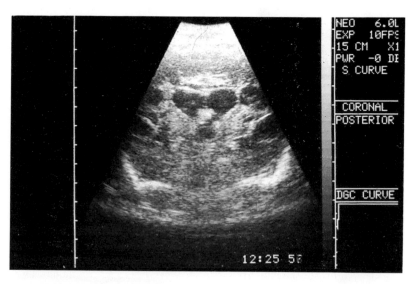

Fig. 14.7 Coronal cranial ultrasound scan showing periventricular leucomalacia with cysts along the lateral ventricle. See page 332.

Subdural haemorrhage.   This results from trauma especially during difficult instrumental delivery (see Chapter 5).

Babies Born to Drug-Dependent Mothers

This is an increasingly recognized problem in many countries. About 70% of babies born to mothers taking heroin or methadone will show signs of withdrawal. Some are only mildly affected, but others have severe symptoms; the babies born to methadone users show more frequent and prolonged signs than those of heroin users. Babies withdrawing from methadone may show signs for up to six weeks.

The likelihood of the baby being affected is related to maternal consumption and how long she has been a drug user. However, some babies born to heavily addicted mothers may be normal while those born to light users may show serious signs of withdrawal. The closer to delivery the last dose was taken, the more likely the baby is to be affected.

Although 70% will show signs of withdrawal, only 40% will have signs severe enough to require treatment. Two-thirds of those showing signs will start to have them in the first 24 hours, 90% by 48 hours and most of the others within the next two days. Initial signs of withdrawal are rare after 10 days of age, but withdrawal signs of barbiturates occur later than those from narcotics. Infants showing mild signs initially may suddenly show severe signs later, but life-threatening illness only occurs within the first week. The mortality is about 3%.

It is important to consider meningitis, hypocalcaemia, and hypoglycaemia in the differential diagnosis.

Signs of withdrawal include the following:

- tremors
- irritability
- hypertonicity
- vomiting
- high-pitched cry
- sneezing
- respiratory distress
- fever
- diarrhoea
- sweating
- mucus secretion
- convulsions
- yawning

Treatment consists of giving a sedative drug. Many recommend chlorpromazine as the drug of choice, given at 2.2 mg/kg/24 h in four divided doses either orally or by injection. Full dosage is given for

SIGN	TIME												
TREMOR													
IRRITABILITY													
HYPERTONICITY/ HYPERACTIVITY													
VOMITING													
HIGH PITCHED CRY													
SNEEZING													
RESPIRATORY DISTRESS													
FEVER													
DIARRHOEA													
SWEATING													
CONVULSIONS													
TOTAL													

Name:

Score baby 6 hourly

Score according to the following scale:

        0 = Absent

        1 = Mild to moderate

        2 = Severe

Fig. 14.8 Clinical score for infants born to drug-dependent mothers. Consider treatment if the score increases above 4 or 5.

two to four days then decreased at two-day intervals if baby's condition (according to clinical score) permits (Fig. 14.5). Some paediatricians use morphine sulphate in the first week as they effectively suppress the signs during the dangerous phase of the illness.

Drug usage is increasing, and many more drugs are used by mothers than in the past. In the USA the use of cocaine has become much more common, sometimes in the form of *crack*. This particularly causes growth retardation and may cause cerebral thrombosis (Chasnoff *et al.*, 1986; Flandermeyer, 1987; Kennard, 1990).

References and Further Reading

Cooke, R.W.I. (1986) Ventriculoperitoneal shunt for post-haemmorhagic hydrocephalus in low birth weight infants. Paper presented to the BPA: York, April.

Cooke, R.W.I. (1987) Determinants of major handicap in post-haemmorhagic hydrocephalus. *Arch. Dis. Child., 62*, 504–506.

Chasnoff, I. (ed) (1986) Drug use in pregnancy. Lancaster, England: MTP.

Chasnoff, I., Burns, K., Burns, W. *et al.* (1986) Prenatal drug exposure: Effects on neonatal and infant growth and development. *Neurobehavioural Toxicology and Teratology, 8*, 357–362.

Clewell, W.H., Johnson, M.L., Meier, P.R. *et al.* (1982). Placement of ventriculo-amniotic shunt for hydrocephalus in fetus. *New Engl. J. Med., 305*, 955.

de Vries, L.S., Dubowitz, L.M.S., Dubowitz, V. *et al.* (1985) Predictive value of cranial ultrasound in the newborn baby: a reappraisal. *Lancet, ii*, 137–140.

Dubowitz, L.M.S., Bydder, G.M. & Mushin, J. (1985 Developmental sequence of periventricular leucomalacia. Correlation of ultrasound, clinical and nuclear magnetic resonance functions. *Arch. Dis. Child., 60*, 349–355.

Flandermeyer, A. (1987) A comparison of the effects of heroin and cocaine abuse upon the neonate. *Neonatal Network*, 42–47.

Kennard, M. (1990) Cocaine use during pregnancy: Fetal and neonatal effects. *Journal of Perinatal and Neonatal Nursing, 3*(4), 53–63.

Papille, L.A., Munswick-Bruno, G. & Schaefer, A. (1983) Relationship of cerebral intrventricular haemmorhage and early childhood neurological handicaps. *J. Pediatr, 103*, 273–277.

Whitelaw, A., Placzek, M., Dubowitz, L. *et al.* (1983) Phenobarbitone for prevention of periventricular haemmorhage in very low birth weight infants. A randomised double blind trial. *Lancet, ii*, 1168–1170.

—15

Care of the Large-for-Gestational-Age Baby

Large-for-gestational-age (LFGA) babies are, by definition, heavier than the 90th centile for gestational age. Some are normal babies at the heavy end of the spectrum with tall and large parents.

Diabetes Mellitus

The common pathological diagnosis among LFGA babies is that their mothers are diabetic or pre-diabetic. These babies have a characteristic appearance which may point to previously unsuspected impairment of glucose tolerance in an asymptomatic mother. About one in every thousand pregnant mothers has diabetes, while about one in a hundred are gestational diabetics.

A generation ago, the achievement of pregnancy in a diabetic was rare and the results in terms of perinatal mortality very poor, with a high stillbirth rate. The perinatal morbidity and mortality in such infants is still higher than in normal pregnancies, but careful control of diabetes during pregnancy has reduced the mortality and morbidity dramatically. In many series perinatal mortality is now less than 5%.

Classically, infants of poorly controlled diabetic mothers (IDM) have a strong resemblance to one another (Fig. 15.1). They are large and fat, tend to lie in the frog position typical of preterm babies and often develop RDS. They have at least a two to three times greater incidence of congenital malformations, most of which are structural, for example, sacral agenesis, than babies of normal pregnancies. It is not clear why these babies have more abnormalities; it is likely that inadequate prepregnancy diabetic control is the main teratogenic factor (Soler *et al.*, 1976; Fuhrman *et al.*, 1983). Glucose seems to be teratogenic in animal experiments, and poor diabetic control is associated with an increased risk of spontaneous abortion.

The large size of the IDM is thought to be secondary to maternal (and hence fetal) hyperglycaemia. Insulin produces fat deposition and stimulates growth. Not all babies of diabetic mothers are LFGA;

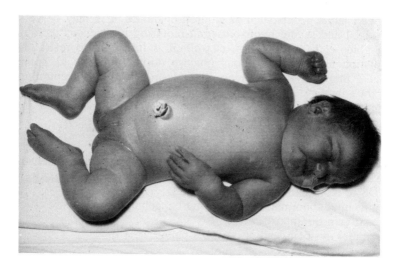

Fig. 15.1 A large-for-gestational-age baby from a diabetic mother

when there is placental insufficiency from complicated diabetes the baby may be small-for-gestational-age (SFGA). There is now good evidence that careful control of blood glucose concentrations in pregnancy (less than 7 mmol/l) results in babies of normal weight, who do not develop hypoglycaemia. Poor maternal metabolic control in the first 6–8 weeks of pregnancy particularly predisposes to the development of congenital malformations; therefore education and counselling of diabetics is necessary before conception, and indeed before a pregnancy is planned. The first prepregnancy clinic for diabetic women was set up in Edinburgh in 1976, and similar clinics are now widespread. They are valuable for focusing on advice about diabetic control as a way of preventing congenital abnormalities, and for more general counselling. There is now evidence that such an approach, by achieving good metabolic control by the time of conception, reduces the risk of malformation.

If there is poor maternal control resulting in sustained fetal hyper-insulinism, the baby is at risk of hypoglycaemia after birth as the blood glucose will fall rapidly. The period of greatest risk is between two and eight hours. It should be anticipated by routine two-hourly monitoring using blood glucose strip estimations and prevented by early feeding. (Detailed management is as for small SFGA babies, see Chapter 6). In some babies whose mothers have received oral hypoglycaemic agents such as chloropropamide, there may be very prolonged and severe hypoglycaemia requiring intravenous therapy with glucose. In a baby who is well, it is important to resist the temptation to give intravenous glucose during the first 12 hours because this will only increase the plasma insulin concentration and thus increase the tendency to hypoglycaemia. Particular problems to which babies born following poorly controlled diabetes are susceptible include:

1 Hypocalcaemia.
2 Hyperbilirubinaemia (due to preterm delivery, polycythaemia, increased red cell breakdown, and traumatic delivery of a big baby).
3 RDS or recurrent apnoeic attacks.
4 Congenital abnormalities (including congenital heart disease).
5 Renal vein thrombosis.
6 Shoulder dystocia leading to Erb's palsy.

With prepregnancy counselling and improved metabolic control, the prognosis for IDM is very good. The overall perinatal mortality varies in recent series between about 23 and 46 per 1000. If the problem of major congenital abnormalities were overcome it would reduce the perinatal mortality rate in this group by half, and be close to that in the non-diabetic population. Ultimately children of diabetic mothers are almost all of normal height, weight and intelligence in later childhood. They do, however, have an increased risk of developing diabetes mellitus themselves. If good, and improving, results are to continue, close cooperation between diabetologist, obstetrician and neonatologist is crucial.

Other Causes

Rarer causes of a baby being LFGA are:

1 *Beckwith syndrome*. These babies are heavy at birth because of a large liver and kidneys (organomegaly). The tongue is also enlarged and protrudes and there is a characteristic transverse crease of the ear lobe. There is often herniation of gut into the base of the umbilical cord or even frank exomphalos or gastroschisis (see Chapter 10). The head circumference is usually on a very much lower centile than length and weight. Hypoglycaemia is common and may be severe; treatment is analogous to the management of hypoglycaemia in

SFGA babies (see Chapter 6). There is an increased risk of having subsequent babies with the syndrome.

2 *Nesidioblastosis of the pancreas.* Persistent hypoglycaemia (beyond about seven days) in a LFGA baby may be due to this diffuse abnormality of the pancreas which causes hyperinsulinism. Ketones will be absent from blood and urine. Very high glucose infusion rates may be necessary to prevent hypoglycaemia. Drugs such as diazoxide can be used to inhibit the excessive insulin release, but, in most cases, subtotal (about 95%) pancreatectomy is necessary. These babies are best managed in specialist centres. It is vital to prevent profound or prolonged hypoglycaemia which may result in severe brain damage or death.

3 *Transposition of the great arteries* (see Chapter 11). It is not clear why these babies are large.

References and Further Reading

Fuhrman, N.K., Reiher, H., Semmler, K. *et al.* (1983) Prevention of congenital malformations in infants of insulin-dependent diabetic mothers. *Diabetes Care*, 6: 219–223.

Gillmer, M.D.G., Oakley, N.W. & Perrson, B. (1984) Diabetes mellitus and the fetus. In *Fetal Physiology and Medicine*, pp. 211–254, eds Beard, R.W. & Nathanielz, P. New York: Marcel Dekker.

Rahman, F.R. & Swift, P.G.F. (1985) Neonatal management of the infant of a diabetic mother. *Practical Diabetes*, 2, 11–15.

Soler, N.G., Walsh, C.H. & Malins, J.M. (1976) Congenital malformations in infants of diabetic mothers. *Quarterly J. Med.*, *178*, 303–313.

Steel, J.M. (1985) The pre-pregnancy clinic. *Practical Diabetes*, 2, 8–10.

Steel, J.M. & Johnstone, F.D. (1986) Prepregnancy management of the diabetic. In *Prepregnancy Care: a Manual for Practice*, pp. 165–182, eds Chamberlain, G. & Lumley, J. Chichester: Wiley.

Stirling, H.F. & Kelnar, C.J.H. (1995) Neonatal diabetes (transient and permanent). In *Childhood and Adolescent Diabetes*, pp. 419–426, ed. Kelnar, C.J.H. London: Chapman & Hall.

Sutherland, H.W. & Stowers, J.M. (eds) (1984) *Carbohydrate Metabolism in Pregnancy and the Newborn*. Edinburgh: Churchill Livingstone.

Vesikari, T., Janas, M. *et al.* (1985) Neonatal septicaemia *Arch. Dis. Child.*, *60*, 542

—16

Infection

Newborn babies are particularly susceptible to infections; sometimes these are caused by microorganisms which are not usually pathogenic. This is because of the relative immaturity of the newborn baby's immune response, and because of vulnerability to certain infections acquired *in utero*.

Infections may be acquired before birth, during delivery or postnatally. The conventional signs and symptoms of infection seen in older children are often absent. Furthermore, infections which in older children are localized to one organ or system are frequently complicated by septicaemia in the newborn, and the rate and spread and deterioration may be extremely rapid.

Defences against Infection

There are a number of specific and non-specific defences which the newborn baby possesses to combat infection. Non-specific defences include the skin, which forms a barrier to invading organisms, phagocytosis by macrophages and the inflammatory response. The specific immune response consists of the production of antibodies in response to a specific antigenic stimulus. An antigen is a substance (e.g. a chemical within an infecting microorganism) which stimulates the production of specific proteins (antibodies) by lymphocytes. The antibodies so formed help to protect the host from possible damage from that antigen. Antibody may be bound to cells (lymphocytes) or may be free in the plasma (humoral antibodies derived from plasma cells, or immunoglobulins). The immunoglobulins are divided into several subclasses according to their properties.

Cellular immunity is effective from birth, hence we can immunize babies with BCG at birth. More research is being done into cellular immunity, and it is probably not as effective in the neonatal period as later in childhood. Humoral immunity develops later than cellular immunity (Fig. 16.1). The newborn baby has a high peripheral lymphocyte count at birth and indeed for the next two or three years.

The IgG subclass of immunoglobulins contains antibodies to most

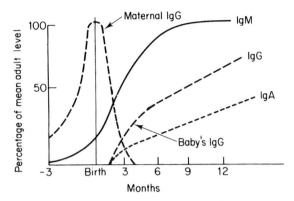

Fig. 16.1 The development of humoral immunity during infancy

bacteria and viruses which the mother has already encountered. Of the various immunoglobulins only IgG can cross the placenta. This is because of its small molecular weight and therefore size, and because of specific binding sites which the molecule possesses. IgG crosses the placenta from the third month of pregnancy onwards, so that in term infants the IgG serum concentrations are similar to those in the mother. This is not so in the preterm infant and is one reason why there is particular vulnerability to infection. These passively acquired antibodies are gradually destroyed over the first three months of extrauterine life. At the same time there is a gradual increase in the baby's own IgG synthesis; IgG levels do not reach those of the adult again until about three years of age. There is, therefore, a physiological trough at about three months of age when maternally acquired IgG is disappearing and the baby's own IgG is being produced only gradually; therefore babies of this age are particularly at risk of infection. Term newborn babies are thus passively protected against such common pathogens as streptococci, pneumococci, meningococci and *Haemophilus influenzae*. They are also protected against tetanus and diphtheria toxins and viruses such as measles, rubella and mumps.

IgM is a larger molecule which does not cross the placenta. It is this immunoglobulin fraction which is responsible for combating Gram-negative bacterial infections, the most common of which is caused by *E. coli*. IgM synthesis begins slowly in the fetus. It starts at about 20 weeks gestation and by term has reached only about 10% of adult levels (less than 20 mg/100 ml). If the fetus has been infected, a high level of IgM is found at birth. It is the low neonatal IgM levels which allow *E. coli* to be such a common and dangerous pathogen for these babies – at no other time of life does *E. coli* commonly cause meningitis. At one time Gram-negative bacteria were the commonest cause of serious neonatal infections, but these have now been taken over by Group B streptococcus (GBS).

IgA does not cross the placenta and is synthesized by babies only after birth. However, it is present in very high concentration in maternal colostrum and breast milk. Some may be absorbed by the baby's intestinal tract, thus protecting breastfed infants (in conjunction with another substance present in breast milk called lactoferrin) from gastroenteritis caused by pathogenic *E. coli*. This is one of the reasons why breastfeeding is so good for the baby: the incidence of gastroenteritis is very much lower in the wholly breastfed infant than in bottle fed babies (see Chapter 7). Lactoferrin is efficient at binding iron, as its name implies; *E. coli* need iron for growth and replication and, therefore, breast milk suppresses the growth of *E. coli*.

Classification of Infections

It is convenient to classify infections in the newborn according to the time at which the infection occurs. Infections can be acquired before birth, and in the neonatal period it is usual to divide them into early or late sepsis, occurring before or after 48–72 hours of birth. In the early period infections are acquired from the birth canal, whereas later ones are from the environment – often from the hands of doctors and nurses.

Antenatally acquired

1 *Viral infections.* Many viruses cross the placenta and some can cause devastating illness in the fetus. Viruses that are known to cause neonatal infections include coxsackie, rubella – which may cause a severe congenital infection with later retinitis, cataracts and brain damage (Miller *et al.*, 1982), – poliomyelitis, cytomegalovirus (Pearl *et al.*, 1986) and HIV (Pinching & Jeffries, 1985).
2 *Protozoal infections.* Toxoplasmosis can cause severe intrauterine infection, with hydrocephalus and severe chorioretinitis. The definitive host for the organism, *Toxoplasma gondii*, is the domestic cat, and women should be encouraged always to wear gloves when dealing

with cat litter or gardening. The disease is much commoner in Europe than in the UK, with about 80% of women having toxoplasma antibodies at booking, compared with only 20% in the UK. This is probably as a result of differences in diet, with Europeans eating undercooked meats. There has been pressure to screen for toxoplasmosis, but this would require repeated, possibly monthly, blood samples. This is not a practical possibility and is therefore not recommended at present. Where toxoplasmosis infection is identified in pregnancy a termination may be considered. Possible drugs for the treatment are spiromycin, to prevent placental transfer of the protozoa, and pyrimethamine. Malaria is another protozoal infection. *Plasmodium falciparum* has been known to cause congenital infection with reduced birthweight and a severe septicaemic illness in the neonatal period.

3 *Bacterial infections.* Syphilis, caused by *Treponema pallidum*, remains a problem in many parts of the world (Rosenberg, 1991). Some other bacteria can infect the fetus without rupture of the membranes having occurred; these include Group B streptococci or *Listeria monocytogenes*, which causes listeriosis with meningitis, pneumonia and septicaemia. Such organisms can also be acquired postnatally.

Acquired during delivery

1 *Ascending vaginal infections.* These occur with prolonged rupture of membranes. This may lead to amnionitis and fetal septicaemia or to a congenital pneumonia following inhalation of organisms.

2 *Gonococcal ophthalmia.* This has become more common again (Snowe & Wilfert, 1973). At one time prophylactic silver nitrate drops were given to all newborn babies. This unfortunately caused chemical conjunctivitis in many babies and, since treatment with systemic and local penicillin proved to be very effective, routine use of the drops was discontinued.

3 *Herpes.* This is usually of type 2 (genital). Acyclovir is the treatment of choice for suspected herpes simplex infection. As the condition is difficult to diagnose it may be necessary to give acyclovir to any unwell baby of a mother who has active herpes, and to withdraw the drug when cultures from the baby are negative. There is a particular clinical problem when the mother has a primary herpes infection with only a fever and flu-like illness. When a newborn baby becomes ill after a mother has had an unexplained flu-like illness, it is safest to start acyclovir treatment and to continue until the results of cultures are available. Neonatal herpes is often a fulminating and fatal infection.

4 *Candidiasis* (thrush) acquired from the mother's vaginal infection (Smith and Congdon, 1985; Johnstone & Marcinak, 1990; Poulsen, 1990).

5 *Listeriosis* (see below).

6 *Group B streptococci* (see below).

7 *Chlamydia* can cause severe ophthalmia and pneumonia (Heggie *et al.*, 1981; Clearkin, 1986).

Postnatally acquired

Examples in this group are *E. coli*, staphylococci, *Klebsiella* sp., *Enterobacter* sp., *Serratia* sp., Group B streptococci.

Prevention of Infection

Prevention of neonatal sepsis is very important:

- Infected or potentially infected babies must be adequately supervised in a separate isolation unit or cubicle. (In some types of infection, e.g. urinary tract infection, isolation is not considered necessary; in contrast gatroenteritis, for instance, is very infectious indeed.)
- Hand-washing before and after handling each baby is the single most important procedure. Basins must be fitted with elbow taps to avoid contamination. It is common practice to use chlorhexidine or an iodine-based disinfectant to rub on to the hands after washing. Disposable paper towels should be used for hand drying. There is no evidence that the wearing of gowns and gloves reduces the spread of infection but disposable gloves must be used during procedures where there is great danger of infecting the baby such as tracheal toilet. Masks are also unnecessary. Anyone with a sore throat or other infectious illness or fever should not be on the unit.
- Floors, incubators and lockers must be cleaned regularly. Dirty nappies and dirty linen should be disposed of separately into colour-coded covered bags.
- Breastfeeding should be encouraged. Careful procedures must be drawn up for human milk banks (see p. 147). Intravenous fluids

and nutrition should be made up in the pharmacy. There must be facilities for aseptic preparation and storage of feeds.

- Crowding infants too closely together should be avoided.
- Antibiotics should be used appropriately and sensibly with good laboratory back-up. Overuse of powerful antibiotics will only lead to the development of resistant organisms.
- Babies admitted from home or other units should be regarded as potentially infected and not admitted to the main unit until proved otherwise.
- Babies must be examined daily by the nursing staff for signs of minor infection, such as a red umbilicus, sticky eyes, septic spots or oral candidiasis.
- There is no evidence that unrestricted visiting by healthy adults and their children increases the infection rate on the nursery. However, all those with an active infection should keep away.

Diagnosis

The diagnosis of neonatal infection is difficult. Fever is not essential for the diagnosis (infected babies are very likely to be hypothermic) and signs are often non-specific, for example poor weight gain or weight loss, reluctance to feed, vomiting, jaundice, lethargy, irritability, tachypnoea, apnoea or collapse. Owing to the rapid spread from a localized infection to generalized septicaemia, delay in diagnosis may be extremely serious. Certainly morbidity and mortality are reduced by early diagnosis and treatment. It is worth remembering that any deterioration after the first two or three days in a previously healthy baby is most likely to be due to infection. For all these reasons, the concept of the infection screen has grown up.

At the first suspicion of infection, the following investigations should be carried out:

- Full white cell count and differential (usually haemoglobin is done at the same time). Neutropenia is a particularly likely finding in septicaemia as much as neutrophilia.
- Platelet count. A low count may be the first sign of septicaemia.
- Blood culture (from a peripheral vein using a 23 gauge butterfly, not from an indwelling catheter). The concentration of C-reactive protein (CRP) rises during infection.
- Fresh, clean sample of urine for culture and sensitivities. A bag

urine specimen is usually obtained, but a suprapubic sample is necessary in a very ill baby.

- Swabs from any obvious infected area. Other swabs may just show organisms which have colonised the baby and do not necessarily show infection.
- In an *ill* baby, CSF should be obtained by lumbar puncture and tested for protein and sugar content, culture and sensitivities. Many units do this routinely as part of an infection screen.
- Blood-gas analysis and biochemical studies (glucose, calcium, urea and electrolytes, bilirubin).

The infection screen must not be thought of as a substitute for full clinical examination of the infant, since local signs may well be present, for example a red umbilicus, a painful, swollen limb in osteitis or a bulging fontanelle in meningitis.

Treatment of Infections

Treatment, like diagnosis, is a matter of urgency. In ill babies antibiotics should be started before the *results* of the investigations are known. There is a choice of antibiotics and each unit needs to use a combination that is suitable for the sensitivities of their common infecting organisms. There is usually a different pattern of infection in early sepsis (48–72 hours) than in late sepsis. Important organisms to be covered in early sepsis are *E. coli*, Group B β-haemolytic streptococcus and *Listeria monocytogenes*. Commonly used regimens are amoxycillin and gentamicin, or amoxycillin and a third generation cephalosporin such as cefotaxime. Similar organisms are seen in late sepsis, but the commonest one is now *Staphylococcus epidermidis* (coagulase-negative staphylococcus). Many of these organisms are resistant to the cephalosporins, but antibiotics which may be used to cover them include flucloxacillin and vancomycin. Again this choice must be made locally after discussion with the microbiologist. A guide to the daily antibiotic dosages for the newborn is given in Table 16.1.

It is important to check plasma gentamicin levels in infants being treated so as to ensure that adequate therapeutic amounts are being given and that toxic levels which might damage the baby's hearing, are not being reached. It is usual to take blood just before an injection and about one hour afterwards. Satisfactory levels should be 5–12 mg/ml (peak) and less than 3 mg/ml (trough). An important rule is that antibiotics should be stopped after 48 hours if there is no bacteriological or clinical evidence of infection.

It is interesting to look back on how the incidence and type of neonatal infections has changed over the past 50 years. The group A streptococcus is still common, as it has been over the past century. In the 1950s and 1960s there was an increase in infections with *Staphylococcus aureus* which occurred in epidemics in nurseries. Later Gram-negative infections were also important, particularly with *E. coli*. Group B streptococcus emerged as an important organism in the 1970s in developed countries, but is still rare in the developing countries. The most important change in the 1980s was the emergence of *Staphylococcus epidermidis* as an extremely common infection in babies receiving intensive care with invasive procedures.

A number of specific conditions, and infections caused by specific organisms or groups of organisms, will now be described in greater detail.

Septicaemia

Septicaemia can be proved by positive blood cultures and may accompany any serious local infection in the neonate, such as meningitis. It may follow a previous infection, or may appear as the first problem by causing collapse in a previously well baby. *E. coli* has now been overtaken by organisms such as Group B β-haemolytic streptococcus and *Staphylococcus epidermidis*. When septicaemia is suspected it is critically important that antibiotics are started as soon as samples for cultures have been obtained.

Meningitis

In the 1980s Group B streptococci replaced *E. coli* as the commonest cause of meningitis in the newborn baby. These two now account for more than 70% of cases. Other causative organisms include *Listeria monocytogenes*, pneumococci, staphylococci and *Candida albicans*. The onset is often insidious with poor feeding, drowsiness and vomiting as the only signs. Convulsions are a late sign, as are a bulging fontanelle or head retraction. Neck stiffness is rare. It is a grave mistake to wait for neurological signs before suspecting meningitis. Lumbar puncture should be performed on any seriously ill baby. If a pathogenic organism which may cause meningitis is grown from a blood culture, a lumbar puncture should be performed even if the baby has been started on antibiotics.

Table 16.1 Daily antibiotic dosage for neonates.

Drug	Route	Preterm infants and term infants less than seven days (/kg/day)	Term infants more than seven days (/kg/day)
Acyclovir	i.v. as 60 minute infusion	15–30 mg divided eight-hourly	15–30 mg divided eight-hourly
Amikacin†	i.v., i.m.	15 mg divided 12-hourly	15–22.5 mg divided 12-hourly
Cefotaxime	i.m.	100 mg divided 12-hourly	150 mg divided eight-hourly
Ceftazidime	i.m., i.v.	50 mg divided 12-hourly	50 mg divided 12-hourly
Cefuroxime	i.m.	30 mg divided 12-hourly	30 mg divided 12-hourly
Chloram-phen-icol†	i.v.	Day 1, 50 mg divided 12-hourly. Then 25 mg divided 12-hourly (may be four-to-six-hourly)	Day 1, 75 mg divided 12-hourly. Then 50 mg divided 12-hourly (may be four-to-six-hourly)
Erythromycin	i.v. (slow)	40–60 mg divided six-hourly	40–60 mg divided six-hourly
Flucloxacillin	i.v., i.m., oral	62.5 mg divided six-hourly	75 mg divided eight-hourly
Fluctyosine†	oral	120 mg divided six-hourly	120 mg divided six-hourly
Fusidic acid	i.v.	20 mg continuous infusion	20 mg continuous infusion
Gentamicin†	i.m.	6 mg divided 12-hourly; 4.5 mg every 18 hours for < 7 days or < 1000 g	7.5 mg divided 12-hourly
Metronidazole	rectal, i.v.	20 mg divided six-hourly	20 mg divided six-hourly
Miconazole	i.v.	30 mg divided 12-hourly	30 mg divided 12-hourly
Netilmicin†	i.m., i.v.	5 mg divided 12-hourly	5 mg divided eight-hourly
Penicillin	i.v., i.m.	100 000 units divided six-hourly (increase in meningitis, Group B β-haemolytic streptococcal infection)	150 000 units divided six-hourly

Table 16.1 Daily antibiotic dosage for neonates.

Drug	Route	Preterm infants and term infants less than seven days (/kg/day)	Term infants more than seven days (/kg/day)
Piperacillin	i.m., i.v.	200 mg divided 12-hourly	200 mg divided 12-hourly
Rifampicin	i.v.	10 mg divided six-hourly	10 mg divided 12-hourly
Vancomycin†	i.v. as 60 minute infusion	30 mg divided 12-hourly	30 mg divided 12-hourly

†Levels need to be assayed.

Remember that normal CSF shows a great variation in the neonate. The fluid is often yellow and this may be due both to the relatively high protein content often following haemorrhage, and to the presence of bilirubin in a jaundiced baby – yellow CSF is not diagnostic of kernicterus and is found at relatively low serum bilirubin levels. Up to 20 cells/µl (if all lymphocytes) may normally occur.

If meningitis is suspected, treatment should be started before culture results are available. A standard regimen is intravenous amoxycillin and a third generation cephalosporin which penetrates CSF well. Gentamicin, though commonly prescribed, does not seem particularly useful in this situation – it does not cross the blood–brain barrier well, and the outcome is not improved by giving the drug intrathecally or into the ventricles.

Chloramphenicol was commonly used in the past, and may still be indicated in particular situations, but blood levels must be monitored to avoid both inadequate dosage and the grey baby syndrome. When the organism and its sensitivities are known, the least appropriate of these drugs may be discontinued.

Meningitis is an extremely serious condition in the newborn with a mortality of approximately 25%. Complications in survivors include subdural effusions, mental retardation, deafness and isolated cranial nerve palsies.

Pneumonia

Congenital pneumonia acquired by the inhalation of infected amniotic fluid presents with respiratory distress during the early hours of life. It is often associated with prolonged rupture of membranes.

Aspiration pneumonia may occur in preterm babies in whom

sucking, swallowing and cough reflexes are poorly developed. It may follow careless tube feeding and is recognized by the sudden onset of choking and cyanosis.

Pneumonia may be due to infection with other specific organisms, for example *Chlamydia* or staphylococci.

Treatment is by oxygen, antibiotics and other supportive treatment as indicated.

Viral respiratory infections do occur in the newborn, and the introduction of respiratory syncytial virus (RSV) into a neonatal intensive care unit, which can cause bronchiolitis, may be very serious.

Gastroenteritis

This is rare in the wholly breastfed baby. Outbreaks are most often due to rotavirus. It is likely that this infection may be asymptomatic in many babies. In some, however, there is rapid deterioration and dehydration. Treatment is by stopping milk feeding and giving oral or intravenous fluid replacement. Antibiotics are not indicated; they do nothing to improve the clinical course and tend to encourage the growth of resistant organisms. The only exception to this rule is in the baby in whom septicaemia has developed.

Necrotizing enterocolitis (NEC)

The cause of this serious illness is still a mystery. There are probably several aetiological factors acting together (Beeby & Jeffery, 1992). We can now identify certain babies as being particularly at risk. They include those who are preterm, weigh less than 2000 g, have suffered perinatal asphyxia or who need intensive care interventions or exchange transfusions. The syndrome is less likely in babies taking milk from the breast or babies fed expressed breast milk (EBM) from a milk bank. It has been shown that even in the babies who receive a mixture of EBM and formula milk, the incidence of NEC is significantly lower than in those fed wholly on formula milk – and significantly higher than those fully fed on breast milk (Lucas & Col, 1990).

It is probable that NEC develops in the following way: a primary insult, such as hypoxaemia, hypoglycaemia or hypothermia, leads to reduced blood flow to the gut. This, perhaps coupled with hypertonic or artificial feeds, produces mucosal oedema and ulceration. In the baby who is not being suckled, the absence of such factors as IgA and lymphocytes in colostrum, plus the colonization of the bowel with Gram-negative organisms such as *E. coli* and *Klebsiella*, leads to invasion of the bowel wall, portal system and bowel lymphatics by these organisms and others such as *Clostridium* and *Bacteroides*. Affected babies become systemically unwell both because of resultant endotoxin release leading to disseminated intravascular coagulation and collapse, and through septicaemia with bowel necrosis and peritonitis. There is recent evidence that cytokines are present in high

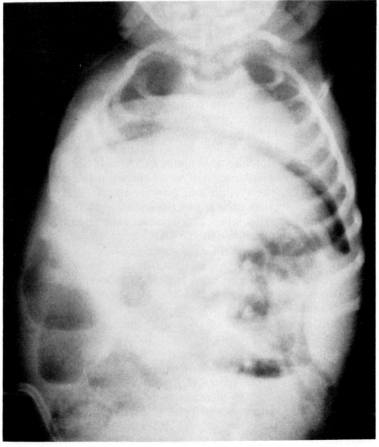

Fig. 16.2 Necrotizing enterocolitis showing dilated loops of bowel

concentrations in the stools, and this indicates that inflammation of the bowel wall is a part of the pathological process.

In the early stages clinical signs are non-specific. Failure of temperature control is an important clue and this is followed by gradual abdominal distension and blood in the stools. Bile-stained vomiting develops, but constipation rather than diarrhoea is usual initially. Unless treatment is started promptly, there is rapid deterioration, collapse and death. Initially, radiographic changes are confined to dilatation of small loops of bowel with or without fluid levels. Later, probably following invasion of the bowel wall by gas-producing organisms, gas is seen within the bowel wall (pneumatosis intestinalis) or the portal tract (Fig. 16.2). Once perforation occurs, free air is seen under the diaphragm in an erect abdominal or lateral decubitus radiograph. The platelet count and plasma sodium concentration are usually low.

Management is initially conservative. The baby must be isolated. Oral feeds should be discontinued and a naso/orogastric tube passed into the stomach and left on continuous drainage with additional regular, gentle aspiration of stomach contents to decompress the bowel. Fluid should be given intravenously. Care must be taken to maintain a normal body temperature. Samples of blood and stool should be sent for culture and antibiotics should then be started. The most effective combination of broad-spectrum antibiotics should be used, such as amoxycillin and gentamicin, or a cephalosporin. Because of the frequent presence of *Bacteroides* and other anaerobic organisms, most paediatricians add intravenous metronidazole. *Klebsiella* species are often found, so the use of an aminoglycoside antibiotic, such as gentamicin, is essential.

As there is considerable loss of fluid from the damaged bowel it is easy to underestimate the volume needed for adequate replacement. Transfusion with plasma or fresh blood (10–20 ml/kg body weight) over one or two hours may help re-establish normal blood pressure and ensure good perfusion of potentially necrotic bowel. Progress should be checked clinically by the baby's general condition and examination of the abdomen including measurements of girth, and radiologically by serial abdominal radiographs.

Surgery should be considered if the urine output drops, if abdominal distension increases, if there is free air in the peritoneal cavity on the radiograph or if there is a palpable abdominal mass. Whether the baby then survives depends largely on the length of necrotic bowel which has to be resected and hence on the amount of viable bowel that is left.

Late complications, of both medical and surgical treatment, include bowel strictures, presenting either as recurrent intestinal obstruction or as recurrent septicaemia, and diarrhoea. This may be due to a secondary lactose intolerance or may follow resection of the terminal ileum (where bile salts are primarily reabsorbed). It is usual to continue intravenous alimentation for one week after the last blood-stained stool. Small epidemics of the condition occur.

The overall survival rate is now about 60–70%.

Urinary tract infection

The only sign of a urinary tract infection in the neonate may be poor weight gain, jaundice or vomiting. This is the only time of life when such infections are commoner in boys than girls. Suprapubic aspiration is the best way to make the diagnosis as there is then no possibility of contamination of the specimen by organisms on the perineum. Septicaemia may supervene if the diagnosis is delayed. The diagnosis of a true urinary tract infection in either sex in infancy is adequate grounds for ultrasound examination of the urinary tract. Micturating cystography is indicated to detect the presence and severity of any reflux.

Hepatitis

Hepatitis may be caused by a number of organisms, for example viruses such as that of serum hepatitis B or C, cytomegalovirus (CMV), rubella or herpes simples, and protozoa such as *Toxoplasma gondii*, or it may be found as a complication of septicaemia with bacteria such as *E. coli*. CMV and rubella may be acquired transplacentally, and hepatitis B may also be acquired during passage down the birth canal.

Characteristically, the baby is jaundiced with pale and heavily bile-stained (dark) urine. The liver is often palpably enlarged. The differential diagnosis from other causes of obstructive jaundice may be extremely difficult (see Chapter 12).

Ophthalmia

The most important organisms causing ophthalmia are *Chlamydia* and, increasingly once more, β-lactamase-producing (i.e. penicillin resistant) strains of the gonococcus, *Neisseria gonorrhoeae*. Purulent ophthalmia, which is a notifiable disease, should not be confused with the common sticky eye, although the latter may progress to ophthalmia. Other significant organisms are *E. coli* and staphylococcus. In all cases of ophthalmia it is worth remembering that the baby should be nursed on its side with the worse affected eye downwards so that infection is not spread needlessly from the infected to the good eye. When treating it is sensible to treat both eyes simultaneously.

Gonococcal and chlamydial infections

In a severe purulent ophthalmia, especially in babies whose mothers have not attended for antenatal care, gonococcal or chlamydial infection should be suspected. This is potentially dangerous and needs extremely vigorous treatment. The organisms may be seen on a smear of the pus. Where gonococci are seen, penicillin drops should be instilled into the eyes every five minutes for the first two hours, then quarter-hourly for 12 hours, half-hourly or 12 hours and so on. It is important during this time to treat with systemic penicillin in addition. Chlamydial infection needs treatment with local tetracycline eye ointment and systemic erythromycin. In both infections the parents should be investigated and treated.

Sticky eye

The fluid that bathes the surface of the eye normally drains down into the nose via the tear duct which leads from the inner canthus of the eye. The tear duct is an extremely fine passage in the newborn baby and is easily blocked by sticky secretions. This results in the sticky eye, which needs cleaning with normal saline while the tear duct is gently massaged towards the nose. If this is not done, the stasis may lead to infection with one of the organisms mentioned above. Such infections are best treated, after a swab has been taken, with chloramphenicol or neomycin eyedrops.

Tetanus

Neonatal tetanus is discussed in Chapter 20.

Breast abscess

Breast abscess is now uncommon in nursing mothers but sometimes occurs in newborn babies. It must not be confused with the common, harmless breast enlargement in the newborn (sometimes confusingly

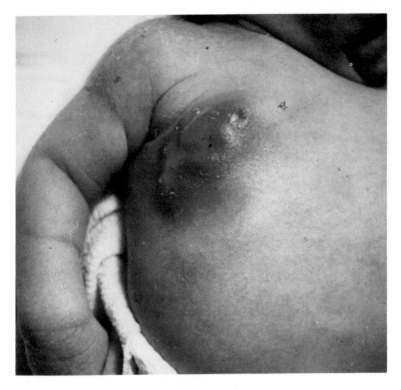

Fig. 16.3 Breast abscess

called mastitis). If a widespread abscess forms over the anterior chest wall (Fig. 16.3) surgical drainage may be necessary.

Omphalitis

The cord is colonised with bacteria shortly after birth, and as the cord separates there is often a little redness of the edge of the skin. Any more widespread erythema is a sign of infection, particularly if there is also a discharge of pus, and should be treated with antibiotics. Severe infection of the umbilicus (see Fig. 16.4) may spread through the umbilical vein to the liver.

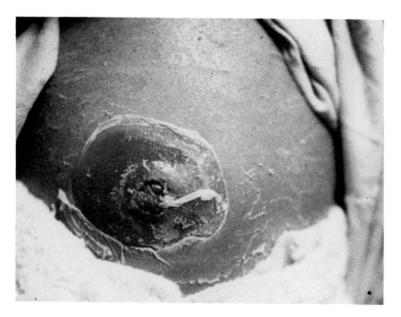

Fig. 16.4 Severe periumbilical infection

Group B β-haemolytic streptococcal (GBS) infection

Infection by this group of organisms has become more widely recognized in recent years. The organisms are commonly found in the maternal birth canal and can be very difficult to eradicate from the vagina by antibiotic treatment. Ascending infection may result in early onset of streptococcal disease in the neonate, since the organisms can pass across the membranes into amniotic fluid. They may be inhaled during passage of the fetus down the birth canal leading to sudden collapse during the first 48 hours of life, with additional signs of respiratory distress (see Chapter 8). In addition, they may cause meningitis during the early weeks of life.

Mortality is still high. As the organisms are relatively penicillin-resistant, treatment must be with high-dose penicillin, see Table 16.1, and gentamicin. Third generation cephalosporins can also be used as the organism is extremely sensitive to these. We do not give penicillin prophylaxis or treat healthy babies colonized with Group B streptococci, although there is a case for giving antibiotics to colonized mothers who have preterm, prolonged rupture of the membranes.

The infection should be suspected in any baby who becomes severely ill within the first 48 hours of life, particularly those with respiratory distress. However, other organisms such as *Klebsiella* may produce similar catastrophic illnesses.

Gram-negative infections

These organisms remain common and important pathogens in the newborn. As well as the commonly recognized infections due to *E. coli* there are reports of infections in newborn babies caused by organisms transmitted in water. This was probably due to the use of incubators with built-in water tanks. It is important to change the water in humidifiers daily to prevent colonization by such organisms.

The most important organism causing such infections is *Pseudomonas aeruginosa* which is particularly likely to affect ill or preterm babies who are being ventilated. Skin lesions looking like red rings are signs of septicaemia, and diarrhoea is sometimes an early sign, but sudden or insidious deterioration in a small or sick baby may be the first warning. Gentamicin is effective against most strains of the organism, but ceftazidime or other drugs may be necessary for resistant types. We now see unusual infections such as *Serratia marcescens* and *Enterobacter* sp. which are becoming a particular problem and are difficult to treat. Infection with *Pseudomonas aeruginosa* seems to be less common than in the past.

Staphylococcal infection

Today infections from *Staphylococcus aureus* appear to be less virulent than in the past. This has been replaced by a remarkable increase in the incidence of infection from *Staphyloccus epidermidis*. Mortality is relatively low but babies may still be extremely ill. A recent problem has been the emergence of types of infection particularly associated with *S. aureus*. These include:

- *Omphalitis.* See above (p. 359). A high incidence of colonization with staphylococci correlates with the incidence of clinical infection. Serious inflammation of the umbilicus with pockets of pus or peeling of the skin is now uncommon (Fig. 16.4).
- *Pustules.* Pustules are the commonest sign of staphylococcal infection in the newborn. They often occur around the neck or in

the axillae. Unlike the pustules in toxic erythema, staphylococcal pustules are rare before the third day of life and contain neutrophils, not eosinophils.

- *Bullous impetigo (pemphigus neonatorum).* Large vesicles, without erythema, containing clear yellow fluid.
- *Scalded skin syndrome* (Ritter's disease, toxic epidermal necrolysis). This is a much more extensive infection of the skin leading to widespread desquamation with raw areas. It is due to an exfoliative toxin produced by certain types of staphylococci (e.g. phage types 71 or 55/71) (Fig. 16.5).
- *Pneumonia.* Staphylococcal pneumonia is now rare in the newborn. It may lead to abscesses or emphysematous bullae. It is common in cystic fibrosis.
- *Septicaemia.* This is now more commonly seen following an invasive procedure, for example the insertion of an umbilical arterial catheter through a contaminated umbilicus. However, any minor infection such as a pustule or paronychia is a potential source of septicaemia and should be taken seriously.
- *Osteomyelitis* or *infective arthritis.* This condition usually presents with pseudoparalysis, and may cause severe damage to bones and joints.
- *Meningitis.* Recurrent staphylococcal meningitis is rare, but should suggest the presence of a midline congenital sinus connecting skin and CSF. It may be necessary to shave the head to seek carefully any sign of a track which could communicate with the subarachnoid space.

Any baby with a proven infection from *Staphylococcus aureus* should be isolated from other babies in the hospital. Hand washing using an antiseptic liquid such as chlorhexidine is important for prevention of cross-infection.

Local treatment may be adequate, for example the treatment of pustules by hexachlorophane powder, and systemic antibiotics are often needed as well, especially in serious infections. Flucloxacillin is the drug of choice as most hospital staphylococci are now penicillin-resistant. A five-day course is adequate for simple pustular lesions, but osteomyelitis may need six weeks treatment or more.

Staphylococcus epidermidis sepsis presents in the same way as other infections, but often produces a milder illness than other types of septicaemia. Depending on the type of organism in the unit, an appropriate antibiotic must be used and these may include flucloxacillin and vancomycin. If an intravenous catheter is in place it is

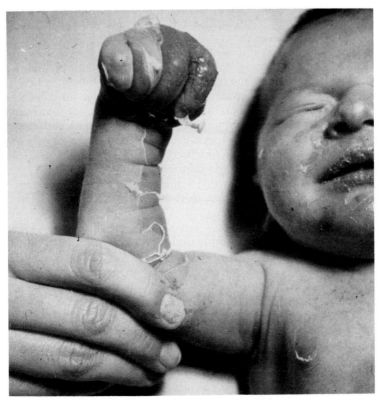

Fig. 16.5 The scalded skin syndrome (toxic epidermal necrolysis)

usually necessary to remove it. Various types of *S. epidermidis* produce slime which sticks to i.v. catheters – this is why the organism is such a problem. It is sometimes possible to sterilize an indwelling catheter by infusing antibiotics down the line, and this may be tried when it is extremely difficult to insert another catheter.

Listeriosis

Listeriosis is an important cause of death in the newborn in many countries where pasteurization of milk is inadequate. The baby is infected from the mother, who is usually a symptom-free carrier.

Sometime previously, she has ingested the bacterium (*Listeria monocytogenes*) in contaminated milk, milk products or undercooked meat. The organism is a Gram-positive rod, and is not difficult to identify on routine culture.

The fetus may be infected transplacentally. This produces septicaemia and often meningoencephalitis with third trimester infections, but usually fetal death and miscarriage if the infection is earlier. The baby may also be infected during passage through the birth canal and this may lead to pneumonia and septicaemia. Jaundice and purpura often occur, with atpyical lymphocytes in the blood. A rash may be present which may be non-specific erythematous macules, or a more florid rash (often called a blueberry muffin rash). There is often associated hepatomegaly and splenomegaly.

Mortality is not high provided that appropriate antibiotic treatment is given promptly. In survivors, there is a risk of mental handicap and hydrocephalus.

The antibiotic of choice is amoxycillin or ampicillin as some strains appear to be penicillin-resistant.

Congenital syphilis

This disease, once common in this country, is still extremely common in many developing countries. The infecting organism, the spirochaete *Treponema pallidum*, infects the fetus by crossing the placenta after the fourth month of pregnancy. The affected baby may be stillborn or may develop a number of characteristic signs of the disease within the first few weeks of life. It is essential that all pregnant women should have serological tests for syphilis. Venereal disease research laboratory (VDRL) and *Treponema pallidum* haemagglutination (TPHA) tests are commonly used.

The clinical signs of congenital syphilis appear after about three weeks and these include snuffles associated with infection of the nasal bones and cartilages, eczema round the mouth with fissures and subsequent scarring at the angles of the mouth (rhagades), hepatosplenomegaly, anaemia, a generalized copper-coloured maculopapular rash with blisters which may be particularly severe over the palms and soles giving rise to 'washerwoman's skin'. There may be general failure to thrive and fever.

It is not uncommon for a syhphilitic mother to give birth to a normal infant. In such a situation, the infant's serum tests such as VDRL will be positive, because of transfer of maternal antibodies. The presence of characteristic symptoms or signs with positive serology, rather than a positive result itself, should therefore be the indication for treatment. However, if the baby's VDRL titre is much higher than the mother's, congenital infection is likely. The IgM specific test may be very helpful; the IgM fluorescent treponemal antibody absorption test (IgM FTA-ABS) indicates that the baby has produced antibodies, as IgM does not cross the placenta. Treatment is with systemic penicillin for 14 days.

Candidiasis (thrush)

This fungal infection is often acquired from the mother's vagina with subsequent re-infection from the mother's or attendant's fingers. It is also common in babies who are on broad-spectrum antibiotics or as a result of careless hygiene and preparation of artificial feeds. Commonly, it presents with white plaques on the tongue or inside the mouth which, unlike milk curds, are difficult to rub off and leave a raw, red bleeding surface underneath. Infection of the perianal, vulval or scrotal skin is also common and may provide a source of re-infection. A candidal napkin rash may often be distinguished from an ammoniacal dermatitis by the fact that it extends into the skin creases and by the presence of satellite lesions around the area of erythema.

In the ill preterm baby receiving intravenous feeding there is a risk that superficial candidiasis may lead to septicaemia which is usually fatal. Topical treatment is with nystatin or miconazole preparations. It is important to treat the nipples of a breastfeeding mother also, if the baby has oral candida. Septicaemia is difficult to treat but amphotericin B, and 5-flucytosine may be used.

Tuberculosis

Very rarely tubercle bacilli are transmitted transplacentally or via infected amniotic fluid from mother to fetus. Less rarely an infant is infected postnatally by a mother with active disease. The incidence of the disease in infants and children in communities with a high rate of adult tuberculosis can be much reduced by immunization with BCG shortly after birth (see Chapter 4). Provided a mother with active disease is started on treatment, she may continue to breast feed her baby. The baby should be immunized with isoniazid-resistant BCG and started on isoniazid to make doubly sure infection does not develop.

Viral infection

Cytomegalovirus (CMV)

This is a virus similar to herpes and is acquired *in utero* causing severe generalized disease in the baby with enlargement of liver and spleen, jaundice, microcephaly with mental retardation, choroidoretinitis and intracranial calcification. The neonate may present with signs of intrauterine growth retardation, microcephaly, respiratory distress or encephalitis. The diagnosis may be confirmed by demonstrating a rising titre of serum complement-fixing antibodies, by culturing the virus from the urine or by finding inclusion bodies in renal tubular cells in the urine. This clinical syndrome is rare, but some surveys have shown that cytomegalovirus can often be grown from the urine of apparently normal newborn babies. The prognosis for these infants is still not certain. When giving a blood transfusion it is now good practice only to give blood which does not contain CMV antibodies.

Congenital rubella

Where in the child and adult, rubella is a mild infection, in the fetus and newborn infant it is an extremely serious disease. If it is acquired during the first four weeks of pregnancy, there is a greater than 50% chance of fetal damage, but most commonly intrauterine death occurs. Over the next few weeks, during the phase of organogenesis, there is about a 25% chance of fetal damage, but when damage does occur it involves many organs in the body. These include the eye, leading to microphthalmos, cataract, glaucoma or choroidoretinitis; the brain, leading to mental retardation or microcephaly; the ear, leading to deafness; and the heart, most commonly resulting in patent ductus arteriosus, pulmonary stenosis, or ventricular or atrial septal defects. In addition, the disease remains active throughout pregnancy and for the early months of extrauterine life so that the infant may be born with osteitis, myocarditis, petechial haemorrhages, anaemia and pneumonia. The virus may be recovered from the urine or throat of an affected infant for several months after birth. The greatest risk of fetal damage occurs, therefore, before the mother knows she is pregnant. In addition, it may follow mild or unrecognized clinical attacks of rubella. When infection occurs after three to four months gestation, there is a less than 2% chance of a fetus suffering damage from congenital rubella, but the baby must always be checked for deafness.

If a woman develops an illness suggestive of rubella during the first trimester of pregnancy, the diagnosis should be confirmed serologically by examination of paired serum specimens. If over the four weeks between the specimens there is a sharp rise in rubella-specific antibody levels, this is clear evidence of a recent infection. It is common practice in this situation to offer a therapeutic abortion, since the fetus is very likely to be born severely handicapped. It is now policy in the UK to immunize all children in the second year of life using the measles, mumps and rubella (MMR) vaccine. Teenage girls should receive immunization with the rubella vaccine if they have not already been immunized in childhood. It is hoped that this policy of vaccination will eradicate the disease, but a very high uptake of the immunization will be necessary for this to happen.

When a woman is found to be rubella susceptible at booking, she should be followed up and offered immunization once the pregnancy is over. Contraceptive advice must be given as it is essential that pregnancy is avoided for the next three months, due to the teratogenic effects of this vaccine.

All babies whose mothers have had serologically confirmed rubella in pregnancy must be followed up carefully. Sometimes there is very little serological evidence of rubella at first in the baby. The IgM specific antibodies may not always be present in an infant with congenital rubella, but deafness may develop after birth. Unfortunately some proven cases of reinfection of the mother from the infected baby, have been reported.

Herpes

See above (p. 347).

Human immunodeficiency virus (HIV)

This virus causes acquired immune deficiency syndrome (AIDS). There is progressive failure of the body's immune system leading to chronic diarrhoea, malnutrition, wasting, increased susceptibility to opportunistic infections with such organisms as toxoplasma, candida and pneumocystis, and death. There is, at present, no cure or vaccine, so it is giving rise to a lot of anxiety.

A baby can be infected with the virus from its mother by transplacental infection, at birth or by breastfeeding (Pinching & Jeffries,

1985). Most infected mothers acquired the virus by sharing needles during i.v. drug use, or as a result of sexual contact with an infected male.

HIV is very prevalent in such areas as the sub-Saharan region of Africa, North America and Thailand. Not all infected patients will develop AIDS. The proportion of babies born to mothers who are themselves infected appears to vary from country to country. It is reported as 60% in Africa, but the European Collaborative Study showed that only 13% are infected. Infection of the baby is identified by finding the presence of the virus, or antibodies persisting longer than 18 months.

There are a number of important issues for pregnancy and the newborn. There is some suggestion that a mother with AIDS is more likely to infect the fetus than one with just HIV infection, and that a termination may need to be considered. Several cases have been reported where a breastfeeding mother has infected her baby. This has occurred after a mother was transfused with infected blood following delivery, and subsequently infected her baby. From recent studies it is reported that breastfeeding may increase the risk of infecting the baby by another 14%; thus nearly a third of breastfeeding babies of HIV-positive mothers may be affected. Therefore breastfeeding cannot be recommended in a developed country where the mother is HIV positive. This would not be true in a developing country where the risks from bottle feeding would be much greater.

It is clearly important for staff to have adequate protection from acquiring HIV from mothers and babies. Since women are not screened for HIV in pregnancy, and it is not possible to identify people from supposed high risk groups, staff should take precautions whenever they come into contact with any blood or blood products. Precautions must also be taken against the risks of needlestick injuries.

The earliest signs of AIDS in infancy are pneumocystis carinii, which can occur from the first month of life. It has now become common practice to treat the baby of an infected mother prophylactically with cotrimoxazole, until the child has been adequately screened for HIV. Infected babies need regular follow-up through childhood to see whether the HIV antibodies disappear. If possible follow-up should be done at a family clinic, so that the medical care for the parents and children is undertaken simultaneously by the same team of people.

Protozoal infections

Congenital toxoplasmosis

Infection in pregnant women may affect the fetus since the protozoon, *Toxoplasma gondii*, is able to cross the placenta. Characteristic features include encephalitis with a raised protein and lymphocyte count in the CSF, choroidoretinitis, jaundice with hepatosplenomegaly, myocarditis and thrombocytopenic purpura. The diagnosis is made by finding a high concentration of toxoplasma antibody in the newborn baby's blood. There is often associated mental retardation and hydrocephalus, and intracranial calcification is classically found on skull radiography.

References and Further Reading

Beeby, P.J. & Jeffery, H. (1992) Risk factors for necrotizing enterocolitis: the influence of gestational age. *Arch. Dis. Child.*, *67*, 432–435.

Clearkin, L.J. (1986) Chlamydial ophthalmia neonatorum. *Midwives Chronicle and Nursing Notes, August*, 174–176.

Davies, P.A. & Gothefors, L.A. (1984) *Bacterial Infections in the Fetus and Newborn*. Philadelphia: W.B. Saunders.

Hanshaw, J.B., Dudgeon, J.A. & Marshall, W.C. (1985) *Viral Diseases of the Fetus and Newborn*, 2nd ed. Philadelphia: W.B. Saunders.

Heggie, A.D., Lumicao, G.G., Stuart, L.A. *et al.* (1981) Chlamydia trachomatis infection in mothers and infants. *Arch. Dis. Child.*, *135*, 507–511.

Johnstone, H.A. & Marcinak, J.F. (1990) Candidiasis in neonatal sepsis. *Neonatal Network 9(6)*, 9–14.

Lucas, A. & Col, T.J. (1990) Breast milk and necrotising enterocolitis. *Lancet*, *336*, 1519–1523.

Miller, E., Cradock-Watson, J.E. & Pollock, T.M. (1982) Consequences of confirmed maternal rubella at successive stages of pregnancy. *Lancet*, *ii*, 781–784.

Pearl, K.N., Preece, P.M., Ades, A. *et al.* (1986) Neurodevelopmental assessment after cytomegalovirus infection. *Arch. Dis. Child.*, *61*, 323–326.

Pinching, A.J. & Jeffries, D.J. (1985) AIDS and HTLV-III/LAV infection: consequences for obstetrics and perinatal medicine. *British Journal of Obstetrics and Gynaecology 92*, 1211–1217.

Poulsen, N. (1990) Candidiasis in the premature infant. *Neonatal Network 8(4)*, 9–14.

Reed, G.B., Claireaux, A.E. & Bain, A.D. (1989) *Diseases of the Fetus and Newborn*, St Louis: Mosby.

Remington, J.S. & Klein, J.O. (eds) (1983) *Infectious Diseases of the Fetus and Newborn Infant*, 2nd ed. Philadelphia: W.B. Saunders.

Rosenberg, A.L. (1991) The return of congenital syphilis. *Neonatal Network*, 9(5), 17–22.

Smith, H. & Congdon, P. (1985) Neonatal systemic candidiasis. *Arch. Dis. Child.*, 60, 365–369.

Snowe, R.J. & Wilfert, C.M. (1973) Epidemic reappearance of gonococcal ophthalmia neonatorum. *Pediatrics, 51*, 110.

Wilson, D. (1988) An overview of sexually transmissible diseases on the perinatal period. *Journal of Nurse-Midwifery*, 33(3), 115–128.

—17

Sudden or Gradual Deterioration

The recognition of a particular disease in a newborn baby is often difficult. This is because many conditions affecting, for example, the brain, heart or lungs may produce the same clinical signs. In particular, infections commonly mimic other illnesses. Making an accurate diagnosis depends on the clinical and laboratory evaluation of a relatively small number of non-specific signs and symptoms. In preterm babies, who are at higher risk, the severity of the disease is often greater yet the clinical features are even less specific than in term babies.

If a baby suddenly deteriorates, it is important to rely on the general principles of resuscitation (see Chapter 3). This will include correcting hypoxaemia with added oxygen and assisted ventilation, correcting acidaemia or hypoglycaemia and, subsequently, treating with antibiotics appropriate for a wide range of possible pathogens.

After initial resuscitation or in the baby who deteriorates insidiously it is very important to make a careful assessment. Treatment (especially antibiotics) should not be started until adequate baseline investigations have been done: arterial blood gases, blood for culture, haemoglobin and full blood count, sugar and electrolytes, lumbar puncture (LP) and urine culture must all be considered. Treatment should not await the results in an ill baby.

The purpose of Table 17.1 is to provide a quick guide to the possible differential diagnoses of some important features of illness in the newborn. Detailed discussions of these conditions will be found elsewhere in this book.

Table 17.1 Possible differential diagnosis of some presenting features of illness in the newborn.

Presentation	Time	Additional symptoms, signs or associated clinical features	Possible cause	Action	See also chapter
Collapse (sudden illness producing a shocked, grey mottled floppy baby)	Usually after first 48 hours	Cyanotic attacks, diarrhoea or vomiting, weight loss, poor sucking, refusing feeds, minor infection	Septicaemia	Infection screen including LP; antibiotics before results are available	16
	< 48 hours	As above	As above. especially Group B β-haemolytic streptococcal infection	As above. High dose antibiotics	16
	< 48 hours	SFGA, baby of diabetic mother	Hypoglycaemia	Intravenous glucose	6, 15
	< 48 hours	Prematurity, RDS	Periventricular haemorrhage (PVH)	Ventilation, transfusion, repeated cerebral ultrasound scans	8
	2–3 weeks	Dehydration, ambiguous genitalia in female	Salt-losing congenital adrenal hyperplasia	Intravenous saline	10
Bleeding	< 48 hours	Umbilical cord	Slipped clamp	Reclamp, transfuse if necessary	13
	48–72 hours	Umbilical stump, melaena	Haemorrhagic disease of newborn (HDN)	Vitamin K transfuse	13

	generally after 48 hours	Gut haemorrhage, small baby, rhesus disease	Necrotizing enterocolitis	Plain abdominal X-ray, antibiotics, cease oral feeds	10
	Any age	Any site	Disseminated intravascular coagulation (DIC)	Treat precipitating illness; fresh frozen plasma	13
Pallor (sudden anaemia)	At birth	Tachypnoea, tachycardia or bradycardia shock in severe cases	Fetomaternal haemorrhage; torn velamentous cord vessel Hydrops fetalis	Immediate clamping of cord transfuse Exchange transfusion, paracentesis, diuretics, ventilation	13
	Any time	Already ill baby	DIC, covert bleeding	Treat precipitating illness; fresh plasma, blood	13
	< 72 hours	Breech or difficult delivery,	Intra-abdominal haemorrhage (adrenal, liver or spleen)	General supportive measures, transfusion	13
	< 72 hours	Severe RDS, history of hypoxia large volumes of intravenous alkali	PVH	Ventilation, transfusion, USS	8
	2nd week	Normochromic blood film, preterm baby	Anaemia of prematurity	Transfusion	6

Table 17.1 Possible differential diagnosis of some presenting features of illness in the newborn. Contd.

Presentation	Time	Additional symptoms, signs or associated clinical features	Possible cause	Action	See also chapter
Fits	< 24 hours	SFGA baby; LFGA baby; baby of diabetic mother	Hypoglycaemia	Intravenous dextrose after confirming with blood glucose test strips	6, 15
	< 48 hours	Cyanotic attacks, difficult or traumatic delivery	periventricular, subarachnoid or subdural haemorrhage, intrapartum asphyxia, Hypoxic ischaemic encephalopathy (HIE)	General resuscitation. Transfuse if necessary	14
	5–8 days	Mother with vitamin D deficiency or hyperparathyroidism	Hypocalcaemia	Calcium and magnesium supplements	14
	1st week	Hypotonia	Organic acidaemias	Check plasma and urine by amino and organic acid chromatography	10, 14
	Any age	Apnoeic attacks, general illness, bulging fontanelle, very rarely neck stiffness	Meningitis, usually Group B β-haemolytic streptococci or *E. coli*	Antibiotics, general measures for resuscitation	16

	Age	Clinical features	Diagnosis	Management	Page
Cyanotic attacks	< 48 hours	Fits, history of traumatic delivery	Subdural haemorrhage, HIE	General resuscitation transfuse if necessary	14
	After 48 hours	vomiting, lethargy, poor sucking	Infection, especially septicaemia	Infection screen, including LP, antibiotics	16
	Any age	preterm baby less than 32 weeks gestation	Apnoeic attacks of prematurity, PVH	Stimulation, theophylline, apnoea alarm	6
	Any age	Murmur, tachypnoea, heart failure	Congenital heart disease	ECG and treatment for heart failure	11
Respiratory distress (tachypnoea/ recession/gasping/ cyanosis)	Birth	Meconium staining of liquor and skin. Fetal distress. SFGA baby	Meconium aspiration	Suck out trachea, appropriate O_2, antibiotics	6
	< 4 hours	Preterm, low Apgar scores	RDS	Appropriate ambient O_2 concentration, respiratory support	8
	Birth	Cyanosis, worsening condition on bag and mask resuscitation	Diaphragmatic hernia	Ventilate, replogle tube, CXR, surgical referral	3

Table 17.1 Possible differential diagnosis of some presenting features of illness in the newborn. Contd.

Presentation	Time	Additional symptoms, signs or associated clinical features	Possible cause	Action	See also chapter
	Birth	Oligohydramnios; characteristic facies; failed resuscitation	Potter's syndrome (renal agenesis, pulmonary hypoplasia)	Fatal	10
	Birth	Nasogastric tube fails to pass down both nostrils	Bilateral choanal atresia	Intubate, ventilate, surgical referral	3, 10
	Birth	Retrognathia, glossoptosis, midline cleft palate	Pierre Robin anomalad	Nurse prone consider inserting airway	10
	Any age	During resuscitation, ventilation	Pneumothorax	Increase inspired O_2 concentration, drain if under tension	3, 8
	< 48 hours	Choking during feed, hydramnios, inability to pass tube into stomach, excessive salivation	Tracheo-oesophageal fistula, oesophageal atresia	Suck out pouch, refer to surgeon	3, 10
	During feed	Choking	Aspiration	Treat pneumonia (oxygen, antibiotics)	8
	Any age	Cyanosis, murmur, abnormal heart size and/or 'ground glass' lung fields on chest X-ray	RDS, TAPVD especially, but many forms of cyanotic CHD	ECG, assessment of oxygenation	11

| On ventilator | Deteriorating hypoxia, struggling | Blocked tube, extubated, tension pneumothorax, worsening pulmonary disease | reintubate, chest drain, increase ventilation | 8 |
| On ventilator | Big baby fighting ventilator | Above causes excluded | Paralyse and sedate | 8 |

—18

The Neonatal Intensive Care Environment

Separation

Pregnancy, birth and the transition into parenthood bring with them major changes, both physical and emotional. The expectation of most parents is that they will have a healthy, term baby to take home a few days after the birth. The delivery of a preterm or small baby is therefore a shock and disappointment. The baby does not resemble the one they imagined; families need to grieve the loss of this imagined child before they can begin to form a relationship with their actual baby.

There is a sensitive period after the birth, in which the parents and newborn infant get to know each other. If they are denied this opportunity, parents may find it more difficult to form an attachment to their baby. A sick or preterm infant may need to be resuscitated immediately following the delivery, or quickly transferred to the neonatal unit. All parents should at least get to see their baby before transfer, and ideally have the opportunity for a cuddle. Instant photographs of the baby should be given to the parents as soon as possible, taken before too many tubes and pieces of equipment are attached. An increasing problem in recent years has been the need to transfer some sick infants to other hospitals for treatment. The mother should also be transferred but this is not always practical or possible.

There is evidence that babies separated from their parents on the neonatal intensive care unit (NICU) for many weeks or months, are more at risk of subsequently being neglected or abused by their parents (Budin, 1907; Klaus & Kennell, 1982). There is no automatic affection between parents and their child, the relationship is built up gradually over the early days, weeks and months of life. It depends on intimate contact and frequent handling, both of which may be denied to families in the NICU owing to circumstances, inhibitions or fear. Staff can do much to encourage such contact between the family and their baby, but must appreciate that it is normal for them to be reluctant to do so in the first few days or even weeks (Townshend,

1987). Very few babies are too sick to be touched or cuddled by their parents.

As well as the physical separation there are also psychological aspects to the issue of separation (Valentin, 1981; Swan Parente, 1982). It is common for parents to exhibit anticipatory grief (Lindemann, 1944), whereby they avoid forming a close relationship with their baby in case it does not survive. Many parents feel that a very small or preterm baby does not look attractive, but dressing them in specially designed clothes can help considerably (Plate IX).

Visiting

Hospital visiting for friends and relatives has, in the past, been severely restricted. The reasons given included prevention of infection and to allow the mother to rest. There is now no doubt that visits by friends and family should be unrestricted, as they can be a source of great comfort and support to the parents. There is no evidence that such a policy increases the incidence of infections providing that people with obvious colds, sore throats and other infections stay away.

A busy NICU looks very frightening to visiting families and it is important to explain what the various pieces of equipment are for. Staff may consider such things as eye shields for babies under phototherapy routine, but to the unprepared family they can be a great shock. Much can be done to make the atmosphere on NICU welcoming and friendly, with pictures on the walls, staff wearing less formal uniforms and the identification of a key nurse for each family. Parents and siblings should be encouraged to bring soft toys, photographs, pictures or mobiles for the baby's cot or incubator. Playgroup or creche facilities are very helpful to families with other children, and one of our aims for the future should be to employ a play specialist for siblings in each unit. Siblings can be involved in the care by doing things such as fetching nappies or drawing pictures for the baby (Troy et al., 1988). The need for support for members of the extended family is sometimes overlooked. It is important they also understand what is happening to the baby, in order that they can then support the parents more effectively (Gyulay, 1975; Blackburn & Lowen, 1986). All NICUs should provide parents' rooms or hostel accommodation so that they can stay overnight whenever necessary; for example, if their baby is particularly ill or unstable, or in preparation for discharge home. They should also have access to a sitting room, bathroom and cooking facilities.

Environmental Neonatology

As we continue to make rapid technological advances in the field of neonatology, so the survival rate of very small and very preterm babies improves. For some the cost of survival is a degree of mental or physical handicap, and it is important that we consider both morbidity and mortality figures when assessing outcomes.

Typically, NICUs are brightly lit, busy, noisy places. During the course of a day a baby will be subjected to numerous episodes of handling, some associated with painful procedures, and virtually all initiating a startle reaction if not apnoeas or bradycardias. There is an increasing awareness amongst neonatal staff that we need to implement baby-centred care, by considering the effects the NICU environment has on them both emotionally and physically. Changes may entail reducing or eliminating a particular stimulus, such as noise, or introducing a positive stimulus, for example baby massage.

Light

Over the past two decades the light intensity in NICU has increased five- to ten-fold, with the average now about 60–90 footcandles (Glass *et al.*, 1985). To enable staff to observe babies adequately, the American Academy of Pediatrics (Gottfried & Gaiter, 1985) recommends a minimum of 100 footcandle intensity. However, a level of just 60 footcandles has been shown to contribute to the development of retinopathy of prematurity (ROP) (Glass *et al.*, 1985), with the risk increasing the smaller the baby. Bright sunlight and the use of phototherapy lamps increases the light intensity even further.

The harmful effects of high levels of lighting can be alleviated to some degree by establishing a day and night pattern (Mann *et al.*, 1986), and dimming lights when their use is not imperative. Care to cover the eyes of all babies under phototherapy and avoiding placing babies in direct sunlight are also beneficial practices.

Positive visual stimuli for babies include brightly coloured pictures or objects with contrasting colours placed in the incubator, or mobiles above the cot. Babies focus on facial features when looking at people, especially mouths and eyes; drawings of faces are often viewed with great concentration.

Noise

According to the British safety standards the mean noise level inside an incubator should not exceed 60 decibels (Hilton, 1987). Most of the equipment alarms are within this limit, but incubator alarms can be as loud as 85 decibels. The main source of noise is from staff and visitors to the unit. Sudden loud noises cause adverse physiological effects such as sleep disturbance, crying, tachycardia, hypoxaemia and raised intracranial pressure (Long *et al.*, 1980). Tapping the incubator or putting an object on to its top heavily, results in a very loud sound for the neonate. Closing the incubator doors can be as noisy as 115 decibels.

A study of infants with reduced light and noise stimulus at night, showed that on discharge from hospital they slept for an average of two hours more per 24 hours, and their weight gain was more than those who did not undergo the day and night patterns (Mann *et al.*, 1986).

Staff must be aware of the noise levels in NICU and take care to reduce them whenever possible. This includes careful positioning of equipment away from the incubator, turning radios down, taking care when closing incubator doors, and not placing objects on top of incubators.

Handling

The reported incidence of the number of times a baby is handled in 24 hours varies dramatically, with an average number of 130 times being cited by Korones (1976). In this study the length of time between handlings ranged from 4.6 to 19.2 minutes. Nursing staff handled the babies most frequently and parents least. Murdoch & Darlow (1984) reported that 93% of bradycardias occurred during or following handling, as did 83% of hypoxaemic episodes and 38% of apnoeas. The most consistent effect of handling is a disturbance of sleep patterns.

It is well accepted that babies need human touch for optimum physiological and emotional development (Weiss, 1979). Numerous different therapeutic tactile stimulation studies have been carried out to assess their effects, benefits and drawbacks (Lacy & Ohlsson, 1993). Baby massage is becoming more widely practiced in neonatal units, as a way of enhancing the parent–child relationship and providing a positive touch stimulus for the baby (Booth *et al.*, 1985; Field *et al.*, 1987). Kangaroo care, where the baby is cuddled naked, except for a nappy, against the parent's skin, beneath the clothing, is also growing in popularity (Plate X). The two main benefits of skin-to-skin contact are improved lactation and the development of a closer relationship between the parent and their baby (Anderson, 1991).

Careful assessment of the need for any handling of sick babies should take place, with the recommendation that minimal handling should apply to as many babies as possible, unless it is positive touch by parents or staff. Procedures should not be carried out routinely, but their necessity must be questioned.

Positioning

The sensorimotor development of preterm babies is affected by their low muscle tone and long periods of static positioning in cots and incubators (Bellefeuille-Reid & Jakubek, 1989). Prolonged and repeated periods of being nursed prone results in externally rotated hips and everted feet, both of which may delay weightbearing and walking (Bottos & Stefani, 1982).

A normal baby will spend much of the last month *in utero* curled up in a flexed position. At this stage myelination of the cerebral cortex and spinal tract occurs. Preterm babies lose the compression effects of the uterus early, and are therefore born with a lack of physiological flexion. Developmental delays may ensue if careful positioning is not implemented to ensure that extension occurs at about 40 weeks gestation, as would normally occur (Fetters, 1986).

Frequent changes in the position of the baby's head will help to reduce flattened, elongated, asymmetrical head shapes. The use of water-filled mattresses has aided this in some units.

Simple interventions will help to achieve normal postures. In the prone position a rolled sheet should be placed under the hips. A horseshoe-shaped roll is placed around the feet extending up the sides of the trunk. These will ensure that the hips are internally rotated, adducted and flexed. Continually lying in the prone position can also cause retraction of the shoulders, which may result in delay in rolling, balancing when sitting, reaching for objects and hand-to-eye coordination. Periods of prone positioning must therefore be mixed with side-lying. In this position a nappy placed under the lower hip rotates the pelvis slightly. A folded sheet placed across

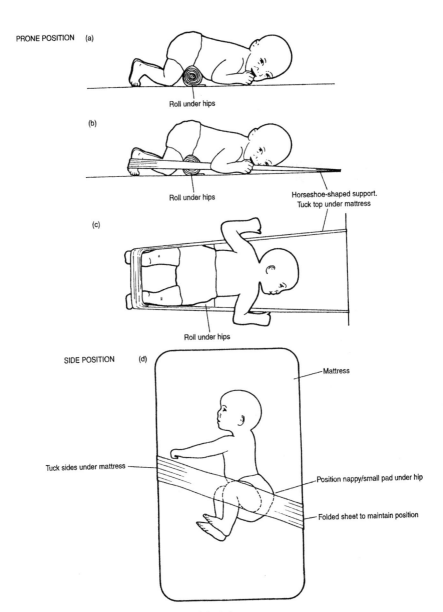

PRONE POSITION   (a)

Roll under hips

(b)

Roll under hips

Horseshoe-shaped support.
Tuck top under mattress

(c)

Roll under hips

SIDE POSITION   (d)

Mattress

Tuck sides under mattress

Position nappy/small pad under hip

Folded sheet to maintain position

Fig. 18.1 Prone positioning and side-lying

the hips and knees maintains this position with the upper leg flexed and rotated onto the mattress.

Pain

Response to painful stimuli shows that babies do feel pain (McGrath & Unruh, 1987; Anand & Hickey, 1987). The extent of their perception at cortical level is difficult to assess, but the evidence available strongly supports the use of analgesia when necessary. Several different methods for assessing pain in the neonate have been suggested, by looking at various physical and physiological responses to pain (Conkin, 1986; Franck, 1986; Beaver, 1987).

Discharge Home

The discharge of a baby from NICU may follow many months of illness. Families inevitably experience a mixture of apprehension and excitement at this time. Careful organization is required, with the primary health care team notified a week or so in advance of the impending discharge, to enable the necessary support networks to be prepared. A pre-discharge meeting for everyone involved with the family is very useful. A liaison health visitor who regularly visits the unit to review each baby's progress and notifies the community staff, is an asset. Feedback of information about the baby's home environment or social circumstances can also help in arranging adequate facilities prior to discharge. A leaflet with information about who to contact if they have any concerns, what medicines their baby needs and general advice, should be given to the parents on discharge (see Appendix).

Waiting until the baby achieves a specific weight or gestation before allowing discharge is unnecessary and costly. Many babies of 1700 g are now discharged home quite safely. The community follow up for these families varies greatly throughout the country. Family Care Sisters have been shown to be very cost-effective in enabling earlier discharge of babies, and reducing re-admission rates by the early detection and treatment of problems (Couriel & Davies, 1988). They use a family-centred approach to care, visiting the family as often as they require offering support and advice to help with the transition from hospital to home. Integration of the baby into the family can be harder than they anticipated, as many babies discharged are quite demanding or may have residual health problems or vulnerabilities. The effect this has on the family dynamics can be immense, and much support is required in order to facilitate integration.

References and Further Reading

Anand, K.J.S. & Hickey, P.R. (1987) Pain and its effects in the human neonate and fetus. *N. Engl. J. Med., 317,* 1321–1329.

Anderson, G.C. (1991) Current knowledge about skin-to-skin (kangaroo) care for preterm infants. *Journal of Perinatology, 10*(3), 216–226.

Beaver, P.K. (1987) Premature infants' response to touch and pain: can nurses make a difference? *Neonatal Network, 6,* 13–17.

Bellefeuille-Reid, D. & Jakubek, S. (1989) Adaptive positioning intervention for premature infants: issues for paediatric occupational therapy practice. *British Journal of Occupational Therapy, 52*(3), 93–96.

Blackburn, S. & Lowen, L. (1986) Impact of an infant's premature birth on the grandparents and parents. *Journal of Obstetric, Gynecologic and Neonatal Nursing, 15*(2), 173–178.

Booth, C.L., Johnson-Crowley, N. & Barnard, K.E. (1985) Infant massage and exercise: worth the effort? *MCN, 10,* 184–189.

Bottos, M. & Stefani, D. (1982) Postural and motor care of the premature baby. *Dev. Med. Child Neurol., 24,* 706–707.

Budin, P. (1907) *The Nursling.* London: Caxton.

Conkin, D. (1986) A multidimensional study of infants' response to painful stimulus. *Pediatric Nursing, 12,* 30–31.

Couriel, J.M. & Davies, P. (1988) Costs and benefits of a community special care baby service. *BMJ, 296,* 1043–1046.

Fetters, L. (1986) Sensorimotor management of the high-risk neonate. *Phys. Occup. Ther. Pediatr., 6,* 217–229.

Field, T., Scafidi, F. & Schanberg, S. (1987) Massage of preterm newborns to improve growth and development. *Pediatric Nursing, 13*(6), 385–387.

Franck, L.S. (1986) A new method to quantitively describe pain behaviour in infants. *Nursing Research, 35*(1), 28–31.

Glass, P., Avery, G. *et al.* (1985) Effect of bright light in the hospital nursery on the incidence of retinopathy of prematurity. *New Eng. J. Med., 313,* 7.

Gottfried, A.W. & Gaiter, J.L. (eds) (1985) *Infant Stress Under Intensive Care: Environmental Neonatology.* Baltimore: University Park Press.

Gyulay, J. (1975) The forgotten grievers. *Am. J. Nurs., 75*(9), 1476–1479.

Hilton, A. (1987) The hospital racket: how noisy is your unit? *Am. J. Nurs., 87,* 59–61.

Klaus, M.H. & Kennell, J.H. (1982) *Parent–infant bonding,* pp. 151–226. St Louis: C.V. Mosby.

Korones, S.B. (1976) Disturbance and infants' rest. In *Report of the 69th*

Ross Conference on Pediatric Research, pp. 94–97, ed. Moore, T.D. Columbus: Ross Laboratories.

Lacy, J.B. & Ohlsson, A. (1993) Behavioral outcomes of environmental or care-giving hospital-based interventions for preterm infants: a critical overview. *Acta Paediatr.*, *82*, 408–415.

Lindemann, E. (1944) Symptomatology and management of acute grief. *American Journal of Psychiatry*, *101*, 141–148.

Long, G.J., Lucey, J.F. & Philip, A.G.S. (1980) Noise and hypoxaemia in the intensive care nursery. *Pediatrics*, *65*, 143–145.

Mann, N.P., Haddow, R., Stokes, L. *et al.* (1986) Effect of night and day on preterm infants in a newborn nursery: randomised trial. *BMJ*, *293*, 1265–1267.

McGrath, P.J. & Unruh, A.M. (eds) (1987) *Pain in Children and Adolescents. Pain Research and Clinical Management*, Vol. 1. Amsterdam: Elsevier.

Murdoch, D. & Darlow, B. (1984) Handling during neonatal intensive care. *Arch. Dis. Child.*, *59*, 957–961.

Swan Parente, A. (1982) Psychological pressures in a neonatal unit. *British Journal of Hospital Medicine*, *27*, 266–268.

Townshend, P. (1987) Impact of intensive care. *Midwives Chronicle*, *1193*, 194–197.

Troy, P., Wilkinson-Faul, D., Smith, A. *et al.* (1988) Sibling visiting in NICU. *Am. J. Nurs.*, *88*(1), 70.

Valentin, L. (1981) The problems of grief and separation in the Special Care Baby Unit. *Nursing Times Nov. 4th*, 11.

Weiss, S.J. (1979) The language of touch. *Nursing Research Journal*, 28(2).

—19

The Grieving Process

There are five recognized stages in the grieving process. They are not sequential, some may occur simultaneously and there will be erratic swings from one to another. They are:

- Shock
- Denial
- Anger
- Equilibrium
- Acceptance

Many things will influence the length of time it takes for the acceptance stage to be reached, and there is often a period of fluctuation between denial and anger. The significance of the level of care and support given by professionals cannot be overestimated in its effects on the family or the course of the grieving process. Bereavement counselling training can prove invaluable to neonatal staff.

It is not just when a baby dies that a family grieves. When a deformed, handicapped or preterm baby is born, the parents grieve for the healthy, mature infant they expected. This process is worsened with the birth, and by the death, of a sick infant, as the parents often resist becoming too attached in case their baby does not survive. Feelings of grief may recur, often unexpectedly, when the parents are reminded of the death by such things as anniversaries, or visiting the hospital where the death occurred.

Babies with Congenital Malformations and other Handicaps

Wherever possible the initial examination of a newborn baby should be carried out in the presence of the parents. Any obvious abnormalities seen at this time must be explained to them sensitively and honestly. The attitude of staff during the early hours of life is critical. Thoughtless remarks, or a misguided wish to protect the parents, may contribute substantially to rejection of the baby, or exacerbate feelings of guilt and distress.

It is sometimes obvious to the midwife or paediatrician that the baby has a congenital abnormality or syndrome likely to result in handicap. Sensitive handling of this situation may enable some degree of preparation of the parents prior to a senior paediatrician confirming the diagnosis and explaining the implications to them. This meeting should be a joint consultation involving the nursing or midwifery staff, to ensure consistency of information given to the parents. In such situations it is important that parents have the chance to cuddle and feed their baby before being told the diagnosis, and ideally whilst being told. If the baby has been named, staff should use the name in all discussions.

Explanations will need to be repeated over the next few days and weeks. Long-term support and follow-up for these families is vital, and will often be co-ordinated by paediatricians. Communication throughout the primary care team is important and the general practitioner, health visitor and community midwife should be informed of any problems as soon as possible.

Genetic counselling should be offered for all these parents, to explain the chances of recurrence and give advice for future pregnancies.

All neonatal units should to have a social worker attached to them. Their support often proves invaluable, with advice on a wide range of topics from finances to funeral and cremation arrangements. In addition to this they offer emotional support to the parents, and provide a link between the unit and community by visiting the family at home when necessary.

Stillbirths and Late Miscarriages

This is a tragic end to pregnancy. It is important for the parents to accept that their baby is a real entity, and it has been found to be of great benefit if they spend time holding and getting to know their dead infant, whom they should be encouraged to name. Photographs and mementos will also help them to acknowledge their child's existence and individuality, although it must be remembered that some cultures reject momentos.

Deaths on the Neonatal Unit

Now that babies of such low birthweight and short gestational age are surviving, it is inevitable that some of them will still die from complications associated with their size or gestation.

The circumstances surrounding each death will be very individual, and should be treated as such. The baby may have been on the unit for several months, a few days or even just a matter of hours. It may have been possible to prepare some families in advance, whilst others may be faced with this tragedy immediately after the birth. Many hospitals have a bereavement room attached to the delivery suite or the neonatal unit, where parents can have some privacy with their baby away from the noise and distractions of intensive care.

Religious, cultural and personal beliefs of the family must be taken into account. Many parents appreciate the presence of a minister or priest from their faith for support. Some religions and faiths have ceremonies such as baptism for Christians, and it is important to arrange these in the neonatal unit if the parents wish.

In all cases a post-mortem examination should be recommended in order to establish the precise cause of death, or to identify abnormalities and features of a particular syndrome. This allows the parents to be given as full an explanation as possible for their baby's death, and where appropriate, preconceptual counselling and antenatal screening to be arranged in future pregnancies. If the importance of, and reasons for, a post-mortem examination are explained in a sensitive manner, most parents will agree to this being carried out. They often fear that their infant may be unsightly or even dismembered following the post-mortem examination, and it is important that reassurance is given over this matter. It should be explained that the post-mortem incision is performed and sutured as carefully as an operation incision. The parents should be offered the opportunity to see their baby again prior to the funeral to dispel these fears.

Staff can do much to help bereaved families form some positive memories of their baby. Sensitive photographs of the baby may not be wanted by parents at the time, but should be kept in the notes and offered again in the future. Similarly, handprints, footprints, identity bracelets and locks of hair may be given. It has been suggested that the parents bath their baby in a strong smelling bath liquid, the smell of which then lingers on the clothes. These clothes when sealed in a plastic bag then offer the parents a scented reminder of their infant for several months. It is important to recognize that there are many religious and cultural differences surrounding death. In some ethnic groups the baby's clothes are deliberately discarded and mementos not kept.

If the parents wish and the baby's condition is suitable, some neonatal units give families the opportunity to take their dying baby home, either for a few hours or even for the whole of terminal care. This depends greatly on the support of specialized community staff who have to be available 24 hours a day. Advantages to one family may be disadvantages to another; for example, some parents welcome the opportunity to provide terminal care at home, whilst others find this a great strain. Home care allows the siblings to be looked after with less disruption to their routines, and produces happier memories of a baby as a part of the family. The period at home may become difficult or distressing to the family, and the parents should have the option of asking for a further period of hospital care at any time.

Follow-up

Parents need to come back and see the paediatrician or obstetrician, to discuss the death of their baby, to talk through their experiences and have the findings of the post-mortem examination explained. They should be given the opportunity to have an early appointment, but a definitive appointment has to wait until the post-mortem examination results are fully available, which may take up to three months. Further appointments can then be made as necessary.

There may be both physical and emotional reasons for not having another pregnancy soon after the death of a baby. It has been suggested that at least six months elapses before embarking on another pregnancy, to allow the grieving process to move towards resolution, and for the mother to be physically fit. However, this advice may be distressing for families who are anxious to have another pregnancy as soon as possible.

The Staff

The environment and type of work of a neonatal intensive care unit involves a high level of stress, and caring for a dying baby causes considerable extra pressures on the staff. Until quite recently we have not paid sufficient attention to supporting staff in such situations, with the consequences of high sickness rates and low morale.

There are many different ways in which this support may be established – for example, by holding multidisciplinary unit meetings to discuss issues; by assigning an independent counsellor to the unit, to work confidentially with individuals or groups; or by organizing relaxation and yoga classes. Although informal networks amongst friends and family ease a lot of tensions, there is still a tremendous amount of work to be done in the field of establishing effective formal support systems, which cater for all grades of staff. Staff support groups have not been as successful as wished. Members of staff often feel threatened by discussing their emotional reactions to death in front of their junior and senior colleagues. Rather than having general support groups, it may be more useful to have meetings to discuss the death of an individual baby. During the discussion of the physical management, it may be possible to raise other relevant issues. Because of the difficulties surrounding this area, an independent counsellor in every neonatal unit would prove invaluable. This person may come from a number of different professions, including psychology or psychotherapy.

Sudden Infant Death Syndrome (SIDS)

The possible tragedy of sudden infant death syndrome (SIDS) is an anxiety for every parent of a preterm baby. SIDS can be defined as a sudden, unexpected and unexplained death in the first 12 months of life. This diagnosis can only be made if a post-mortem examination has failed to reveal an adequate cause of death.

Incidence and risk factors

SIDS occurs in approximately 2 children per 1000 live births, but the incidence has declined dramatically recently. There are enormous variations worldwide; it is particularly common in the South Island of New Zealand (rate approx. 6.3/1000), and much lower in Hong Kong (rate approx. 0.3/1000) (Lee *et al.*, 1989).

There are many theories for the causation of SIDS, and its aetiology is thought to be multifactorial. Overheating and sleeping in the prone position are each independently associated with an increased risk of SIDS. The studies from Bristol in addition to those from the Netherlands, New Zealand and Hong Kong, resulted in a recommendation that babies should not be placed in a prone sleeping position

(Nelson *et al.*, 1989; Fleming et al., 1990). This appears to have resulted in the dramatic reduction in the incidence of SIDS.

It is more common in male babies, those born preterm and particularly those of very low birthweight. Babies with chronic lung disease and oxygen dependancy are also at greater risk. The incidence of SIDS is increased in the less advantaged families, those who do not breastfeed, those who smoke and drug using mothers. It is important to recognize that SIDS may occur in a family with no risk factors, and over half occur in social classes 1 to 3 with very few or no known risk factors. It is more common in the winter months and there is a peak incidence at two to five months of age.

Infection may well play a part since many children have minor signs, such as snuffles or diarrhoea, in the few days before the death. New methods are being developed of alerting parents and professionals to early signs of serious illness in a baby. Whereas a single sign may not be important on its own, it may become very significant when added to other signs. In Cambridge, a scoring system has been developed, called Baby Check (Morley *et al.*, 1991), which it is hoped will be effective in alerting families early, where a medical opinion needs to be sought. This is now widely used. Parents should also be encouraged to use the Child Health Record provided, which includes some health education information.

Parents often ask about the risk of recurrence of SIDS, and the estimated relative risk in subsequent siblings is thought to be increased three-fold. The Care of the Next Infant (CONI) project, which monitors subsequent siblings following a baby dying from SIDS, has proved very successful in supporting and reassuring families and the professionals caring for them. Where several babies have died within a family and inherited metabolic disorders have been discounted, suffocation or other methods of infanticide must be considered.

Home monitoring

The use of apnoea monitors at home has been discouraged. The simple monitors with an air-filled capsule attached to the stomach, or a mattress sensitive to respiratory movements, have proved very sensitive for the detection of apnoea of preterm babies in neonatal units. It is common for preterm babies to have periods of apnoea during sleep, but this usually resolves by the equivalent of 32 weeks gestation. Babies who die from SIDS may make breathing movements up to the moment of death, therefore monitors which detect a cessation of breathing movements may not be expected to be effective in a baby who is about to die from SIDS.

Many parents see apnoea monitors used on their babies in neonatal units and naturally request one to take home on discharge. They may be distressed when this is refused and a careful explanation about their ineffectiveness in detecting SIDS must be given. Apnoea alarms can be bought by members of the public, and it has been suggested that their use frequently leads to increased parental anxiety due to the number of false alarms, caused by normal sleep apnoea, shallow breathing or a badly positioned sensor in a healthy baby. Trials are at present being made of saturation monitors for home use; these would detect a drop in oxygen saturation. Such monitors would be effective in cases of obstructive apnoea, where the baby was becoming cyanosed but still making breathing movements. They are at present very expensive, but might become cheaper if sold in large quantities. Their efficacy remains to be proved.

Advice to parents

In order to reduce the risk of SIDS it is important that the home circumstances should be as good as possible. Breastfeeding should be strongly encouraged (Ford et al., 1993) and parents should be advised to stop smoking in the house, as passive smoking has been linked to an increased risk of SIDS (Mitchell et al., 1993). The recent implementation of advice concerning clothing and sleeping position appears to have dramatically reduced the incidence of SIDS, and parents therefore need to be given clear advice. The Foundation of Sudden Infant Deaths has produced an advisory leaflet covering these topics, and all parents should be given this information. All babies should be put down to sleep on their backs or sides, not prone. Babies placed on their sides need to be positioned carefully to ensure that they do not roll on to their stomachs. The prone position is used in neonatal units because it does have advantages for preterm babies with respiratory difficulties, and they are usually monitored at this stage. This advantage has disappeared by the time the baby is ready for discharge, and this apparent discrepancy needs to be carefully explained to the parents.

The baby should be appropriately dressed according to the temperature of the room, size and age of the baby. The parents should be advised more specifically about how many layers of clothing or blankets is appropriate, by the midwife or health visitor. The use of baby duvets should be discouraged, especially in young babies who may become overheated, and for the same reasons babies should not be swaddled tightly in blankets when sleeping. The parents should be encouraged to seek medical advice early if they feel that their baby is unwell.

All parents should be taught how to resuscitate their baby if they become apnoeic (see Appendix).

Audit

It is crucial that each neonatal unit should collect sufficient information to audit its performance and the outcome of the babies. Clinical audit is seen to be imperative and there has been a long tradition of examining perinatal mortality very carefully. Basic information such as the birthweight and gestation of all admissions to special and intensive care units should be kept. Major clinical events such as diagnosis and special treatments, for example endotracheal tubes or the treatment of retinopathy or prematurity, must also be collected. The mortality data by the birthweight and gestation of the baby can be analysed cumulatively and displayed visually on a computer in the neonatal unit. This allows the nursing and medical staff to estimate the risk of death for a given baby. This not only allows the professional staff to understand the outcome of their work, but also enables them to answer the parents questions more effectively.

A task for the future will be routine standardized collection of morbidity data for the survivors of neonatal care. In order to allow statistics to be compared, this should be done on a population basis not information obtained from just one unit. The examination of survivors at frequent intervals during childhood to estimate the disability rate is very time consuming and difficult. New methods of estimating morbidity are being developed using questionnaires addressed to health visitors, general practitioners and parents. More detailed examinations can be done on those children identified as having a problem by the questionnaire.

All audit should be based on the audit cycle. The plan is to analyse clinical procedures, to improve the procedures as a result of the analysis and then to check that this has been effective when in practice. This completion of the audit cycle is difficult to achieve and must be constantly in mind. Audit for its own sake without improving practice is not useful.

References and Further Reading

Cunningham, C. (1982) *Down's Syndrome: an Introduction for Parents*. London: Souvenir Press.

Fleming, P.J., Gilbert, R., Azaz, Y. *et al.* (1990) Interaction between bedding and sleeping position in the sudden infant death syndrome: a population based case control study. *BMJ*, *301*, 85–59.

Ford, R.P.K., Taylor, B.J., Mitchell, E.A. *et al.* (1993) Breast feeding and the risk of sudden infant death. *Int. J. Epidemiol.*

Kluber-Ross, E. (1989) *On Death and Dying*. London: Tavistock.

Lee, N.N.Y., Chan, Y.F., Davies, D.P. *et al.* (1989) Sudden infant death in Hong Kong: confirmation of low incidence. *BMJ*, *298*, 721.

Mitchell, E.A., Ford, R.P.K., Stewart, A.W. *et al.* (1993) Smoking and the sudden infant death syndrome. *Pediatrics*, *91*, 893–896.

Morley, C.J., Thornton, A.J., Cole, T.J. *et al.* (1991) Baby Check: a scoring system to grade the severity of acute illness in babies under 6 months old. *Arch. Dis. Child.*, *66*, 100–106.

Nelson, E.A.S., Taylor, B.J. & Weatherall, I.L. (1989) Sleeping position and infant bedding may predispose to hyperthermia and the sudden infant death syndrome. *Lancet*, *i*, 199–201.

Redshaw, M., Rivers, M. & Rosenblatt, D. (1985) *Born Too Soon*. Oxford: Oxford University Press.

Rosen, H. (1988) *Unspoken Grief – Coping with Childhood Sibling Loss*. Lexington Books.

SANDS (1991) *Guidelines for Professionals: Miscarriage, Stillbirth and Neonatal Death*. London: SANDS.

Varley, S. (1985) *Badger's Parting Gifts*. Collins Picture Books.

Worden, W. (1983) *Grief Counselling and Grief Therapy*. London: Tavistock.

—20

Perinatal Care in Developing Countries

This chapter cannot provide a comprehensive review of babies throughout the world, but it would be wrong to forget that most babies in the world are born without the benefits of sophisticated medicine. Adherence to simple principles of neonatal care could dramatically improve survival.

Of all low birthweight infants born worldwide, 95% are in developing countries; the rate is even higher for SFGA babies, at 98%.

Many of the principles of perinatal care in the industrialized nations apply equally to those countries that are still developing. However, in those parts of the world where the infant mortality rate is the same as that in the UK a century ago, and where the money available per head is often less than 70p (or 1 US dollar) per year, priorities must clearly be very different.

Prevention is especially important. Efforts must be concentrated against malnutrition and infection, the two biggest killers in developing countries. But progress can only be made if local customs are taken into account. In addition, political instability and war will undermine even the most sophisticated medical programme.

In many developing countries children make up nearly 50% of the population, yet a high proportion of them will not live to reach adult life. When parents see that their children will survive, they appear more likely to accept family planning advice, and reduce the size of their families. Increasing the interval between births improves the health of the mother and allows her to care for her children better. Before family planning advice will be acceptable in such communities, it is probably essential to reduce the infant mortality rate. Only then can parents accept family planning, and the perinatal mortality will eventually fall.

Even in developed countries, where the perinatal mortality rate has fallen greatly, there are still considerable differences between social classes. In Africa and Asia, 75% of the population is dispersed in rural areas, where perinatal mortality is higher, but unfortunately, most doctors work in the towns. In many countries periurban slums and shanties are expanding at an alarming rate, and there may be little access to health care.

Antenatal Care

It is difficult to establish the relationship of maternal diet to the outcome of pregnancy (see also Chapter 2). Experience from occupied countries during the Second World War, where the population suffered severe undernutrition, showed that their babies tended to be shorter and lighter, and had an increased chance of being born early. The rate of growth in man is greatest and most critical during fetal life and the first year of life, by which time most brain growth has occurred. Thus it is very important to improve maternal and therefore fetal nutrition as well as infant nutrition. Birthweight is a major determinant of infant mortality. The underweight fetus is usually born into an environment which is totally unsuitable for subsequent satisfactory growth. In areas where undernutrition is common, there is evidence that supplementation of total energy will improve the baby's birthweight. However, food supplementation can be expensive, and the results from carefully supervised feeding trials may be better than can be achieved in national programmes. Protein supplementation, which is more expensive, may not be as effective.

Prenatal care is good preventive medicine and is therefore very worthwhile. In order to reduce infant mortality we need to know more about the nature, aetiology and prevention of low birthweight in developing countries. Anaemia needs to be recognized and treated; it may be caused by many factors such as malnutrition, malabsorption, hookworm or haemolysis. Iron and folate supplements should be considered. Osteomalacia may lead to bone deformities, resulting in difficulties during labour and calcium deficiency in the fetus. This not only needs detection and treatment with vitamin D supplements in adult life, but good nutrition during childhood. Chronic parasitization with malaria (parasites crossing the placenta) can cause poor fetal growth. This problem is a part of the general need to provide better mosquito and malaria control, and underlines the importance of the development of a vaccine for the condition. Another example of treatment during pregnancy which can lead to immense benefits for the newborn is tetanus vaccination. Two or three injections during pregnancy can irradicate this disease.

Good antenatal care needs careful planning – it is not realistic to expect women to travel long distances to clinics. Local clinics need to be set up to provide basic care and to detect women at high risk of abnormalities in pregnancy and labour. Mothers may need to be encouraged to move to a hospital if a serious condition is detected. Some countries have been successful in developing teams of health care workers who can be simply trained to provide a basic care and screening service.

Labour

It is important to recognize that a very large proportion of women in some parts of the world are delivered by traditional birth attendants (TBAs). Some programmes have aimed to improve the knowledge and skills of these TBAs, so that they can care for pregnant women and conduct labour more safely, by detecting abnormalities. This has been done in areas where it does not seem likely that sufficient trained midwives can be provided in the near future. Elaborate equipment is usually neither possible nor desirable. The local 'wise women' or TBAs should be educated in simple sterile techniques including hand washing, and such procedures as episiotomies and stitching. In this way, it is usually possible to make use of the positive features of the culture to good effect, while discouraging harmful customs such as packing the vagina with rock salt or dressing the umbilical cord with animal dung. The Sudan and India are good examples of places where such progress has been made.

Trained midwives should recognize that a most important factor in reducing perinatal (and also maternal) mortality is the prevention of prolonged labour. This can be due to cephalopelvic disproportion (not uncommon in communities where there is widespread rickets and osteomalacia leading to a deformed pelvis). Some prolonged labours will be due to malpresentation, but an important and common cause is abnormal uterine action and this may be easily recognized and treated without sophisticated apparatus or drugs. The principles of management involve early recognition of inert labour (by doing a vaginal examination as soon as the patient presents and subsequently at least every four hours), an active first stage which should be no longer than six to 12 hours and, finally, avoiding delay in the second stage. Progress is assessed both by dilatation of the cervix and by the level of the presenting part in relation to the pelvic brim. The cervix normally dilates at about 1 cm per hour. If a simple tool like a cervicograph is used it is easy to detect at once when action needs to be taken so a midwife may seek a doctor's help. The addition of an

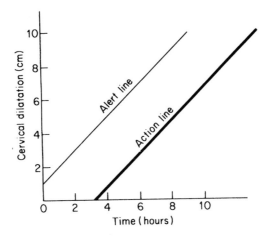

Fig. 20.1 A cervicograph. From Phillpot & Castle (1972) by permission of the authors and editor

alert line to the cervicograph (Fig. 20.1) has proved a simple and effective way of detecting primigravidae with reduced pelvic size and inefficient uterine action in many parts of the world, and it is especially valuable in rural areas where there are fewer doctors and X-ray facilities. The patient's cervical dilatation is plotted successively on the cervicograph. If the rate of dilatation is too slow, the plot will cross the alert line. Arrangements are then made to transfer the patient to a central obstetric unit so that the active management can be started as soon as possible. This usually involves stimulating the uterus by oxytocin for as long as there is progress in the absence of fetal distress. For a detailed account of the use of such guidelines, see Philpott (1979).

Fetal distress has to be detected without sophisticated monitoring equipment. It is usually adequate for a midwife to listen to fetal heart rate through a Pinard's fetal stethoscope to detect danger signs. In addition, observations of fetal movements may be very useful. It has been noticed that fetal movements stop about two days before the death of the fetus. If, therefore, the mother subjectively counts less than 10 movements per day, the fetus should be considered in danger of imminent demise.

This will not necessarily prevent deaths due to intrapartum asphyxia. If there is a delay in the second stage, methods of speedy delivery, such as ventouse or the careful use of forceps, should be considered. Ruptured uterus is still a high cause of mortality and morbidity in many parts of the world, and urgent referral should be considered where there are signs of obstructed labour. Every rural area should be served by a unit where caesarean section can be performed safely.

Birth

If a baby is born asphyxiated, the principles laid down in Chapter 3 apply. Only simple equipment is required: a laryngoscope, endotracheal tube, some form of suction and an operator who understands the principles of what is required. It is important to realize that air is perfectly good for resuscitating the baby; 100% oxygen is not required. The first line of resuscitation is a bag and mask, or simple apparatus such as that described by Milner (Milner, 1991). Mouth-to-mouth resuscitation in parts of the world where HIV infection is particularly prevalent, is no longer acceptable.

A control must be maintained of both the volume of air administered and its pressure (less than 30 cm water). Simple pressure monitoring equipment can be made cheaply and easily. Perhaps the most important thing is the teaching of the difference between blue and white asphyxia, thereby reducing greatly the incidence of iatrogenic problems. Resuscitation may be greatly aided by receiving the baby on to a suitably firm surface on which the head may be easily extended.

Care of the umbilical cord is a matter frequently surrounded by traditional practices in many communities. The high incidence of neonatal mortality from tetanus acquired following cutting of the cord with an unclean instrument, or treatment of the cord with cow dung may be reduced greatly. This is best done by immunizing pregnant mothers with tetanus toxoid during the last trimester of pregnancy. This produces IgG antibody response which passively protects the neonate from acquired tetanus. Secondly, education must be given in cord care: this means giving either packs containing a blade (which TBAs are instructed to boil before use), some swabs and a simple tie, or rubber bands, which are cheap and effective.

The delivery room itself needs no special facilities. It may be a simple hut heated by a stove and humidified by evaporating water from a wet cloth. The baby is particularly at risk from heat loss immediately after the birth, even in the tropics, and it is important to dry and swaddle the baby immediately. The first bath should be delayed for at least a day.

Feeding

The best prophylaxis against subsequent infant mortality from infective diarrhoea and protein-energy malnutrition is breastfeeding. It is particularly unfortunate that commercial advertising in the developing countries, coupled with a not unnatural desire in mothers to mimic more sophisticated women in urban areas or the developed world, has led to a decline in breastfeeding. In urban areas the rate of breastfeeding is much lower than in rural areas, particularly amongst the wealthier families. In many parts of Asia and Africa, however, the majority of women are still breastfeeding their babies at nine months of age, and often continue for up to two years (Muhudhia *et al.*, 1989).

The advantages of breastfeeding are set out in Chapter 7. Protection against infection and the establishment of adequate intervals between births are particularly important advantages in the developing countries. Frequent suckling and prolonged lactation postpone the return of menstruation and ovulation, because prolactin is released from the anterior pituitary gland in response to suckling and inhibits ovulation in the ovary. Supplementary milk or other foods significantly reduces the contraceptive effect of breastfeeding.

Children who are breastfed suffer fewer episodes of infection than those who are artificially fed. In rural Africa, Asia or South America, infection resulting from the inability of the parents to make up or keep feeds in a sterile way is a major cause of infant death. Their inability to afford the expensive powdered milks also means that they may make them up in too dilute a concentration, thereby leading to protein-energy malnutrition and an even greater susceptibility to infection. Inadequate lactation is very uncommon in these mothers, but where it does occur wet nursing is often undertaken. There are taboos against this practice in many countries, and a potential risk of transmission of infections, including HIV. Cup and spoon feeding of freshly expressed milk (Fig. 20.2) is considered a safer alternative to bottle feeding, and is routinely used in special care units in developing countries (Armstrong, 1987; Musoke, 1990).

An important advance was the introduction of the indwelling plastic nasogastric tube for feeding infants too ill or too immature to suck. Such tubes are cheap, easy to place in position after a little

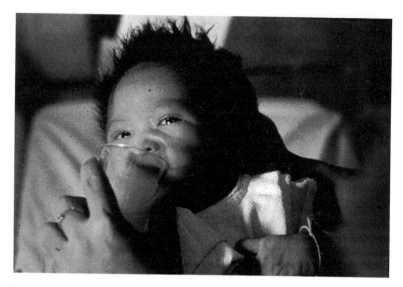

Fig. 20.2 Cup feeding. Reproduced by permission of World Health Organization

practice and straightforward in use provided simple precautions are taken. The intrinsic anti-infective qualities of breast milk (lactoferrin, secretory IgA, polymorphs and lymphocytes) are irreplaceable. If formula milk has to be used there are huge benefits in adding raw expressed breast milk to it, as it has been well established that this reduces the risk of infection in newborn babies (Narayanan *et al.*, 1982). For this reason, breastfeeding should be continued for as long as possible and this will also have the important effect of spacing pregnancies adequately since, as we have seen, the mother is less likely to conceive whilst fully breastfeeding her baby.

From about four to six months of age other foods should increasingly be given to supplement the breast milk.

General Neonatal Care

It is often not realized that even in the tropics babies need to be kept warm at night as the temperature can fall very sharply. The principles of the neutral thermal environment apply (see Chapter 6), but in many ways temperature control becomes more difficult in developing countries as incubators can be positively dangerous. This is because they are a potent source of infection if not looked after properly. They are expensive to buy in the first place and resources are better spent elsewhere; they are complex pieces of equipment, which frequently go wrong and are expensive in time, money and trained personnel to put right. An alternative way which has been formally evaluated for maintaining adequate temperature control, is to use heated water mattresses (Tunell & Sarman, 1986). Although these are still expensive, though not as costly as incubators, they have been found to be more effective as they remain warm for longer if there is an interruption in the electrical supply, and are also more easily maintained (Sarman *et al.*, 1989). One good heat source for these babies is their own mother, which has the additional advantage of promoting the mother–infant relationship, a field in which the developing countries are far in advance of the West.

When a baby is nursed in a cot it is important that it is deep so that there are no draughts over the sides. Additional heat can be provided by one or two guarded electric light bulbs under or over the cot. These simple, locally made incubators have not been properly evaluated, but have the advantage of being produced locally, and being easily serviced. Perspex heat shields are relatively inexpensive and simple to make locally and considerably cut down evaporative heat loss. Expanded bubble plastic packing material is an extremely cheap way of providing good insulation when wrapped around a baby. As indicated in Chapter 4, situations in which the baby is particularly at risk from heat loss include immediately after birth, during nappy changing, and bathing.

When to use antibiotics and which antibiotic to use are difficult problems in communities where there are absent or inadequate bacteriological services. A good rule of thumb is that any deterioration of the baby's condition after about 48 hours of life is due to infection, and the threshold for the use of antibiotics in a given clinical situation must be low. It is important to discuss the appropriate use of antibiotics with the local microbiologist. A knowledge of the local bacterial flora and common pathogens is important when selecting the drugs to be used. A regimen used in one country may be inappropriate in another. Common drugs used include penicillin, gentamicin and chloramphenicol. Chloramphenicol when used for short courses in appropriate dosage (50 mg/kg per day for the first 48 hours, then 25 mg/kg per day) is a relatively safe drug as well as being very effective against a wide range of bacterial infections. The incidence of the 'grey baby' syndrome when the drug is correctly used is low, but blood levels are monitored in developed countries.

The treatment of conjunctivitis in tropical countries is important. Any purulent discharge should be assumed to be gonococcal and treated with systemic and topical penicillin. Silver nitrate (Credé) drops are potentially dangerous as they become concentrated due to evaporation in high temperatures and cause chemical burns. Sulphacetamide or collodial silver drops are both cheap and effective and may be used for non-gonococcal infections.

In the management of jaundice, it is not necessary to have sophisticated phototherapy units. Reflected sunlight will often provide very adequate phototherapy, although care must be taken not to allow the baby to be burned.

There are few specific tropical diseases of infancy. However, diphtheria, tetanus, whooping cough, polio and measles are still common, dangerous and largely preventable by an active immunization programme. Chronic malaria is a widespread cause of babies being born small. It is useful to give the baby BCG at birth although the amount of protection does not always seem to be as great in developing countries as in the developed world. This may also protect against atypical mycobacterial infections which are common. Polio vaccine is essential. If it is to be given effectively it must be kept cool. The cold chain that ensures preservation of the virus from manufacture to administration is essential.

Treatment of established neonatal tetanus is by high doses of penicillin, heavy sedation (sufficient to abolish the spasms) and tube feeding; paralysis and ventilatory support are used in some sophisticated units. Anti-tetanus serum (ATS) also has a place. Mortality rates remain high.

Future Priorities

In every country children are more likely to die in the neonatal period than at other times of life. It is important that greater attention is paid to pregnancy, birth and the early neonatal period if the perinatal mortality rate is to be improved.

There is no doubt that the high perinatal mortality rate in many developing countries is associated with a high incidence of low birthweight babies (less than 1500 g). This is largely due to intrauterine growth retardation rather than preterm delivery, and is probably related to the low standard of nutrition and health in the community as a whole. Priority must be given to improving nutritional standards.

Mothers and babies particularly at risk of serious disorders should be identified early and transferred to an appropriate centre for care. Local customs should be encouraged except when they are harmful, and education of TBAs in the principles of modern midwifery is particularly valuable. Mothers should be educated in the importance of antenatal care, but it may be particularly difficult to build up their confidence if the person giving advice is foreign or westernised.

Breastfeeding must be actively encouraged as a means of preventing infant malnutrition, infection and death, and as a way of spacing pregnancies adequately. Available resources must be spread in the most effective possible way: priority cannot be given to babies who are very preterm, severely malformed, injured or retarded. Much can be done with simple, cheap and locally made aids such as light bulbs as an overhead source of heat, and careful attention to risks of hypothermia, by wrapping babies adequately. Many 'disposable' items such as feeding and suction catheters and endotracheal tubes can be used several times if they are resterilized on each occasion. This is much cheaper than throwing them away after only their first use. It is important that sophisticated equipment, such as incubators and ventilators, are not bought unless they can be adequately serviced. It is important not to simply copy what is useful in a sophisticated neonatal unit. In addition, the Western practice, still too widespread, of separating mothers from their babies and bottle feeding should be strongly discouraged.

It is unfortunate that the implementation of any medical programme for improving perinatal care depends as much on political stability and political decisions as on strictly medical implications. It is this which most limits progress in many developing countries at present.

References and Further Reading

Armstrong, H.C. (1987) Breastfeeding low birthweight babies – advances in Kenya. *J. Human Lactation*, *3*(2).

Cutting, W.A.M. & Ludlam, M. (1984) Making the best of breast feeding. *Family Practice*, *1*, 69–78.

Ebrahim, G.J. (1977) *Care of the Newborn in Developing Countries.* London: Macmillan.

Appendix

Normal Values in the Newborn

Blood

pH	7.3–7.4
Pa_{CO_2}	4.6–6.0 kPa (35–45 mmHg)
Pa_{O_2}	7.3–12.0 kPa (55–90 mmHg)
Bicarbonate	18–25 µmol/l
Base excess	−7 to −2 mmol/l
Ammonia	50–100 µmol/l (may be higher in preterm or jaundiced babies)
Calcium	1.9–2.7 µmol/l (tendency to lower values in preterm babies)
Creatinine	9–62 µmol/l (day 2) (higher in cord blood)
Electrolytes	
Sodium	135–150 mmol/l (may be lower in preterm babies)
Potassium	4.0–6.0 mmol/l
Chloride	95–105 mmol/l
Glucose	2.0–6.0 mmol/l (lower in the first few hours)
Immunoglobulins	
IgA	none–0.5 g/l ⎫
IgM	less than 0.2 g/l ⎬ cord blood
IgG	4–15 g/l ⎭
Iron	20–50 µmol/l
Magnesium	0.7–1.2 mmol/l
Osmolality	280–305 mosmol/kg water
Phenylalanine	< 0.37 mmol/l

Protein
  Total   50–70 g/l
  Albumin   30–40 g/l
  Globulins   10–30 g/l

T_4 125–275 nmol/l   ⎫ Higher than older child normal
TSH   <3 mu/l   ⎬ range during first week of life.
                                   ⎪ Decreases to normal range by
                                   ⎭ 8.10 days

Urea   3.4–8.4 mmol/l

Haemoglobin (capillary blood levels are 2–3 g/dl higher than those of
blood obtained by venepuncture)

day 1	16–20 g/dl	1 month	11–17 g/dl
1 week	13–23 g/dl	3 months	10–14 g/dl

Packed cell volume   Reticulocytes
  day 1   52–58%   day 1   2–8%
  2 weeks   46–54%   1 week   0.5–5%
  3 months   35%   1 month   0–0.5%

White cell count   Platelets (see also Chapter 13)
  day 1   6–35 × 10^9/l   day 1   350 × 10^9/l
  1 week   8–16 × 10^9/l   2 weeks   300 × 10^9/l
  1 month   6–14 × 10^9/l   3 months   250 × 10^9/l

Neutrophils   Fibrinogen   1–3.5 g/l
  day 1   50–80%
  day 4   35–60%
  3 months 25–45%

Urine

Creatinine clearance   0.6–1.1 ml/s/1.73 m^2
VMA   up to 10 μmol/24 hours

Cerebrospinal fluid

Glucose   3.8–5 mmol/l
Total protein   100–1200 mg/l (higher in preterm babies)
Cells   up to 20/μl (lymphocytes)

Categories of Babies Receiving Neonatal Care

There should be four levels of care; level 1 intensive care (maximal intensive care), level 2 intensive care (high dependency intensive care), special care and normal care.

Definitions of neonatal care

Level 1 intensive care (maximal intensive care)

Care given in an intensive care nursery which provides continuous skilled supervision by qualified and specially trained nursing and medical staff. Such care includes support of the infant's parents.

Level 2 intensive care (high dependency intensive care)

Care given in an intensive or special care nursery which provides continuous skilled supervision by qualified and specially trained nursing staff who may care for more babies than in Level 1 intensive care. Medical supervision is not so immediate as in Level 1 intensive care. Care includes support of the infant's parents.

Special care

Care given in a special care nursery, transitional care ward or postnatal ward which provides care and treatment exceeding normal routine care. Some aspects of special care can be undertaken by a mother supervised by qualified nursing staff. Special nursing care includes support and education of the infant's parents.

Normal care

Care given by the mother, or mother substitute, with medical or neonatal nursing advice if needed.

Clinical categories of neonatal care

Level 1 intensive care (maximal intensive care)

Level 1 intensive care should be provided for babies:

1 Receiving assisted ventilation (including intermittent positive airway pressure, intermittent mandatory ventilation and constant positive airway pressure), and in the first 24 hours after its withdrawal.

2 Of less than 27 weeks gestation for the first 48 hours after birth.

3 With birthweight of less than 1000 g for the first 48 hours after birth.

4 Who require major emergency surgery for the pre-operative period and postoperatively for 48 hours.

5 On the day of death.

6 Being transported by a team including medical and nursing staff.

7 Who are receiving peritoneal dialysis.

8 Who require exchange transfusions complicated by other disease processes.

9 With severe respiratory disease in the first 48 hours of life requiring an FiO_2 of > 0.6.

10 With recurrent apnoea needing frequent intervention, e.g. over five stimulations in eight hours or resuscitation with IPPV two or more times in 24 hours.

11 With significant requirements for circulatory support, e.g. inotropes, three or more infusions of colloid in 24 hours, or infusions of prostoglandins.

Level 2 intensive care (high dependency intensive care)

Level 2 intensive care should be provided for babies:

1 Requiring total parenteral nutrition.

2 Who are having convulsions.

3 Being transported by a trained skilled neonatal nurse alone.

4 With arterial line or chest drain.

5 With respiratory disease in the first 48 hours of life requiring an FiO_2 of 0.4–0.6.

6 With recurrent apnoea requiring stimulation up to five times in an eight-hour period or any resuscitation with IPPV.

7 Who require an exchange transfusion alone.

8 Who are more than 48 hours postoperative and require complex nursing procedures.

9 With tracheostomy for the first two weeks.

Special care

Special Care should be provided for babies:

1 Requiring continuous monitoring of respiration or heart rate, or by transcutaneous transducers.
2 Receiving additional oxygen.
3 With tracheostomy after the first two weeks.
4 Being given intravenous glucose and electrolyte solutions.
5 Who are being tube fed.
6 Who have had minor surgery in the previous 24 hours.
7 Who require terminal care but not on the day of death.
8 Being barrier nursed.
9 Undergoing phototherapy.
10 Receiving special monitoring (for example frequent glucose or bilirubin estimations).
11 Needing constant supervision (e.g. babies whose mothers are drug addicts).
12 Being treated with antibiotics.

Resources required for neonatal care

Staffing

The BPA recommendation and the Neonatal Nurses Association guidelines for staffing are as follows, but are subject to local conditions and are not, as yet, founded on research on dependency levels. On presentation of appropriate research findings, these may require amending.

Nursing staff

Trained Nurses hold RGN, RM, RSCN or EN. Qualified Nurses hold a certificate in Intensive Care of the Newborn, e.g. English National Board Course 405, 409, 904, 904A certificate or Joint Board of Clinical Studies certificate, i.e. 400, 401, 402.

Maximal intensive care (Level 1 intensive care).   5.5 nurses whole time equivalent (wte) qualified and trained per cot.

High dependency intensive care (Level 2 intensive care).   3.5 nurses (wte) qualified and trained per cot.

Special care.   1.0 nurses (wte) qualified per cot.

Neonatal transport.   Additional provision of staff will be required by centres offering transport to sick infants.

Medical staff

Maximal intensive care (Level 1 intensive care).   Minimum medical staffing should consist of both an experienced paediatric registrar and a senior house officer on duty and available in the intensive care area at all times, with an appropriately trained consultant in charge.

High dependency intensive care (Level 2 intensive care).   An experienced senior house officer on duty and available in the high dependency area at all times, with a more senior member of staff on call and a consultant paediatrician in charge.

Special care.   Minimum medical staff for 24 hour cover: an appropriately experienced senior house officer on duty, an experienced more senior member of staff on call and a consultant paediatrician in charge.

Neonatal transport.   Additional provision of staff will be required by centres offering to transport sick infants.

Equipment

The BPA recommends the following equipment:

Maximal intensive care (Level 1 intensive care).   The following equipment should be available for each baby:

Intensive care incubator or unit with overhead heating (1)
Respiratory or apnoea monitor (1)
Heart rate monitor (1)
Intravascular blood pressure transducer or surface blood pressure recorder (1)
Transcutaneous Po_2 monitor or intravascular oxygen transducer or saturation Po_2 monitor (1)
Transcutaneous Pco_2 monitor (1)
Syringe pumps (2)
Infusion pumps (2)
Ventilator (1)
Continuous temperature monitor (1)

Phototherapy unit (1)
Ambient oxygen monitor (1)
Facilities for frequent blood gas analysis using micromethods
Facilities for frequent biochemical analysis including glucose, bilirubin and electrolytes by micromethods
Facilities for autopsy by an appropriately trained paediatric pathologist
Access to equipment for visualisation of organs such as the brain
Access to equipment for radiological examination
Access to transport incubator with transport ventilator.

High dependency intensive care (Level 2 intensive care). Same as Level 1 intensive care but without a ventilator.

Special care. The following equipment should be available for each baby who may need it:

Incubator or cot adequate for temperature control (1)
Ambient oxygen analyser (1)
Apnoea alarm (1)
Heart rate monitor (1)
Infusion pump (1)
Phototherapy unit (1)
Ventilator to be used for short-term ventilation (1)
Access to frequent blood gas analysis using micromethods
Access to biochemical analysis (including glucose, bilirubin and electrolytes) by micromethods
Facilities for autopsy by an appropriately trained paediatric pathologist
Access to equipment for radiological examination
Access to transport incubator with transport ventilator

Special care may take place on a postnatal ward, particularly in an area specially set aside for the purpose.

Units providing Level 2 intensive care or special care only should have the availability of equipment for maintaining babies in optimal condition prior to transfer.

Drug Dosages

Drug dosages are discussed in the appropriate chapter but this table also provides a useful summary of those most commonly used.

Drug	Dose	Route	Comments
Acyclovir	7.5 mg/kg/dose 8 hourly for 7–10 days	i.v. infusion	
	100 mg\dose 5 times a day for 7–10 days	Oral	Oral absorption has not been tested in neonates
Amikacin	Loading dose: 10 mg/kg	i.v. bolus	Bloods levels: 1 hour post dose 15–20 mg/l Pre-dose less than 8 mg/l
	Maintenance dose: 7.5 mg/kg/dose 12 hourly		Check blood levels during concurrent indomethacin therapy; dosage may need to be reduced until good urine output returns
Aminophylline	Loading dose: 6.2 mg/kg	i.v. infusion over 20 minutes	Blood levels: 6–12 mg/l 30 minutes after short infusion, any time during a continuous infusion
	Maintenance dose: 4.4 mg/kg/dose 24 hourly		Levels may be higher if clinically indicated
Amoxycillin	30 mg/kg/dose 12 hourly Meningitis – increase dose to 60 mg/kg	i.v. bolus or oral	

	Dose	Route	Notes
	Alternatively: 100 mcg/kg/dose 24 hourly for 6 days		
Iron	5.5 mg elemental iron 24 hourly	Oral	Elixir sodium iron edetate 5.5 mg elemental iron in 1 ml sytron
Magnesium sulphate	50 mg (0.2 mmol magnesium)/kg/dose 6–8 hourly as necessary	i.v. infusion i.m. injection	i.m. injection is very painful Watch for hypotonia – reversible with calcium gluconate
Mannitol	Cerebral oedema: 250 mg/kg/dose 8 hourly for 3 doses	i.v. infusion over 30 minutes	
Metoclopramide	100 mcg/kg/dose 8 hourly	Oral or i.v. bolus	
Metronidazole	7.5 mg/kg/dose 12 hourly	Oral or i.v. infusion over 20 minutes	
Miconazole	15 mg/kg/dose 12 hourly	i.v. infusion	
	Oropharyngeal Candida: 2.5 mg oral gel 12 hourly after feeds	Oral	

Drug	Dose	Route	Comments
	12 hourly 2% miconazide nitrate to nappy area	Topical	
Morphine	Acute pain: 100 mcg/kg/dose over 30 minutes		Monitor blood pressure Facilities for resuscitation and naloxone must be immediately available
	Chronic pain: 50-200 mcg/kg/ dose over 30 minutes followed immediately by 10 mcg/kg/h gradually increasing to 50 mcg/kg/h if necessary	i.v. infusion	
Naloxone	Analgesic: 80 mcg/kg/dose 4 hourly	Oral	This oral dose occasionally used in narcotic withdrawal
	40 mcg/ stat. Further doses may be necessary	i.v. bolus or i.m.	i.v. – onset of action faster than i.m., duration 3–4 hours i.m. – onset of action 3–4 minutes, duration 18 hours
Pancuronium	50–100 mcg/kg/ dose	i.v. bolus	Use with caution in severe renal impairment as duration of action may be prolonged

Paraldehyde	0.1–0.2 ml/kg/ dose mixed with 0.1 ml hyaluronidase injection. May be repeated after 30 minutes	i.m. injection	Plastic syringes may be used if dose is given immediately, otherwise glass syringes
	0.1–0.3 ml/kg/ dose mixed with equal quantity of arachis oil	Rectal	
Phenobarbitone	Loading dose: 20 mg/kg/dose. A further loading dose may be given if necessary	i.v. infusion over 30 minutes (maximum rate 1 mg/kg/min or	Blood levels: 20–40 mg/l at least 2 hours after end of 30-minute infusion
	Maintenance dose: 3–4 mg/kg/dose 24 hourly	oral	
Piperacillin	100 mg/kg/dose 12 hourly	i.v. bolus	

Drug	Dose	Route	Comments
Potassium phosphate	0.5 mmol phosphate/dose 12 hourly increasing to 1 mmol phosphate 12 hourly if necessary	i.v. infusion or oral	i.v. infusion – maximum 4 mmol potassium in 100 ml. Maximum rate 0.5 mmol potassium/kg/h Oral phosphate supplement use sodium acid phosphate 1 mmol/1 ml oral solution
Rifampicin	Tuberculosis: 5–10 mg/kg/dose 24 hourly	Oral	
	Indications other than tuberculosis: 5 mg/kg/dose 12 hourly	i.v. infusion over 2–3 hours	
Sodium bicarbonate	Mmol of bicarbonate required = base deficit (mmol/l) × weight (kg) × 0.3	i.v. infusion or i.v. bolus	Half correction
Spironolactone	1.2 mg/kg/dose 12 hourly	Oral	
Theophylline (Choline theophyllinate)	Loading dose: 6.2 mg/kg		Blood levels: theophylline 6–12 mg/l 1–2 hours post dose
	Maintenance dose: 1.1 mg/kg/dose 6 hourly	Oral	

Tolazoline	Stat: 1–2 mg/kg/dose	i.v. bolus
	Maintenance: 1–2 mg/kg/h	i.v. infusion
Trimethoprim	Treatment: 4 mg/kg/dose 12 hourly	i.v. bolus or oral
	Prophylaxis: 2 mg/kg/dose 24 hourly	
Vancomycin	15 mg/kg/dose 12 hourly	i.v. infusion over 1 hour
	11 mg/kg/dose 6 hourly	Oral
	2.5 mg/dose 24 hourly. Seek advice from microbiologist	Intrathecal injection

Blood levels: peak (1 hour after end of 1 hour infusion) 20–30 mg/l
Trough 5–10 mg/l

CSF levels: Peak no greater than 50 mg/l
Trough less than 10 mg/l

Neonatal Special Care Chart

Hospital Name _____

Name: No: DOB :

Date														
Time														

> 38°C

Temp
38 / 37.5 / 37 / 36.5 / 36 / 35 / 34 / 33 / 32 / 31

≤ 31°C

> 170

Heart rate
170 / 160 / 150 / 140 / 130 / 120 / 110 / 100

< 100

B.P.

> 100

Resp. rate
100 / 90 / 80 / 70 / 60 / 50 / 40 / 30 / 20

< 20

Colour
Recession
Grunting

Weight
Type mls/Kg
Cont mls/hr
Int (....hrly)
(....mls)
Supplements
Vits/iron

TcPO₂
PH
PO₂
PCO₂
HCO₃
BE
TcPO₂
Hb/PCV
U&E/Ca
D.Stix/B.sugar
SeBILI

Intake 24hr
Aspiration
Urine vol
Urine S.G.
Bowels

Comments on progress

	Name			Details of baby i.e. Name, Number. DOB.
Date				Each day should be separated by a vertical red line
Time				

Temp	> 38°C			Incubator, skin and rectal temperatures may be recorded in different colour codes
	38			
	37.5			
	37			Temperatures of greater than 38°C and less than 31°C should be recorded in numerical form
	36.5			
	36			
	35			
	34			
	33			
	32			
	31			
	≤ 31°C			

Heart rate	> 170			
	170			
	160			
	150			
	140			Heart rates of greater than 170 and less than 100 beats per minute should be recorded in numerical form
	130			
	120			
	110			
	100			
	< 100			
B.P. →				Systolic and diastolic blood pressure recordings

Resp. rate	> 100			
	100			
	90			
	80			
	70			Respiratory rates greater than 100 and less than 20 breaths per minute should be recorded in numerical form
	60			
	50			
	40			
	30			
	20			
	< 20			

Colour				P = Pink C = Cyanosed J = Jaundice
Recession				0 = None + = Mild + + = Moderate + + + = Severe
Grunting				0 = None + = Mild + + = Moderate + + + = Severe
				} Spare for the recording of other observations e.g. Abdominal girth

Weight				Daily weight
Type mls/Kg				Feed -- Type and amount in mls/Kg/day A = Artificial milk B = Breast milk
FEED Cont mls/hr				Feed -- Continuous (mls/hr) and whether N/G or N/J G = Gastric J = Jejunal
Int (....hrly)				Feed -- Intermittent...Interval between feeds hrs and mode (T = Tube / Bo = Bottle / Br = Breast)
(....mls)				...mls in each feed
Supplements				Feed supplements e.g. Caloreen
Vits/iron				Vitamins = V Iron = I
				} Spare Other feed / Other medication

TcPO$_2$				Transcutaneous PO$_2$ recordings noted by nursing staff
PH				
PO$_2$				
PCO$_2$				Blood gas recordings.
HCO$_3$				N.B. Source of blood must be stated e.g. Capillary, Radial etc
BE				
TcPO$_2$				Transcutaneous PO$_2$ at the time of blood sampling for correlation
Hb/PCV				Haemoglobin/packed cell volume
U&E/Ca				Urea and electrolytes, and serum calcium
D.Stix/B.sugar				Blood glucose
SeBILI				Serum bilirubin
				} Spare for the recording of other laboratory investigations

Intake 24hr				Separate fluid charts required for hourly recordings
Aspiration				Gastric aspirates
Urine vol				Urine volumes
Urine S.G.				Urine specific gravities
Bowels				Bowel function

Comments on progress				

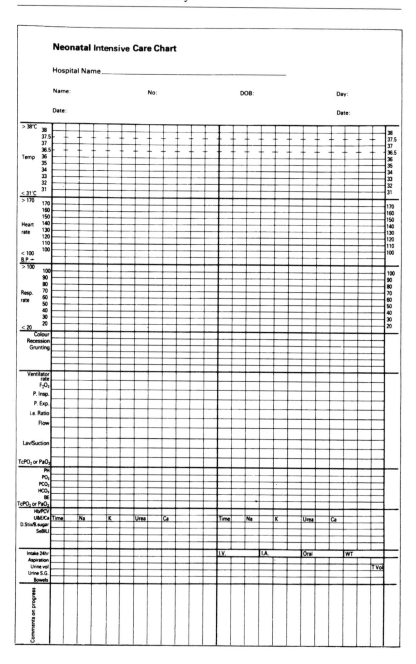

	13	14	15	
				Details of baby i.e. Name, Number, DOB, Day of life
				Date at beginning and the end of the 24 hr chart
				Time of recordings

Temp				
> 38°C				
38				
37.5				Incubator, skin and rectal temperatures may be recorded in different colour codes
37				
36.5				
36				Temperatures of greater than 38°C and less than 31°C should be recorded in numerical form
35				
34				
33				
32				
31				
≤ 31°C				

Heart rate				
> 170				
170				
160				
150				
140				Heart rates of greater than 170 and less than 100 beats per minute should be recorded in numerical form
130				
120				
110				
100				
< 100				

B.P. → | | | | Systolic and diastolic blood pressure recordings

Resp. rate				
> 100				
100				
90				
80				
70				Respiratory rates greater than 100 and less than 20 breaths per minute should be recorded in numerical form
60				
50				
40				
30				
20				
≤ 20				

Colour				P = Pink	C = Cyanosed	J = Jaundice	+++ = Severe
Recession				0 = None	+ = Mild	++ = Moderate	+++ = Severe
Grunting				0 = None	+ = Mild	++ = Moderate	
				Spare for the recording of other observations e.g. Abdominal girth			
				Positioning L = Left R = Right B = Back F = Front			

Ventilator rate				Ventilator rate
F₁O₂				Fractional inspired oxygen concentration
P. Insp.				Peak inspiratory pressure
P. Exp.				Positive end expiratory pressure or continuous positive airways pressure
i.e. Ratio				Inspiratory to expiratory time ratio
Flow				Total flow of gas to ventilator
				Spare space for other ventilator recording e.g. Inspiratory gas temperature
Lav/Suction				Bronchial lavage/endotracheal suction
				Spare space for other recordings e.g. Secretions C = Clear Y = Yellow + = Scanty ++ = Moderate +++ = Profuse
				e.g. Hourly transcutaneous PCO₂ (TcPCO₂) recording noted by nursing staff
TcPO₂ or PaO₂				Hourly transcutaneous or arterial PO₂ (delete as appropriate) recording noted by nursing staff

Changes in ventilator settings should be indicated in red by the medical staff

	Time		Na	
PH				
PO₂				
PCO₂				Blood gas recordings
HCO₃				N.B. Source of blood must be stated e.g. UAC, radial, capillary etc
BE				
TcPO₂ or PaO₂				Transcutaneous or arterial PO₂ (delete as appropriate) at the time of blood sampling for correlation
Hb/PCV				Haemoglobin/packed cell volume
U&E/Ca	Time		Na	Urea and electrolytes, and serum calcium - space for two timed samples
D.Stix/B.sugar				Blood glucose
SeBILI				Serum Bilirubin
				Spare for the recording of other laboratory investigations

Intake 24hr				Separate fluid charts required for hourly recordings
Aspiration				Gastric aspirates
Urine vol				Hourly urine volumes
Urine S.G.				Hourly urine specific gravities
Bowels				Bowel function

24 hr urine output _____ mls

Comments on progress

e.g. pneumothorax
chest drain insertion
etc., etc.

Useful Names and Addresses

Asian Women's Resource Centre
134 Minet Avenue
Harlesden
London NW10
Tel: 0181–9616549

Association for Children with Heart Disorders
35 Upper Bank End Road
Holmfirth
Huddersfield
West Yorkshire HD7 1EP
Tel: 01484–685431

Association for Post-Natal Illness
25 Jerdan Place
Fulham
London SW6 1BE
Tel: 0171–386 0868

Association for Spina Bifida and Hydrocephalus (ASBAH)
ASBAH House
42 Park Road
Peterborough PE1 2UQ
Tel: 01733–555988

Association of Breastfeeding Mothers (ABM)
Order Dept
Sydenham Green Health Centre
26 Holmshaw Close
London SE26 4TH
Tel: 0181–778 4769 (for recorded list of UK counsellors)

Association of Paediatric Nurses
c/o Miss D MacCormack
Children's Hospital
Western Bank
Sheffield S10 2TH
Tel: 01742–7111

Baby Life Support Systems (BLISS)
(Charity raising money for neonatal units)
17–21 Emerald Street
London WC1N 3QL
Tel: 0171–831 9393

British Heart Foundation
57 Gloucester Place
London W1H 4DH
Tel: 0171–935 0185

British Institute for Brain Injured Children
(Teaches programmes of stimulation therapy)
Knowle Hall
Knowle
Bridgewater
Somerset TA7 8PJ
Tel: 01278–684060

British Paediatric Association
5 St Andrews Place
Regents Park
London NW1 4LB
Tel: 0171–486 6151

Child 2000 – National Council for Child Heath
(Previously National Rubella Council)
Bray Business Centre
Weir Bank
Bray on Thames
Berkshire SL6 2ED
Tel: 01628–770011

Child Poverty Action Group (CPAG)
4th Floor
1–5 Bath Street
London EC1V 9PY
Tel: 0171–253 3406

Children's Liver Disease Foundation (CHILD)
40–42 Stoke Road
Guildford GU1 4HS
Tel: 01483–300565

Cleft Lip and Palate Association (CLAPA)
1 Eastwood Gardens
Kenton
Newcastle-upon-Tyne NE3 3DQ
Tel: 0191–285 9396

Coeliac Society
PO Box 220
High Wycombe
Buckinghamshire HP11 2HY
Tel: 01494–437278

Cruse – Bereavement Care
Cruse House
126 Sheen Road
Richmond
Surrey TW9 1UR
Tel: 0181–940 4818

Cry-sis
B.M. Cry-sis
London WC1N 3XX
Tel: 0171–404 5011 (for local contact number)

Cystic Fibrosis Research Trust
Alexandra House
5 Blyth Road
Bromley
Kent BR1 3RS
Tel: 0181–464 7211

Cytomegalovirus Support Group
69 The Leasowes
Ford
Shrewsbury
Shropshire SY5 9LU
Tel: 01743–850055

Down Syndrome Association
153–155 Mitcham Road
Tooting
London SW17 9PG
Tel: 0181–682 4001

Foundation for the Study of Infant Deaths
(Cot Death Research and Support)
35 Belgrave Square
London SW1X 8QB
Tel: 0171–235 0965
        0171–235 1721 (24 hour helpline)

Gingerbread
(For one parent families)
35 Wellington Street
London WC2E 7BN
Tel: 0171–240 0953

Haemophilia Society
123 Westminster Bridge
London SE1 7HR
Tel: 0171–928 2020

Heartline Association
40 The Crescent
Bricket Wood
St Albans
Hertfordshire AL2 3NF
Tel: 01923–670763

Invalid Children's Aid Association
126 Buckingham Palace Road
London SW1W 9SB
Tel: 0171–730 9891

Joint Breastfeeding Initiative
Alexandra House
Oldham Terrace
Acton
London W3 6NH
Tel: 0181–992 8637

La Leche League (Great Britain) Ltd
(Breast feeding advice and support)
B.M. 3424
London WC1N 6XX
Tel: 0171–404 5011
    0171–242 1278 (24 hours)

Meet-A-Mum Association (MAMA)
(Help and support for mothers with postnatal depression)
58 Malden Avenue
South Norwood
London SE25 4HS
Tel: 0181–656 7318

Multiple Births Foundation
Queen Charlotte's + Chelsea Hospital
Goldhawk Road
London W6 0XG
Tel: 0181–748 4666 ext 5201

Naevus Support Group
58 Necton Road
Wheathampstead
Hertfordshire AL4 8AU
Tel: 01582 832583

National Association for Hospital Play Staff
Thomas Coram Foundation
40 Brunswick Square
London WC1
Tel: 0171–278 2424

National Association for Maternal and Child Welfare (NAMCW)
Suite 25
Strode House
46–48 Osnaburgh Street
London NW1 3ND
Tel: 0171–383 4541

National Association for the Welfare of Children in Hospital (NAWCH)
Argyle House
29–31 Euston Road
London NW1 2SD
Tel: 0171–833 2041

National Centre for Down Syndrome
Room 154
Birmingham Polytechnic
Westbourne Road
Birmingham B15 5TN
Tel: 0121–454 3126

National Childbirth Trust (NCT)
(Education for parenthood)
Alexandra House
Oldham Terrace
London W3 6NH
Tel: 0181–992 8637

National Council for One Parent Families
255 Kentish Town Road
London NW5 2LX
Tel: 0171–267 1361

National Deaf Children's Society
45 Hereford Road
London W2 5AH
Tel: 0171–229 9272

National Eczema Society
Tavistock House East
Tavistock Square
London WC1H 9SR
Tel: 0171–388 4097

National Meningitis Trust
Fern House
Bath Road
Stroud
Gloucester GL3 3TJ
Tel: 01453–751738
　　01453–755049 (24 hour helpline)

National Perinatal Epidemiology Unit (NPEU)
John Radcliffe Infirmary
Oxford OX2 6HE
Tel: 01865–224876

National Society for Brain-damaged Children
35 Larchmere Drive
Hall Green
Birmingham

National Society for Phenylketonuria and Allied Disorders
Worth Cottage
Lower Scholes
Pickels Hill
Keighley
West Yorkshire BD22 0RR
Tel: 01535–44865

National Society for the Prevention of Cruelty to Children (NSPCC)
67 Saffron Hill
London EC1N 8RS
Tel: 0171–242 1626

Neonatal Nurses Association
Room 7
A Block
Forest House
Berkeley Avenue
Nottingham NG3 5AF
Tel: 01602–602494

**NIPPERS (National Information for Parents of Prematures –
Education, Resources and Support)**
c/o The Sam Segal Perinatal Unit
St Mary's Hospital
Praed Street
London W2 1NY
Tel: 0171–725 1487

Prader–Willi Syndrome Association (UK)
30 Follett Drive
Abbots Langley
Hertfordshire WD5 0LP
Tel: 01923–67543

Prenatal Diagnosis Group
Dr Alan McDermott
(Editor of newsletter)
South Western Regional Cytogenetics Centre
Southmead Hospital
Westbury-on-Trym
Bristol BS10
Tel: 01179–505050

REACH
(The Association for Children with Hand or Arm Deficiency)
13 Park Terrace
Crimchard
Chard
Somerset TA20 1LA
Tel: 01460–61578 (24 hours)

Research Trust for Metabolic Diseases in Children
53 Beam Street
Nantwich
Cheshire CW5 5NF
Tel: 01270–629782

Royal National Institute for the Blind (RNIB) and
Royal National Institute for the Deaf
224 Great Portland Street
London W1N 6AA
Tel: 0171–388 1266

Royal Society for Mentally Handicapped Children and Adults (MENCAP)
Mencap national centre
123 Golden Lane
London EC1Y 0RT
Tel: 0171–454 0454

SENSE
(National Deaf–Blind and Rubella Association)
311 Gray's Inn Road
London WC1X 8PT
Tel: 0171–278 1005

Sickle Cell and Thalassaemia Information Centre
St Leonard's Hospital
Nuttall Street
London N1 5LZ
Tel: 0171–739 8484 ext 4646

SOFT UK
Support Organization for Trisomy 13 (Patau Syndrome)
Tudor Lodge
Redwood
Ross-on-Wye
Herefordshire HR9 5UD
Tel: 01989–67480

SOFT UK
Support Organization for Trisomy 18 (Edward Syndrome)
48 Froggatts Ride
Walmley
Sutton Coldfield
West Midlands B76 8TQ
Tel: 0121–351 3122

Spastics Society
12 Park Crescent
London W1N 4EQ
Tel: 0171–636 5020
      01800–626 216 (helpline 1.00 pm to 10.00 pm daily)

STEPS
(National Association for Families of Children with Congenital Abnormalities of the Lower Limbs)
15 Statham Close
Lymm
Cheshire WA13 9NN

Stillbirth and Neonatal Death Society (SANDS)
28 Portland Place
London W1N 4DE
Tel: 0171–436 5881

Stillbirth and Perinatal Death Association
37 Christchurch Hill
London NW3 1LA
Tel: 0171–794 4601

Tracheo-Oesophageal Fistula Support (TOFS)
St George's Centre
91 Victoria Road
Netherfield
Nottingham NG4 2NN
Tel: 01602–400694

Twins and Multiple Births Association (TAMBA)
59 Sunnyside
Worksop
Nottinghamshire S81 7LN
Tel: 01909–479250

Tamba Bereavement Support Group
32 Denton Court Road
Gravesend
Kent DA12 2HS
Tel: 01474–567320

Gestational Assessment

For best results the assessment should be carried out when the baby is between 4 and 48 hours of age. The assessments are least accurate when the baby is ill or older (quick postnatal maturation of the skin alters the accuracy of the external criteria).

1 Dubowitz score

This has proved a reliable method of assessing the gestational age of a baby in the early days of life (see p. 74). With practice it is quick to perform and accurate to within about two weeks either way provided the baby is examined at least a few hours after delivery and is not ill.

Score each external sign and neurological criterion (pp. 440–44). Add up the scores obtained. Read off the baby's gestational age from the vertical axis of the chart on p. 443 where the total score (horizontal axis) meets the diagonal line.

External (superficial) Criteria

EXTERNAL SIGN	SCORE				
	0	1	2	3	4
OEDEMA	Obvious oedema hands and feet: pitting over tibia	No obvious oedema hands and feet: pitting over tibia	No oedema		
SKIN TEXTURE	Very thin, gelatinous	Thin and smooth	Smooth: medium thickness. Rash or superficial peeling	Slight thickening. Superficial cracking and peeling esp. hand and feet	Thick and parchment-like; super-ficial or deep cracking
SKIN COLOUR (Infant not crying)	Dark red	Uniformly pink	Pale pink: variable over body	Pale. Only pink over ears, lips, palms or soles	
SKIN OPACITY (trunk)	Numerous veins and venules clearly seen, especially over abdomen	Veins and tributaries seen	A few large vessels clearly seen over abdomen	A few large vessels seen indistinctly over abdomen	No blood vessels seen
LANUGO (over back)	No lanugo	Abundant; long and thick over whole back	Hair thinning especially over lower back	Small amount of lanugo and bald areas	At least half of back devoid of lanugo
PLANTAR CREASES	No skin creases	Faint red marks over anterior half of sole	Definite red marks over more than anterior half; indentations over less than anterior third	Indentations over more than anterior third	Definite deep indentations over more than anterior third
NIPPLE FORMA-TION	Nipple barely visible; no areola	Nipple well defined; areola smooth and flat diameter <0.75 cm.	Areola stippled, edge not raised; diameter <0.75 cm.	Areola stippled, edge raised diameter >0.75 cm.	
BREAST SIZE	No breast tissue palpable	Breast tissue on one or both sides <0.5 cm. diameter	Breast tissue both sides; one or both 0.5–1.0 cm.	Breast tissue both sides; one or both >1 cm.	
EAR FORM	Pinna flat and shapeless, little or no incurving edge	Incurving of part of edge of pinna	Partial incurving whole of upper pinna	Well-defined incurving whole of upper pinna	
EAR FIRMNESS	Pinna soft, easily folded, no recoil	Pinna soft, easily folded, slow recoil	Cartilage to edge of pinna, but soft in places, ready recoil	Pinna firm, cartilage to edge, instant recoil	
GENITALIA MALE	Neither testis in scrotum	At least one testis high in scrotum	At least one testis right down		
FEMALE (With hips half abducted)	Labia majora widely separ-ated, labia minora protruding	Labia majora almost cover labia minora	Labia majora completely cover labia minora		

(Adapted from Farr et al., *Develop. Med. Child Neurol.* (1966) **8**, 507)

Neurological Criteria

NEURO LOGICAL SIGN	SCORE					
	0	1	2	3	4	5
POSTURE						
SQUARE WINDOW	90°	60°	45°	30°	0°	
ANKLE DORSI FLEXION	90°	75°	45°	20°	0°	
ARM RECOIL	180°	90–180°	<90°			
LEG RECOIL	180°	90–180°	<90°			
POPLITEAL ANGLE	180°	160°	130°	110°	90°	<90°
HEEL TO EAR						
SCARF SIGN						
HEAD LAG						
VENTRAL SUSPENSION						

Some notes on techniques of assessment of neurological criteria

Posture.   Observed with infant quiet and in supine position. Score 0: arms and legs extended; 1: beginning of flexion of hips and knees, arms extended; 2: stronger flexion of legs, arms extended; 3: arms slightly flexed, legs flexed and abducted; 4: full flexion of arms and legs.

Square window.   The hand is flexed on the forearm between the thumb and index finger of the examiner. Enough pressure is applied to get as full a flexion as possible, and the angle between the hypothenar eminence and the ventral aspect of the forearm is measured and graded according to diagram. (Care is taken not to rotate the infant's wrist while doing this manoeuvre).

Ankle dorsiflexion.   The foot is dorsiflexed on to the anterior aspect of the leg, with the examiner's thumb on the sole of the foot and other fingers behind the leg. Enough pressure is applied to get as full flexion as possible, and the angle between the dorsum of the foot and the anterior aspect of the leg is measured.

Arm recoil.   With the infant in the supine position the forearms are first flexed for five seconds, then fully extended by pulling on the hands, and then released. The sign is fully positive if the arms return briskly to full flexion (Score 2). If the arms return to incomplete flexion or the response is sluggish it is graded as Score 1. If they remain extended or are only followed by random movements the score is 0.

Leg recoil.   With the infant supine, the hips and knees are fully flexed for five seconds, then extended by traction on the feet, and released. A maximal response is one of full flexion of the hips and knees (Score 2). A partial flexion scores 1, and minimal or no movement scores 0.

Popliteal angle.   With the infant supine and his pelvis flat on the examining couch, the thigh is held in the knee–chest position by the examiner's left index finger and thumb supporting the knee. The leg is then extended by gentle pressure from the examiner's right index finger behind the ankle and the popliteal angle is measured.

Heel to ear manoeuvre.   With the baby supine, draw the baby's foot as near to the head as it will go without forcing it. Observe the distance between the foot and the head as well as the degree of extension at the knee. Grade according to diagram. Note that the knee is left free and may draw down alongside the abdomen.

Graph for reading gestational age from total score (Dubowitz method)

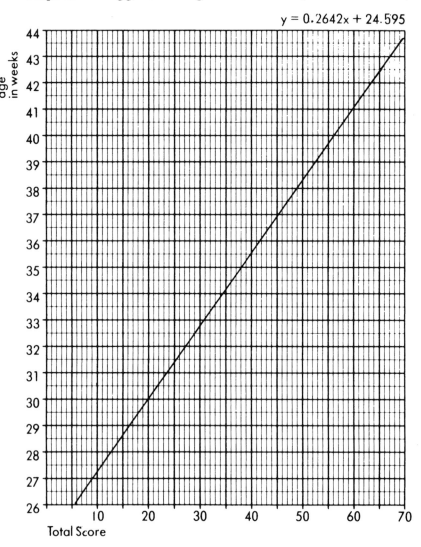

$$y = 0.2642x + 24.595$$

Scarf sign.   With the baby supine, take the infant's hand and try to put it around the neck and as far posteriorly as possible around the opposite shoulder. Assist this manoeuvre by lifting the elbow across the body. See how far the elbow will go across and grade according to illustrations. Score 0: elbow reaches opposite axillary line; 1: elbow between midline and opposite axillary line; 2: elbow reaches midline; 3: elbow will not reach midline.

Head lag.   With the baby lying supine, grasp the hands (or the arms if a very small infant) and pull slowly towards the sitting position. Observe the position of the head in relation to the trunk and grade accordingly. In a small infant the head may initially be supported by one hand. Score 0: complete lag; 1: partial head control; 2: able to maintain head in line with body; 3: brings head anterior to body.

Ventral suspension.   The infant is suspended in the prone position, with examiner's hand under the infant's chest (one hand in a small infant, two in a large infant). Observe the degree of extension of the back and the amount of flexion of the arms and legs. Also note the relation of the head to the trunk. Grade according to diagrams.

If the score for an individual criterion differs on the two sides of the baby, take the mean.   For further details see Dubowitz *et al.*, 1970.

2 Parkin, Hey and Clowes score

This is quicker to perform but may not be quite so accurate.

Skin texture.   Tested by picking up a fold of abdominal skin between finger and thumb, and by inspection.

0 Very thin with a gelatinous feel.
1 Thin and smooth.
2 Smooth and of medium thickness, irritation rash and superficial peeling may be present.
3 Slight thickening and stiff feeling with superficial cracking and peeling especially evident on the hands and feet.
4 Thick and parchment-like with superficial or deep cracking.

Skin colour.   Estimated by inspection when the baby is quiet.

0 Dark red.
1 Uniformly pink.
2 Pale pink, though the colour may vary over different parts of the body, some parts may be very pale.

3 Pale, nowhere really pink except on the ears, lips, palms and soles.

Breast size.   Measured by picking up the breast tissue between finger and thumb.

0 No breast tissue palpable.
1 Breast tissue palpable on one or both sides, neither being more than 0.5 cm in diameter.
2 Breast tissue palpable on both sides, one or both being 0.5–1 cm in diameter.
3 Breast tissue palpable on both sides, one or both being more than 1 cm in diameter.

Ear firmness.   Tested by palpation and folding of the upper pinna.

0 Pinna feels soft and is easily folded into bizarre positions without springing back into position spontaneously.
1 Pinna feels soft along the edge and is easily folded but returns slowly to the correct position spontaneously.
2 Cartilage can be felt to the edge of the pinna though it is thin in places and the pinna springs back readily after being folded.
3 Pinna firm with definite cartilage extending to the periphery and springs back immediately into position after being folded.

Score each external sign in turn. Add them up. Read off the baby's gestational age on the following chart:

Score	Gestational age	
	days	weeks
1	190	27
2	210	30
3	230	33
4	240	34.5
5	250	36
6	260	37
7	270	38.5
8	276	39.5
9	281	40
10	285	41
11	290	41.5
12	295	42

References and Further Reading

Brazelton, T.B. (1984) *Neonatal Behavioural Assessment Scale*, 2nd ed., Spastics International Medical Publications. London: Blackwell.

Dubowitz, M.S. & Dubowitz, V. (1977) *Gestational Age of the Newborn*, Reading, MA: Addison-Wesley.

Dubowitz, L., Dubowitz, V. & Goldberg, C. (1970) Clinical assessment of gestational age in the newborn infant. *J. Pediatrics 77*, 1.

Parkin, J.M., Hey, E.N. & Clowes, J.S. (1976) Rapid assessment of gestational age at birth. *Archives of Disease in Children, 51*, 259.

The Ten Steps to Successful Breastfeeding

In 1989 WHO and UNICEF issued a Joint Statement describing how maternity facilities can encourage and support breast feeding. It is called 'Protecting, Promoting and Supporting Breastfeeding. The Special Role of Maternity Services', and is the basis for the 'Baby Friendly Initiative'.

The 'Ten Steps', which summarise the main recommendations of the Joint Statement, are as follows:

Every facility providing maternity services and care for newborn infants should:

1 Have a written breastfeeding policy that is routinely communicated to all health care staff.

2 Train all health care staff in skills necessary to implement this policy.

3 Inform all pregnant women about the benefits and management of breastfeeding.

4 Help mothers initiate breastfeeding within a half-hour of birth.

5 Show mothers how to breastfeed, and how to maintain lactation even if they are separated from their infants.

6 Give newborn infants no food or drink other than breast milk, unless *medically* indicated.

7 Practise rooming-in – allow mothers and infants to remain together 24 hours a day.

8 Encourage breastfeeding on demand.

9 Give no artificial teats or pacifiers (also called dummies or soothers) to breastfeeding infants.

10 Foster the establishment of breastfeeding support groups and refer mothers to them on discharge from the hospital or clinic.

Guidelines for Infant Resuscitation

It is important to call for help as soon as possible, if you find the baby is not breathing.

(a) If you are in a house with a telephone, take the baby into the room the telephone is in. Dial 999. *Do not stop resuscitating* the baby – put the receiver on the floor, continue breathing for the baby, then pick the receiver up and talk to the operator. Keep doing this until the operator has repeated your name and address correctly.

(b) If you are in a house without a telephone, shout out of a window for help from a neighbour or person passing by. Ask them to telephone for an ambulance, while you continue with resuscitation. *Make sure* they know your address.

(c) If you are alone, without a telephone, and cannot get anyone to help, *take the baby with you* to the nearest telephone. You will need to stop every 10–20 seconds to continue resuscitating the baby.

If you think the baby is not breathing

1 *Look* for movements of the chest or abdomen (tummy).
2 *Listen* for breathing sounds.
3 Touch the cheek, abdomen or feet to see if the baby moves.
4 *Talk* to the baby.

If there are no signs of breathing

5 *Pick* the baby up, and give three sharp pats on the back.

Do not shake the baby or hit hard – you may cause an injury.

If there is no response

1 *Clear* the baby's mouth of any mucus or vomit, using your little finger.
2 *Lie* the baby on its back on a firm surface (e.g. table or floor).
3 *Tilt* the baby's head back slightly, and *hold* the chin up. (Fig. A)

Check to see if the baby is breathing

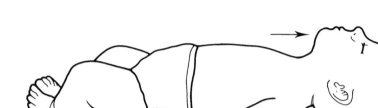

Fig. A

If there are no signs of breathing

1 Take a normal breath in.
2 Cover the baby's *mouth and nose* with your mouth.
3 Blow gently into the baby – just enough to make the chest rise.

Do not blow very hard – you may damage the baby's lungs.

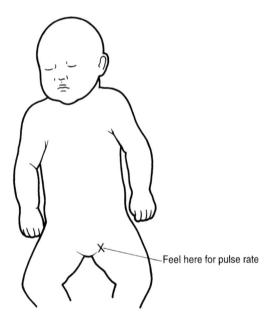

Feel here for pulse rate

Fig. B

4 Take your mouth away from the baby after each breath – the baby's chest will fall again.

Repeat this every 2–3 seconds for about 10 breaths.

Check to see if the baby is breathing.

If the baby is still not breathing you may need to start heart massage

1 Feel for a pulse at the top of the inside of the leg, in the groin. (Fig. B).
2 If the pulse rate is more than about 60 beats a minute, you do not need to start heart massage. Keep breathing for the baby, stopping after every 10 breaths to check for breathing and count the pulse again.
3 If you cannot feel a pulse, or the rate is less than about 60 beats a minute you need to start heart massage, as follows:

a Draw an imaginary line between the baby's nipples.

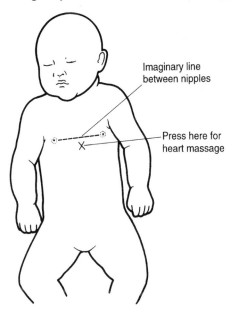

Imaginary line between nipples

Press here for heart massage

Fig. C

b Place your two fingers just below the middle of this line on the chest. (Fig. C)

c Gently press down on this point, about 2–3 cm, and release the pressure immediately.

d Repeat this about twice every second (120 times a minute).

You still need to breathe for the baby whilst doing heart massage – give the baby one breath, then press five times on the chest.

Keep repeating this sequence.

Stop every minute to check the pulse and see if the baby is breathing.

Do not stop resuscitation until the baby starts breathing normally.

When the baby starts to breathe again

1 Wrap the baby in a blanket to keep warm.
2 Turn the baby onto its side.
3 *Do not leave the baby.*
4 Keep checking to see that breathing continues.
5 Wait until help arrives.

Index